Fundamentals of Health Care Administration

Shelley C. Safian, Ph.D.

PEARSON

Boston   Columbus   Indianapolis   New York   San Francisco   Upper Saddle River
Amsterdam   Cape Town   Dubai   London   Madrid   Milan   Munich   Paris   Montréal   Toronto
Delhi   Mexico City   São Paulo   Sydney   Hong Kong   Seoul   Singapore   Taipei   Tokyo

Publisher: Julie Levin Alexander
Publisher's Assistant: Regina Bruno
Editor-in-Chief: Marlene McHugh Pratt
Executive Editor: Joan Gill
Program Manager: Faye Gemmellaro
Editorial Assistant: Stephanie Kiel
Development Editor: Alexis Ferraro, iD8-TripleSSS Media Development, LLC
Director of Marketing: David Gesell
Marketing Manager: Katrin Beacom
Senior Marketing Coordinator: Alicia Wozniak
Marketing Specialist: Michael Sirinides
Project Management Team Lead: Cindy Zonneveld
Project Manager: Yagnesh Jani
Full-Service Project Management: Saraswathi Muralidhar, PreMediaGlobal
Senior Operations Specialist: Nancy Maneri-Miller
Senior Media Editor: Matt Norris
Media Project Manager: Lorena Cerisano
Creative Director: Andrea Nix
Senior Art Director: Maria Guglielmo-Walsh
Interior Design: Marta Samsel
Cover Designer: Suzanne Duda
Cover Image: kentoh/Shutterstock
Chapter Opener Banner: alphaspirit/Shutterstock
Composition: PreMediaGlobal
Printing and Binding: LSC Communications
Cover Printer: LSC Communications
Text Font: 10/12 Times LT Std

Credits and acknowledgments for material borrowed from other sources and reproduced, with permission, in this textbook appear on the appropriate page within the text.

Notice: Care has been taken to confirm the accuracy of information presented in this book. The authors, editors, and the publisher, however, cannot accept any responsibility for errors or omissions or for consequences from application of the information in this book and make no warranty, express or implied, with respect to its contents.

Library of Congress Cataloging-in-Publication Data

Safian, Shelley C., author.
   Fundamentals of health care administration / Shelley Safian. —First edition.
      pages cm
   Includes bibliographical references and index.
   ISBN-13: 978-0-13-306563-3
   ISBN-10: 0-13-306563-4
      1. Health services administration.   2. Public health administration.
I. Title.

   RA971.S24 2013
   362.1—dc23

                                                2013029409

16

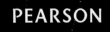

ISBN 10:   0-13-306563-4
ISBN 13: 978-0-13-306563-3

CONTENTS

Fundamentals of Health Care Administration is a foundational text to introduce future health care professionals to the scope of responsibilities of managing a health care facility. It is written to prepare students for their ensuing in-depth study of the health care industry and to begin building their critical thinking and analysis skills.

The health care industry is growing quickly and ever-changing. Health care leaders of the twenty-first century need to combine business knowledge, hospitality knowledge, technical knowledge, and health care knowledge to manage a successful organization. Those individuals who bring this full scope to the job will find a vast number of opportunities, ranging from a single physician's office to a chain of clinics, a network of hospitals, home health and hospice agencies, assisted living and skilled nursing facilities, in addition to the burgeoning industry of continuing care communities.

Each chapter addresses a different aspect of this tremendous scope: finance, human resources, risk assessment, crisis management, compliance, audits (internal and external), quality assessment and control, food-service operations, marketing and advertising, performance improvement, and legal and ethical concerns.

ORGANIZATION OF THE TEXT

The first chapter includes a bulleted list of required knowledge and skills from an actual job description for a health care administrator. The following chapters of the text directly reference specific skills from that job description, highlighted by the heading, "*When You Are the Administrator . . .* " The intent is to connect the dots between learning and then applying knowledge on the job.

Each chapter incorporates examples, including short selections from federal government documents, to illustrate concepts presented. The text strategically breaks down complex concepts into bulleted lists or steps, so students can digest one key piece of information at a time. The chapter review sections provide a variety of assessment methodologies, including multiple choice, matching, short answer, and true/false. The end-of-chapter reviews also include "*When You Are the Administrator . . . Critical Thinking and Analysis*" case study assignments that encourage students to envision themselves in their future career by engaging their critical thinking and assessment skills. Appendixes, provided to support and extend learning, include: real-life case studies from the U.S. Department of Justice and the Office of the Inspector General; a list of additional Internet resources for further research; compliance plan contents and guidance for physician practices drawn directly from the Federal Register; and a tool kit for creating a crisis management plan from the World Health Organization.

CONCEPTUAL APPROACH

This text is written in a way that communicates directly with the student. For example, instead of stating "*health care administrators would . . .*" the text reads, "*you, as the administrator, would . . .* " This approach supports the student in visualizing himself or herself on the job, using the concepts presented in a concrete manner. This approach addresses the common student concern, "Why do I need to learn this?"

All chapters in the text are directly tied to specific knowledge and skills required in the real-life job description for a health care administrator.

The goal of this text is to reach all students in any educational environment. The information is broken into bite-sized pieces, encouraging them to completely understand each part before proceeding to the next. Additional information, such as websites, allow each chapter to target opportunities for extended learning beyond the chapter itself.

In addition, each chapter focuses on fundamentals that support success in future coursework within the health care administration /health care management curriculum. For example, Chapter 3 covers various ways organizations finance the provision of health care services. After completion of this chapter, when the student enrolls in a dedicated health care finance course, he or she will have the crucial foundational knowledge to better understand that next higher level of learning. In a similar fashion, Chapter 14 introduces students to legal and ethical concepts as they relate to health care in preparation for the more intensive health care law and ethics course they will take later on in their program.

Evaluating, analyzing, and thinking critically can be challenging. Therefore, the text provides students with as much support as possible by including topics, scenarios, and case studies to be used as the foundation for classroom discussions, online discussion forums, or other graded assignments.

SUPPLEMENT PACKAGE/ANCILLARY MATERIALS

- Instructor's Resource Manual
- PowerPoint Slides
- MyTest

Consistent pedagogical elements appear in each chapter to facilitate instruction and learning.

LEARNING OBJECTIVES

A list of the primary skills students should have acquired after completing the chapter appears at the beginning of each chapter.

LEARNING OBJECTIVES

Upon completion of this chapter, you should be able to:

- Define commonly used terms, abbreviations, and acronyms.
- Recount the benefits of creating and implementing a strategic plan.
- Identify the components of a strategic plan.
- Recognize the value of staff buy-in.
- Understand how to evaluate and modify the plan, as needed.

KEY TERMS

buy-in
executive summary
long-term goals
mission statement
objective
psychographics
short-term goal
strategic goal
strategic plan
SWOT analysis

KEY TERMS, ABBREVIATIONS, AND ACRONYMS

A list of the essential vocabulary students need to know appears at the beginning of each chapter. These terms appear in bold on first introduction, and are defined in the margin and comprehensive glossary.

SUPPLEMENTAL TERMS AND ABBREVIATIONS

Additional terms or abbreviations are italicized and explained within the context of the text.

- *Emergency or trauma centers* are health care facilities that are open 24 hours a day/365 days a year to provide services to those who require immediate (unscheduled) medical attention based on a single situation or circumstance. For example: trauma care (e.g., injuries from a car accident; fall); acute medical conditions (e.g., heart attack, labor and delivery); psychiatric emergency (e.g., emotional crisis, severe shock); and so on. These facilities will often employ physicians and staff specially trained in emergency medicine or trauma medicine. Independent facilities may be known as *urgent care centers*. On the other hand, *emergency departments* (ED) are more often a part of an acute care hospital. *Community or regional hospitals*, as their name implies, are focused on providing services

WHEN YOU ARE THE ADMINISTRATOR . . .

As the administrator, you will need to be able to:

- Structure and execute a cohesive strategic plan designed to ensure the effective and efficient delivery of services.
- Analyze data to identify trends of improvement or areas of concern and maintain processes designed to follow up on areas of concern.

"WHEN YOU ARE THE ADMINISTRATOR…"

Beginning in Chapter 2 and building off of the list of job skills presented in Chapter 1, this feature presents a list of the specific job responsibilities of the administrator as they pertain to the content presented in the chapter.

INTRODUCTION

This entrance into each chapter provides an overview of what will be covered in the chapter so as to mentally prepare the student for the knowledge and skill that is about to be presented to them.

INTRODUCTION

A health care facility is a living thing. Whether a one-physician office, a fifty-bed assisted living facility, or a 500-bed medical center, a **strategic plan** establishes the identity of the facility, defines its purpose, and illuminates its **objectives**. This is the map that shows *"You Are Here"* as well as *"This Is Where You Are Headed"* and *"How to Get There"* for one department or the entire organization. Needless to say, this is a comprehensive document and for it to provide benefits and value to your facility, it requires the critical investigation of every aspect of how this facility defines the term *success*.

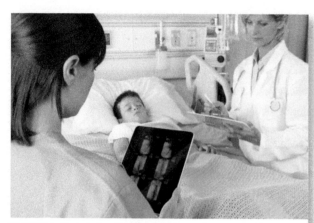

FIGURE 6-3   Timely sharing of patient information contributes to more effective treatments, therefore reducing readmissions.
Photo credit: Monkey Business Images/Shutterstock.

FIGURES

Full-color photographs, line art, and graphs are presented throughout to illustrate key concepts.

BOX 6-1	Eligible Professionals

Medicare EPs
- Doctors of medicine or osteopathy
- Doctors of dental surgery or dental medicine
- Doctors of podiatric medicine
- Doctors of optometry
- Chiropractors
- Medicare Advantage (MA) hospitals
- Critical access hospitals
- Subsection (d) hospitals that are paid under the Hospital IPPS

Medicaid EPs
- Physicians
- Nurse practitioners
- Certified nurse-midwives
- Dentists
- Physician Assistants (PAs) in PA-led federally qualified health centers (FQHC) or those in rural health clinics (RHC)
- Children's hospitals (no Medicaid volume required)
- Acute care hospitals (Including CAHs) with at least 10 percent Medicaid patient volume

Source: U.S. Government Health Information Technology Web Site.

BOXES

Feature boxes vary from actual reprints of case studies to government guidance to tie chapter content together.

TABLE 3-4   Government Grant Opportunities

Opportunity Title	Agency
The Eldercare Locator	Administration for Community Living
Bureau of Democracy, Human Rights and Labor (DRL)–Request for Proposals for International Labor Rights Programs in Cameroon and Pakistan	Bureau of Democracy, Human Rights and Labor
USSOCOM BAA (U.S. Special Operations Command–Broad Agency Announcement)	Department of the Army–USAMRAA
Rural Health Information Technology (HIT) Workforce Program	Health Resources and Services Administration
Disaster Preparedness for Effective Response (PREPARE)	Philippines USAID–Manila
Electronic Data Methods (EDM) Forum: Second Phase (U18)	Agency for Health Care Research and Quality
Land Use Change and Disease Emergence	Thailand USAID–Bangkok
Rapid Hepatitis C Virus Screening and Referral	Substance Abuse and Mental Health Services Administration
STD Surveillance Network (SSuN)	Centers for Disease Control and Prevention
Enhancing Opioid Treatment Program Patient Continuity of Care through Data Interoperability	Substance Abuse and Mental Health Services Administration
Rapid Response to Pakistanis Affected by Disasters–Phase Two (RAPID II)	Agency for International Development
Dental Reimbursement Program	Health Resources and Services Administration
Agriculture and Food Research Initiative–Childhood Obesity Prevention	National Institute of Food and Agriculture
MCH (Maternal and Child Health) Navigator Program	Health Resources and Services Administration
National Farmworker Jobs Program Grants	Employment and Training Administration
MCH Knowledge to Practice Program	Health Resources and Services Administration
Health Promotion and Disease Prevention Research Centers: Special Interest Project Competitive Supplements (SIPS)	Centers for Disease Control and Prevention
FY14 Farm to School Grant Program	Food and Nutrition Service
Maternal and Child Health (MCH) Nutrition Training Program	Health Resources and Services Administration

Source: Grants.gov.

TABLES

Tables within the chapters further illustrate chapter concepts.

A review section at the end of each chapter reinforces key concepts and provides opportunity for additional critical thinking opportunities.

SUMMARY

The chapter summary is a brief restatement of key points in the chapter.

CHAPTER REVIEW QUESTIONS

Multiple-choice, true/false, short answer, and matching questions are provided to assess student learning of key concepts presented within the chapter.

CHAPTER REVIEW

SUMMARY

A strategic plan is a comprehensive document, and for it to provide benefits and value to your facility, it requires the critical investigation of every aspect of how this facility defines the term *success*. This document will enable you to organize and evaluate every activity to ensure that each works as an effective building block in the structure of your organization. Strategic plans are complex tools that are intended to provide a guide for the future of the organization. A thorough analysis of all the elements included in the plan is necessary to have a strategic plan of value.

Strategic goals are the statements of how the organization will accomplish the objectives and, eventually, the mission. The mission statement presents the ultimate objective. Once the plan is complete and the team feels that it represents the facility's objectives and clearly defines what must be done to accomplish them, it is ready to implement. This should be done in two steps: obtaining consensus and delegating action-oriented assignments.

Annual updates should be scheduled for the plan so as to provide the organization the opportunity to learn from the observations of the implementation so far, and benefit from the results of putting theory into action.

REVIEW QUESTIONS

MULTIPLE CHOICE

Choose the most accurate answer.

1. When administration seeks "buy-in" from staff members, it means they are looking for
   a. an investment in the company.
   b. consensus from the staff.
   c. staff to chip in cash to pay for a new project.
   d. enrollment in a payroll deduction plan.

2. A market overview includes
   a. pharmaceutical representatives.
   b. unique features of the facility.
   c. psychographic profiles.
   d. a mission statement.

6. Which of the following describes secondary research?
   a. Surveying the patients
   b. Downloading statistics from NCHS
   c. Reading an article in JAMA
   d. b and c only

7. An all-encompassing long-term goal is known as the _____ statement.
   a. buy-in
   b. action
   c. mission
   d. demographic

8. The executive summary includes all of the following

WHEN YOU ARE THE ADMINISTRATOR...
CRITICAL THINKING AND ANALYSIS

Every chapter includes case studies, articles, or scenarios for the students to engage their critical thinking skills to analyze and evaluate real life situations and project themselves into scenarios they may encounter in their future careers. This not only encourages critical thinking skills but also encourages students to get a true feel for what their future career will entail.

WHEN YOU ARE THE ADMINISTRATOR . . .

Critical Thinking and Analysis

Case Study #1

Clinical Public Health Group Mission

The Veterans' Administration, Clinical Public Health Group has a strategic plan that includes this mission:

"We improve the health of Veterans through the development of sound policies and programs related to several major public health concerns. This includes HIV infection, hepatitis C infection, seasonal influenza, smoking and tobacco use cessation, health-care associated infections, and other emerging public health issues.

Our primary focus is the health of Veterans. In order to achieve this goal, we work with Veterans and their families, organizations that represent and support Veteran health care needs, and the variety of providers who deliver clinical, preventive, and support services to Veterans.

Our mission is accomplished through a variety of efforts, including: education and outreach, policy development, clinical demonstration projects, quality improvement initiatives, population based surveillance, performance measurement, clinical practice guidelines, and research."

Source: Clinical Public Health Group, United States Department of Veterans Affairs.

How would you use this mission statement to create an outline for a strategic plan? Come up with at least three action steps that you could include in a strategic plan to accomplish at least one of these visions.

INTERNET CONNECTIONS

Websites with content directly connected to the learning for the specific chapter are provided at the end of each chapter.

INTERNET CONNECTIONS

U.S. Department of Health and Human Services Strategic Plan 2010–2015

The US Department of Health and Human Services (DHHS), an agency of the federal government, also has to create a strategic plan. This is published on the internet and available for download.
http://www.hhs.gov/secretary/about/priorities/strategicplan2010-2015.pdf

American Hospital Association Strategic Plan 2012/2013

The American Hospital Association has posted its strategic plan on this International Hospital Federation website. Read through their vision, mission, values, and goals.

http://www.ihf-fih.org/en/IHF-Newsletters/Articles/February-2011/Hospitals-and-Health-Services-Worldwide-News/Americas/American-Hospital-Association-Strategic-Plan-2011–2013

Practical Techniques for *Strategic Planning* in *Health Care*

An article from the Health Information Management Systems Society (HIMSS) in conjunction with the American College of Physician Executives created this 4-page summation of strategic planning for health care organizations.
http://www.himss.org/files/HIMSSorg/content/files/Code%2039-Practical%20Techniques%20for%20Strategic%20Planning_ACPE_2010.pdf

ACKNOWLEDGMENTS

It truly takes a village to create a text, and I have great esteem for everyone who worked with me on this project.

- My deepest thanks to Joan Gill, my executive editor, and Pam Jeffries, account manager, for welcoming me into the Pearson family and supporting me throughout this endeavor.
- Alexis Breen Ferraro, developmental editor, earned my great appreciation as she supported my vision and helped me create a quality text.
- Stephanie Kiel, editorial assistant, has my gratitude for the support she provided to ensure that this text met its goals.
- Leslie Gibson helped me firm up my confidence and confirm my *i*'s were dotted and my *t*'s were crossed.
- Harriet and Jack Safian, my parents, who instilled in me the love of learning and the true value of sharing knowledge.

REVIEWERS

The feedback and insights provided by the following educators and health care professionals was invaluable. Thank you to:

Kristin Hawthorne,
CCI Training Center

Antionette Woodall,
Remington College Allen School

Christine Jerson,
Lakeland Community College

Kim Kubricky,
Bryant and Stratton College

Mia Marie Young,
Independent Education Consultant

Shawn Matheson,
Independence University

Emmanuel Touze,
Keiser University

Shiela Rojas,
Santa Barbara Business College

Sherry-Lynn Amaral,
Miller-Motte College

THE BALANCE OF GOOD ADMINISTRATION

LEARNING OBJECTIVES

Upon completion of this chapter, you should be able to:

- Define commonly used terms, abbreviations, and acronyms.
- Identify the responsibilities of a health care administrator.
- Enumerate the differences of the perceptions of health care by clinical professionals and administrative professionals.
- Evaluate the impact of the facility's ability to provide services needed by its patient population.
- Describe the various aspects of health care utilization.

KEY TERMS

administrator
clinician
complementary alternative
    medicine (CAM)
compliance
mortality
noninvasive procedure
patient population
preventive care
strategic plan
teletherapy
utilization

INTRODUCTION

The health care industry has been evolving at a tremendous rate and will continue to do so for the next several decades. Baby boomers, currently the largest segment of the population (by age), are moving into the final third of their lives. As you can see in Table 1-1 ■, approximately one-quarter (24.9 percent) of the population of the United States is 55 years of age or older, and almost 13 percent are 65 years of age or older. The Social Security Administration (SSA) has calculated that of the 77 million baby boomers in the country, approximately 10,000 individuals are filing for social security benefits every day. At this point in their lives, these individuals are retiring from work—an action that results in fewer health care workers available to care for patients. Simultaneously, aging bodies require more attention and treatment, resulting in an increase in the number of patients who need time and consideration from health care professionals.

These facts about this segment of the population become even more important when you look at the other side of the scale. As the number of elderly is steadily increasing, the birth rate is slowly declining. The National Center for Health Statistics (NCHS) and the Centers for Disease Control and Prevention (CDC) report that the number of births in the United States for July 2011 to June 2012 was one percent lower than the same period one year earlier. According to these statistics, both fertility and birth rates have been declining every year since 2007.

Complying with local, state, and federal laws and regulations, establishing accepted ethical dynamics, implementing standards of care for every diagnosis, accessing state-of-the-art tools with which all staff work, integrating technological enhancements, and enabling the training required for a staff of excellence are all necessary to provide properly for each and every person who comes to the organization for help to become healthy and stay healthy. Health care providers

TABLE 1-1   Population by Age [Both Sexes]: 2011

AGE	BOTH SEXES	
	Number	Percent
All ages	306,110	100.0
Under 55 years	229,947	75.1
55 to 59 years	19,554	6.4
60 to 64 years	17,430	5.7
65 to 69 years	12,160	4.0
70 to 74 years	9,254	3.0
75 to 79 years	7,088	2.3
80 to 84 years	5,719	1.9
85 years and over	4,957	1.6
Under 55 years	229,947	75.1
55 years and over	76,163	24.9
Under 60 years	249,501	81.5
60 years and over	56,609	18.5
Under 62 years	256,776	83.9
62 years and over	49,333	16.1
Under 65 years	266,931	87.2
65 years and over	39,179	12.8
Under 75 years	288,345	94.2
75 years and over	17,764	5.8

Numbers shown in thousands.

Source: U.S. Census Bureau, Current Population Survey, Annual Social and Economic Supplement, 2011.

TABLE 1-2   Medical and Health Services Managers

PERCENT CHANGE IN EMPLOYMENT, PROJECTED 2010–2020	
Medical and Health Services Managers	22%
Total, All Occupations	14%
Management Occupations	7%

Note: All Occupations includes all occupations in the U.S. economy.

Source: U.S. Bureau of Labor Statistics, Employment Projections program.

and facilities—whether a one-physician office, a huge hospital conglomerate, or every size in between—must find a way to balance all of the complex components necessary to provide services. Health care administrators, also called health care managers, office managers, and practice managers, are needed to oversee all of these elements and ensure the implementation of every one of the factors required for providing quality care to patients. Similar to the conductor of an orchestra, it is the administrators who provide the guidance and organization who will establish the environment as one that is harmonious and in tune with good health: the good health of the patients, the staff, and the facility itself.

The Bureau of Labor Statistics estimates that the job outlook for medical and health services managers is higher than average, with an estimated 22 percent job growth projection from 2010 to 2020 (Table 1-2 ■). You can certainly understand how an increased need for more medical and health services managers will have a domino effect, resulting in the need for additional physicians, facilities, and procedure rooms.

ADMINISTRATIVE AND CLINICAL PERSONNEL

Any health care facility, from a small free clinic to a massive hospital corporation, is composed of two groups that enable them to function: the clinicians and the administrators. These two critical groups, at times, have an ongoing conflict with each other stemming from their perspectives of what is needed to provide continuing health care services.

Clinicians are those professionals who provide diagnostic, preventive, and therapeutic care for patients. Physicians (e.g., internists, radiologists, pathologists), nurses, therapists, and technicians are examples of the front line professionals of health care—the practitioners of medicine. Without them, patients would not get the assistance and support necessary to get better from illness or injury and it would be more challenging to stay healthy in the first place.

Administrators are the professionals who provide management and support to the clinicians. Ensuring financial health for the organization so salaries can get paid, equipment can be purchased and maintained, and laws are complied with to avoid costly governmental fines and penalties are all parts of an administrator's contribution. That x-ray the physician needs in order to diagnose the patient and the scalpel in the hand of the surgeon are available thanks to the hard work done by the administrator.

The clinicians and the administrators are two halves of a health care organization that are both absolutely required to make the organization whole. However, sometimes they each feel the other does not understand what they do or how hard they work. Probably the most difficult aspect of this conflict is that clinicians are responsible for helping the sick become healthy. They often deal, literally, with life and death. A successful administrator must learn to balance the needs of the clinical staff while keeping the organization as a whole running smoothly and with stability.

ADMINISTRATOR'S RESPONSIBILITIES AND SKILL SETS

As the superintendents of the entire facility, administrators are responsible for ensuring that the highest quality of service is provided on the clinical side while keeping the provision of these clinical services in harmony with the business side. In other words, health care administrators must ensure that the facility delivers health care services in an efficient and effective way. Administrators

clinician
individual trained to work directly with the care of patients in a health care environment.

administrator
individual with the responsibility to oversee the workings of an organization and the provision of the services and products provided.

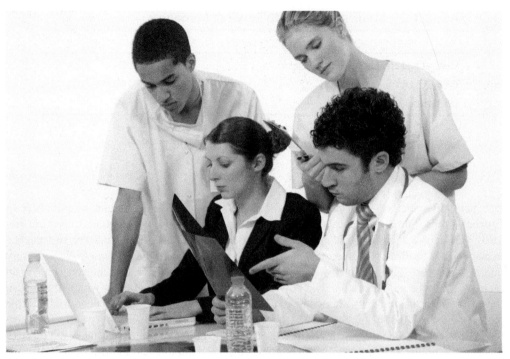

FIGURE 1-1   When administrators and clinicians work together and understand each other, they can create a healthy environment for both patients and staff.
Photo credit: auremar/Fotolia.

work to safeguard the financial security of an organization and keep a watchful eye on maintaining the greater good of the entire facility. It is their responsibility to ensure that medical and preventive services are provided and to maintain the monies required to keep it all going.

Larger organizations are more likely to establish an administrative department with a director and several assistant administrators. Assistant administrators are typically charged with oversight of a specific department such as physical therapy, health information and medical records, nursing, or surgery. Depending upon the departmental structure of the administrators, some facilities will require a clinical background, such as nursing administrator or chief of surgery, in addition to the managerial and business skills (Figure 1-1 ■). However, this clinical requirement is not absolute.

Smaller facilities often hire executive administrators, also known as office managers or practice managers, to supervise specific aspects of daily operations, as well as to manage staff, finances, equipment procurement and maintenance, legal and ethical **compliance**, and patient care.

Essentially, all health care administrators in the twenty-first century must be prepared to handle multiple aspects of the business of health care:

- *Technological innovations.* Technology is frequently entwined into the modernization of both the business aspects and the clinical aspects of health care delivery. Technology has a great impact on diagnostic techniques, such as digital imaging, therapeutic methodologies such as robotic surgery, and administrative functions related to the use of electronic health records and electronic claim creation and submission (Figure 1-2 ■).
- *Compliance strategies.* A clear understanding of legal and ethical compliance strategies and an ability to implement them in accordance with the regulatory agencies and the applicable laws and statutes is required. After a government audit determines noncompliance, the fines and penalties assessed can be high, especially when stacked on top of the repayment of the overage to the third-party payer calculated at treble—meaning that three times the amount of the overpayment must be returned by the facility. This unexpected amount of money to be paid out can cripple, if not shut down, a facility.
- *Organizational behavior.* The facility as a whole has its own culture and this culture affects the behavior of those within. Administrators must be well-versed in the creation and implementation of policies and procedures to provide the foundation for a smooth-running, efficient company that treats its staff and patients with respect.

compliance
observance of laws and policies; behaviors and actions directly following rules and regulations.

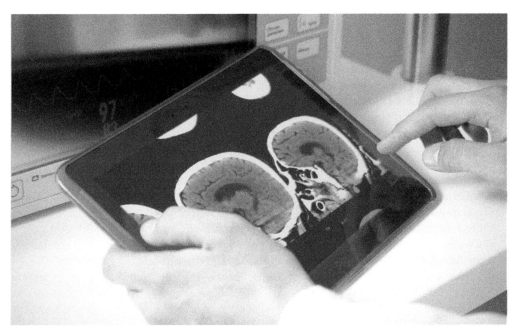

FIGURE 1-2 Technology is an integral part of health care in the twenty-first century. All staff members will have some form of technology involved in their job description.
Photo credit: © sudok1/Fotolia.

- *Health care financing.* Everyone knows that, without money, nothing can be accomplished. Health care services may be provided to a patient for free, at a reduced cost, or at full price. However, the amount paid by the patient has little to do with the money required to provide those services. Staff members need to be paid for their work; supplies and equipment must be purchased from the manufacturers. Budgets must be created, revenue streams need to be consistent, and financial obligations must be met.
- *Human resources.* A health care provider may employ tens or hundreds of staff members. These individuals must be recruited, evaluated, vetted (have credentials and experience confirmed), trained and oriented, and lots more. Those employed by a health care facility are almost always educated professionals with proven skills that fulfill very specific job requirements. This means that the hiring process must be completed with great diligence.
- *Health information management.* Documentation is mandated throughout all processes of providing health care services, and this documentation must be organized, kept to legal standards, and be made available as needed for continuity of care as well as reimbursement and statistical and research compilation. Technology is engrained in this area, with electronic health records (electronic medical records) and patient management systems that handle billing and reimbursement. These electronic systems make the storage, access, and protection of these files much easier, while technology changes the level of training required of the personnel that manage the data.
- *Facility (physical) management.* Administrators must also understand and be able to supervise, negotiate, and oversee the physical environment of health care providers. Whether a suite of offices or a free-standing building, evaluation for a lease or purchase, maintenance of the physical aspects such as power (electricity), ventilation (air conditioning and heating), security, and even parking are all part of the equation.

An administrator's job description will typically include:

- Assessment and identification of specific services, facilities, equipment, and personnel needed to address the current and future health care needs of the community and the funding required to provide such services
- Structure and execution of a cohesive **strategic plan** designed to ensure the effective and efficient delivery of services
- Research, analysis of data, and determination of recommendations for the addition, expansion, or reduction of specialized services currently provided by the organization

strategic plan
the process of determining direction and guidance for the accomplishment of goals.

- Creation of a balanced budget along with strategic planning to maintain fiscal health for the organization
- Supervision of the activities of all departments, including clinical, human resources, finance (including accounts receivable and payable), operations, maintenance, housekeeping, marketing, admissions, and scheduling
- Analysis of data to identify trends of improvement or areas of importance to the patient populations, and ensure the message is clearly communicated through marketing, advertising, and public relations vehicles, as appropriate
- Provision of leadership and promotion of effective and efficient integration of services in a worker-friendly environment
- Promotion of clinical excellence using evidence-based health care principles
- Verification of clinical practice guidelines and quality indicators to ensure patient safety and quality of care
- Oversight and confirmation of professional and staff development
- Creation and implementation of plans for compliance with all federal and state regulations and laws ensuring the participation of all staff and all departments
- Performance of risk assessments prior to enactment of any improvement plans or expansion plans
- Design and application of crisis management plans for dealing with any extraordinary situation
- Coordination of organization-wide performance improvement activities, including maintenance of performance improvement documentation to support credentialing
- Creation and enactment of specific patient assessment reporting parameters in accordance with organizational and accreditation standards
- Analysis of data to identify trends of improvement or areas of concern and maintenance of processes designed to follow up on areas of concern
- Tracking of data for Joint Commission quality initiatives

patient population
the group of individuals accepting health care services from a specific organization.

The next step in understanding the purpose and importance of all of the above responsibilities and skills required of a health care administrator is to also understand who relies (or will rely) on your organization for health care services (your **patient population**) and specifically what these people need, or will need, from your practice or facility.

All of these elements, and more, must be attended to so the facility can be healthy enough to properly care for its patient population. Smaller facilities, such as a small group practice, will have a narrower scope of services and a shorter roster of personnel, but the administrator still needs to keep all of these components in balance. Larger facilities will typically provide the administrator with staff to permit the delegation of tasks. Even in this case, you, as the administrator, will need to understand the full scope of all undertakings for which your department is responsible. Each of the chapters in this book will enable you to learn about all of these disciplines to support your personal development of these skill sets, providing you with a strong foundation for a successful career.

UTILIZATION OF HEALTH CARE SERVICES

utilization
the use of something; operation and employment of resources, including staff time, staff expertise, as well as equipment and supplies.

The need for health care services has actually expanded over recent decades and even centuries. Health care **utilization**—the way individuals use the resources of the health care industry—has changed, as well. Research continues to enhance what we know about the human body and what it needs to thrive. This knowledge is then applied to the development of new treatments and services that more effectively and efficiently care for every aspect of the body, in each stage of development. For example, the expansion of preventive medicine services and techniques that enable the early detection of some diseases, such as cancer, has dramatically lengthened the lifespan of the average person. These breakthroughs have significantly increased the number and types of services provided by the health care industry and have made a tremendous impact on the health and well-being of men, women, and children (Figure 1-3 ■).

Summarized data from the 2010 National Health Interview Survey (NHIS)—a multipurpose health survey conducted by the Centers for Disease Control and Prevention's (CDC) National Center for Health Statistics (NCHS)—show some interesting patterns:

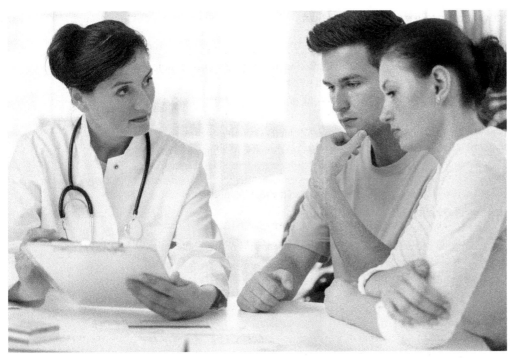

FIGURE 1-3   Information must be gathered and analyzed to determine what services your patient population will need, while information on existing services must be disseminated so patients know what options are available.
Photo credit: Alexander Raths/Fotolia.

- Of all adults aged eighteen years and over surveyed:
  - 61 percent were in excellent or very good health
  - 27 percent were in good health
  - 12 percent were in fair or poor health
- With regard to continuity of health in this same group of adults

  . . . of those who stated they had excellent or very good health in 2010:

  - 78 percent were about the same as a year ago (2009)
  - 19 percent had improved
  - 3 percent were worse

  . . . of those who stated they had good health in 2010:

  - 71 percent were about the same as a year ago (2009)
  - 19 percent had improved
  - 9 percent were worse

  . . . of those who stated they had fair or poor health in 2010:

  - 53 percent were about the same as a year ago (2009)
  - 16 percent had improved
  - 31 percent were worse than last year
- When asked about contact with health care professionals in 2010:

  - 66 percent had last contact within the previous six months
  - 15 percent had last contact more than six months ago/less than one year ago
  - 8 percent had last contact more than one year ago/less than two years ago
  - 6 percent had last contact more than two years ago/less than five years ago
  - three percent had last contact more than five years ago
  - 1 percent had no contact at all

Significant factors in the evolution of health care services directly affect the population's need for, and use of, health care resources (Table 1-3 ■). Some of these elements are discussed in the following sections.

TABLE 1-3   Factors that Affect Overall Health Care Utilization

Factors that may decrease health services utilization	Factors that may increase health services utilization
Decreased supply (e.g., hospital closures, large numbers of physicians retiring)	Increased supply (e.g., ambulatory surgery centers, assisted living residences)
Public health/sanitation advances (e.g., quality standards for food and water distribution)	Growing population
Better understanding of the risk factors of diseases and prevention initiatives (e.g., smoking prevention programs, cholesterol lowering drugs)	Growing elderly population: • more functional limitations associated with aging • more illness associated with aging • more deaths among the increased number of elderly (which is correlated with high utilization)
Discovery/implementation of treatments that cure or eliminate diseases	New procedures and technologies (e.g., hip replacement, stent insertion, MRI)
Consensus documents or guidelines that recommend decreases in utilization	Consensus documents or guidelines that recommend increases in utilization
Shifts to other sites of care may cause declines in utilization in the original sites: • as technology allows shifts (e.g., ambulatory surgery) • as alternative sites of care become available (e.g., assisted living)	New disease entities (e.g., HIV/AIDS, bioterrorism)
Payer pressures to reduce costs	New drugs, expanded use of existing drugs
Changes in practice patterns (e.g., encouraging self-care and healthy lifestyles; reduced length of hospital stay)	Increased health insurance coverage
Changes in consumer preferences (e.g., home birthing, more self-care, alternative medicine)	Consumer/employee pressures for more comprehensive insurance coverage
	Changes in practice patterns (e.g., more aggressive treatment of the elderly)
	Changes in consumer preferences and demand (e.g., cosmetic surgery, hip and knee replacements, direct marketing of drugs)

Source: Centers for Disease Control and Prevention. Retrieved from: Health Care in America: Trends in Utilization—Centers for Disease.

Expanded Life Span

Admittedly, people living longer speaks well for the quality and availability of health care in the United States. In 1960, the life expectancy in the United States was 69.77 years. This has increased to 78.09 years in 2009.[1] The longer the final third of an individual's lifespan lasts, the more health care services he or she will require because, as people age, their body systems need more frequent care and maintenance (Figure 1-4 ■).

mortality
death.

During this same course of time (1960–2009), infant **mortality** rates plummeted from 26 deaths per 1,000 live births to 6.6 deaths per 1,000 live births.[1] This proves the value of good prenatal care as well as the benefit of health care services specifically designed for neonates and infants, especially for those born prematurely and with low birth weights.

These statistics, among others, clearly illustrate that the patient population is growing and requires an attentive and specialized health care system. This system needs to be specific enough to address the needs of the individual patient, while being flexible enough to be ready to provide a wide variety of preventive, diagnostic, and therapeutic services—whatever the patient needs, whenever the patient needs it.

Preventive Care and Screenings

preventive care
health care services intended to keep a patient healthy and avoid illness, disease, or injury.

Research has proven the long-term benefits of applying **preventive care** and screenings. Preventive care, just as the term suggests, actually aims to prevent (stop) a patient from becoming ill. Familiar examples include the varicella vaccine to prevent development of chicken pox or the taking of aspirin to prevent a future heart attack. Screenings are used to catch an illness in its

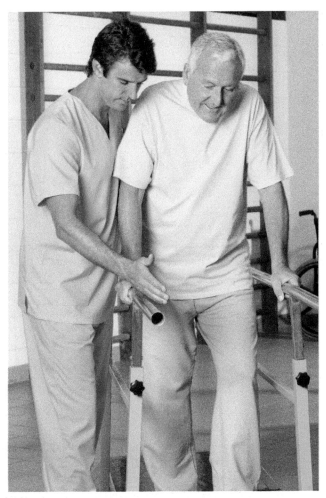

FIGURE 1-4   As people live longer, more services will be needed to keep them healthy and functional.
Photo credit: Tyler Olsen/Fotolia.

earliest stages, making treatment less invasive, less costly, and more supportive of a better prognosis for the patient. Examples include an annual physical with blood tests that might uncover a problem with the patient's thyroid, or a screening mammogram that might find a tiny malignant lesion before it metastasizes (spreads). According to the National Cancer Institute at the National Institutes of Health, the number of patients who die from breast cancer has been dramatically reduced in women aged forty to seventy-four who have had screening mammograms.

The U.S. Preventive Services Task Force[2] works continuously to recommend screenings for purposes of early diagnosis as well as preventive care services, most often based on age or previous/other diagnoses. For example, in June 2009, the task force strongly recommended, and continues to recommend, that all pregnant women, during their first prenatal checkup, be screened for hepatitis B virus infection. In January 2012, the recommendation was put forth for clinicians to screen children aged six years and older for obesity. Should a child be found to be obese (20 percent or higher above normal weight), the recommendation continues for the clinician to offer them, or refer them for, behavioral modification to encourage understanding and progress in long-term weight control. The research shows that the earlier healthy behaviors are established in an individual, the more sustainable they are, therefore leading to a healthy lifestyle for the rest of their lives and reducing the risk of the development of obesity-related conditions.

The benefits of preventive and screening health processes are vast (Figure 1-5 ■). The impact of a flu vaccination is far more than the comparison between the cost of the vaccine serum versus the cost of the treatment necessary after the patient develops the flu. Should an individual get sick, he or she, along with family members, must deal with the illness itself as well as the resulting economic impact of possible lost wages. Businesses must suffer lost productivity from an

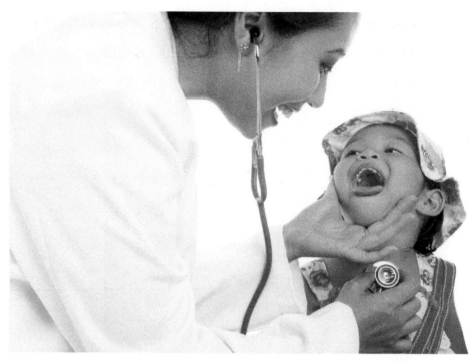

FIGURE 1-5 Preventive health care services benefit everyone—from the oldest patient to the youngest.
Photo credit: Paulus Nugroho R/Fotolia.

employee who calls in sick. And someone must pay the cost of the health care services to support the patient's return to good health.

With this picture of the impact of a flu shot in your mind, now think about the impact of preventive medicine and screenings for early diagnosis and treatment for other conditions, such as breast cancer or heart disease. Getting a colonoscopy may be uncomfortable and embarrassing for twenty-four hours for the patient, but this discomfort and the cost of the test are nothing when compared to the impact and cost of caring for a patient with colon cancer.

The next step in prevention is upon us, as the U.S. Food and Drug Administration (FDA) has already approved three vaccines to prevent cancer: a hepatitis B virus vaccine (hepatitis B can cause liver cancer); a vaccine that works to prevent human papillomavirus (HPV) (the virus that causes approximately 70 percent of cervical cancer cases); and another vaccine designed to help treat some men diagnosed with metastatic prostate cancer. Clinical trials are ongoing to develop treatment vaccines against additional types of malignancies.

The passing of the Affordable Care Act provides new opportunities for patients to take advantage of preventive health care innovations (Box 1-1 ■). Those patients with a new health insurance plan or insurance policy beginning on or after September 23, 2010, must have the following preventive services covered, without having to pay a copayment, coinsurance, or contribution to their deductible, when these services are provided within the policy's network.

Complementary Alternative Medicine (CAM)

Acupuncture and herbal remedies have been used in various cultures and countries around the world for thousands of years, yet it has only been within the last decade or so that western (modern) medicine has begun to acknowledge the value of alternative medicine (Figure 1-6 ■). Many third-party payers are covering these services, including acupuncture and massage therapy.

According to the National Center for Health Statistics, more than half of all adults in the United States participating in their survey used some type of alternative medicine methodology during the year immediately prior to the survey.[3] The survey's description of **complementary alternative medicine (CAM)** provided 27 varieties of health care including acupuncture, homeopathic treatments, chiropractic care, massage therapy, hypnosis, yoga, tai chi, biofeedback, deep-breathing exercises, megavitamin therapy, and folk remedies. Some of these are detailed in Table 1-4 ■.

complementary alternative medicine (CAM)
a term used to represent the use of theories and practices not considered to be included in conventional medicine: acupuncture, chiropractics, and physical therapies are included in this grouping.

BOX 1-1	Preventive Services for Adults Covered under the Affordable Care Act

1. *Abdominal Aortic Aneurysm* one-time screening for men of specified ages who have ever smoked
2. *Alcohol Misuse* screening and counseling
3. *Aspirin* use for men and women of certain ages
4. *Blood Pressure* screening for all adults
5. *Cholesterol* screening for adults of certain ages or at higher risk
6. *Colorectal Cancer* screening for adults over 50
7. *Depression* screening for adults
8. *Type 2 Diabetes* screening for adults with high blood pressure
9. *Diet* counseling for adults at higher risk for chronic disease
10. *HIV* screening for all adults at higher risk
11. *Immunization* vaccines for adults—doses, recommended ages, and recommended populations vary:
    - Hepatitis A
    - Hepatitis B
    - Herpes Zoster
    - Human Papillomavirus
    - Influenza (Flu Shot)
    - Measles, Mumps, Rubella
    - Meningococcal
    - Pneumococcal
    - Tetanus, Diphtheria, Pertussis
    - Varicella
12. *Obesity* screening and counseling for all adults
13. *Sexually Transmitted Infection (STI)* prevention counseling for adults at higher risk
14. *Tobacco Use* screening for all adults and cessation interventions for tobacco users
15. *Syphilis* screening for all adults at higher risk

Source: Healthcare.gov.

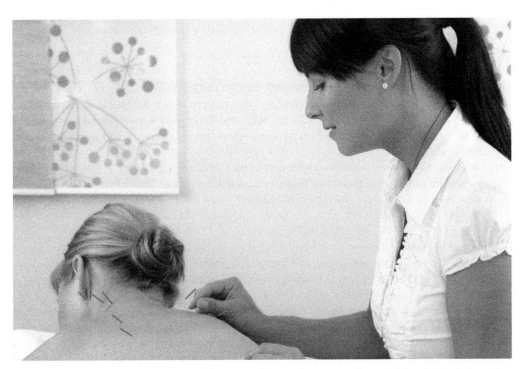

FIGURE 1-6 More and more patients are taking advantage of available alternate health care services, such as this patient receiving acupuncture.
Photo credit: Trish23/Fotolia.

TABLE 1-4   Some Types of Complementary Alternative Medicine (CAM)

Mind and Body Medicine

Mind and body practices focus on the interactions among the brain, mind, body, and behavior, with the intent to use the mind to affect physical functioning and promote health. Many CAM practices embody this concept—in different ways.

- Meditation techniques include specific postures, focused attention, or an open attitude toward distractions. People use meditation to increase calmness and relaxation, improve psychological balance, cope with illness, or enhance overall health and well-being.

- The various styles of yoga used for health purposes typically combine physical postures, breathing techniques, and meditation or relaxation. People use yoga as part of a general health regimen and also for a variety of health conditions.

- Acupuncture is a family of procedures involving the stimulation of specific points on the body using a variety of techniques, such as penetrating the skin with needles that are then manipulated by hand or by electrical stimulation. It is one of the key components of traditional Chinese medicine and is also among the oldest healing practices in the world.

- Other examples of mind and body practices include deep-breathing exercises, guided imagery, hypnotherapy, progressive relaxation, qi gong, and tai chi.

Manipulative and Body-Based Practices

Manipulative and body-based practices focus primarily on the structures and systems of the body, including the bones and joints, soft tissues, and circulatory and lymphatic systems. Two commonly used therapies fall within this category:

- Spinal manipulation is practiced by health care professionals such as chiropractors, osteopathic physicians, naturopathic physicians, physical therapists, and some medical doctors. Practitioners perform spinal manipulation by using their hands or a device to apply a controlled force to a joint of the spine. The amount of force applied depends on the form of manipulation used. The goal of the treatment is to relieve pain and improve physical functioning. Spinal manipulation is among the treatment options used by people with low-back pain—a very common condition that can be difficult to treat.

- The term massage therapy encompasses many different techniques. In general, therapists press, rub, and otherwise manipulate the muscles and other soft tissues of the body. People use massage for a variety of health-related purposes, including to relieve pain, rehabilitate sports injuries, reduce stress, increase relaxation, address anxiety and depression, and improve general well-being.

Source: NCCAM Pub No.: D347. Date created: October 2008. Last updated: July 2011.

There is scientific evidence that some patients with chronic pain can benefit from CAM and gain relief without paying the price of dealing with surgery and/or narcotics. Those suffering with low-back pain, arthritis, headache, neck pain, and fibromyalgia have been documented as finding pain relief from procedures such as acupuncture, herbal remedies, and spinal manipulation, to name a few.

Including any of these methodologies on the list of health care resources available to your patient population benefits the entire industry as much as it does individual patients and the economy as a whole.

Reduction of Inpatient Procedures

Health care researchers and professionals have made tremendous advancements with surgical techniques that reduce the emotional and financial burden of a hospital stay. More procedures and treatments are being performed in outpatient and physician offices now, than ever before, as shown in Table 1-5 ■.

Laparoscopic procedures that can be performed in an outpatient setting reduce more than just the cost of the procedure. Recovery time is shortened because the invasion to the body is much smaller, enabling patients to get back to work and their normal lives more quickly. All of these factors make it easier for a patient to have procedures completed sooner, and therefore support good health, as opposed to waiting for the time and money to be right. Some conditions will continue to get worse during this waiting time and require more health care resources to resolve the condition, costing more time and more money.

TABLE 1-5   Use of Health Care Services: United States, 1990–2000

Year	Office-based physician visits	Hospital outpatient department visits	Hospital emergency department visits	Short-stay hospital discharges
1990–1991	2,777			122
1992–1993	2,925	236	356	119
1994–1995	2,643	256	364	117
1996–1997	2,865	271	349	114
1998–1999	2,931	296	375	117
2000	3,004	304	394	114

Source: Centers for Disease Control and Prevention, National Center for Health Statistics, National Ambulatory Medical Care Survey (NAMCS), National Hospital Ambulatory Medical Care Survey (NHAMCS), and National Hospital Discharge Survey (NHDS).

In recent years, the development of natural-opening surgery has progressed. This type of procedure enters the body via the nose, mouth, vagina, or anus, eliminating the need for any surgical incisions. Again, this methodology ensures even faster recovery time, less time off from work and away from family, and, overall, is less traumatic for the patient.

Enhancement of Emergency Medicine

Over the last few decades, emergency medical technicians (EMTs) and paramedics have been supplied with more training and are now able to provide certain life-saving methodologies, including the administration of medications. EMTs and paramedics are typically the first to arrive at the scene of an automobile accident, a woman in labor, an individual suspected of having a heart attack or stroke, or someone who slipped and fell, possibly suffering spinal damage. These health care professionals are specially trained to quickly assess the nature of the patient's condition, determine any current medications or preexisting medical conditions that may be relevant, and provide needed medical treatments to stabilize the patient's condition for safe transport to a facility.

There is no doubt that a patient in a health crisis can only benefit from proper medical treatment as soon as possible. There are circumstances when care provided by an EMT during that ten-minute ride to the hospital can make a dramatic difference in the patient's prognosis—and sometimes between life and death (Figure 1-7 ■).

Innovations in Pharmaceutical Treatments

It can be very easy to lose sight of the tremendous benefits of medication—tiny pills and injections. The pharmaceutical industry has contributed significantly to the well-being of the general public, acting as preventive and therapeutic agents toward good health.

Some medications prevent the recurrence of disease, such as imatinib mesylate (trade name: Gleevec), a medication that interferes with the progression of chronic myeloid leukemia (CML) and meclizine hydrochloride (trade name: Bonamine), a medication that prevents motion sickness and vertigo.

Other medications are therapeutic, encouraging the resolution of an illness or condition. For example, tetracycline hydrochloride (trade name: Tetralan) is an antibiotic used to inhibit gram-positive and gram-negative bacteria, particularly chlamydial infections and mycoplasmal infections. Eprosartan mesylate (trade name: Teveten) is used to treat hypertension.

Pharmaceutical innovations have done a great deal to improve the health of millions of individuals, in some cases preserving quality of life and, in other cases, prolonging life. In addition, many individuals would rather opt for health care that required only taking medication versus undergoing surgery (Figure 1-8 ■). Pharmaceutical options enable the health care industry as a whole, and health care facilities individually, to again expand the scope of care to be provided, increasing the number of individuals who can be helped, and reducing the negative impact on the overall economy.

Improved Noninvasive Procedures

Technology has provided us with more benefits than text messaging and instant video updates. The numerous methodologies that can be used to see inside a patient's body and observe what is

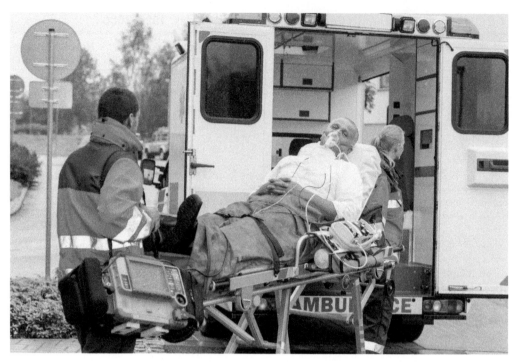

FIGURE 1-7 Improved training for EMTs and more sophisticated equipment in ambulances support better prognoses for patients requiring emergency care.
Photo credit: CandyBox Images/Fotolia.

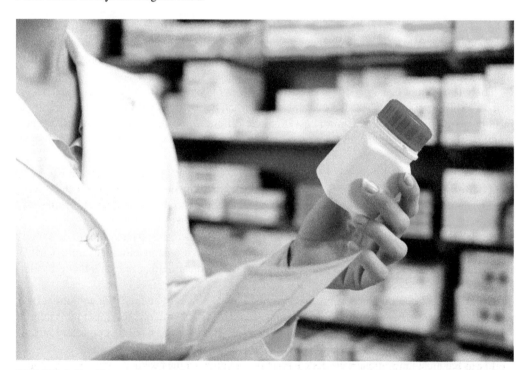

FIGURE 1-8 Pharmaceutical innovations are crucial, noninvasive health care treatments.
Photo credit: Kzenon/Shutterstock.

noninvasive procedure
a health care procedure that does not physically enter the body.

going on, without anesthesia or surgical incisions, are known as **noninvasive procedures**. These various types of investigative approaches are additional ways that health care professionals can diagnose and treat patients at a lower cost and with less interference to the patient's everyday life. Digital imaging, such as CT scans, MRI, ultrasonography, computed tomographic angiography (CTA), magnetic resonance arthroscopy (MRA), myelography, venography, and so much

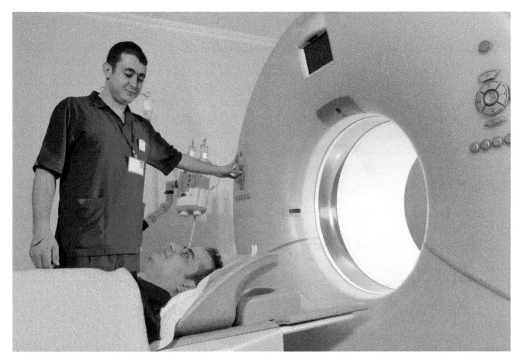

FIGURE 1-9 Imaging technology has dramatically improved the ability for a physician to see inside a patient, without any trauma, to determine an accurate diagnosis.
Photo credit: Konuk/Shutterstock.

more, has increased the detail and clarity of images, thereby giving the radiologist a greater opportunity to accurately determine the condition (Figure 1-9 ■). Safe passage for digital images to travel instantly through cyberspace gives a patient the benefit of an expert in another state or another country who can provide interpretation and recommendations.

In addition, radiation oncology services, including **teletherapy** and brachytherapy, enable noninvasive treatment for the eradication of malignant cells. Nuclear medicine procedures used for both diagnosis and treatment can also provide patients with noninvasive benefits.

teletherapy
the provision of health care services and/or consultation without direct patient contact.

What does this information mean to you as a health care administrator? It all adds up to an increase in potential patient rosters, an increase in the types of services that your facility may consider providing, and the expanded scope of knowledge needed to properly manage the personnel, equipment, patient load, and financial requirements for them all.

THE ROLE TO THE COMMUNITY AND THE ROLE OF THE COMMUNITY

Every health care facility has a responsibility to its community. Physician's office, walk-in clinic, acute-care hospital all serve as visual reminders within the community of their primary purpose of caring, nurturing, and protecting the people within. Emotionally, they are representative of a mother to her child, ever present to heal pain, disease, injury, or better yet, to prevent the illness altogether. From the application of a bandage on a small wound to heart transplant surgery, the bottom line is that this type of result is what the community expects from its health care providers. It is not realistic, but it is inherent in the public consciousness.

At the same time, the community has its own responsibilities to its health care providers. A bit more distanced, this support may come in the form of the approval of zoning, getting out of the way of an ambulance, or simply paying their share of the cost, as required. To take it one step further, a community fully supportive of its health care partners would also honor its responsibility for being proactive with preventive care so a reduction in the severity of illness will benefit everyone.

CHAPTER REVIEW

SUMMARY

A successful health care administrator needs to have managerial understanding of human resources, technology, financing, risk assessment, regulation compliance, and scope of services being provided and those that should be considered. Advances in preventive health care services, complementary alternative medicine methodologies, reduced need for inpa~~~~ ~~~~ions for many procedures, and advances in pharma~~~~als~~~~ emergency medicine have all contributed to long~~~~~~~~ives for your patient population. You will need to ~~~~te an~~~~alyze

the way your patient population makes use of the health care resources your facility has to offer them, and then consider ways that you can provide additional help.

As you make your way through this text, you will notice that each chapter will address one or more of the requirements ~~~~ ~~~~ the bulleted list of the job description provided to you ~~~~~~~~s chapter. The plan is that by the time you reach the ~~~~xt, you will have built a strong foundation for a suc~~~~~~~~er in health care.

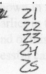

Handwritten notes:
1. A   11
2. D   12
3. C   13
4. B   14
9 C   15
6 D   16
7   17
8   18
9   19
10   20
21
22
23
24
25

REVIEW QUESTIONS

MULTIPLE CHOICE

Choose the most accurate answer.

1. Clinicians are the professionals whose primary responsibility is
    a. diagnosing and treating patients.
    b. ensuring the facility is financially stable.
    c. hiring support staff.
    d. analyzing data to determine addition of services.

2. Which of the following tasks is performed by a clinician?
    a. Procurement of x-ray machines
    b. Maintenance of x-ray machines
    c. Hiring of x-ray technicians
    d. Interpretation of an x-ray of the patient's knee

3. Health care administrators must supervise all of the following EXCEPT
    a. professional credential confirmation.
    b. accounts receivable and payable.
    c. determination of a patient's diagnosis.
    d. housekeeping and maintenance personnel.

4. From 1960 to 2009, the life span of people living in the United States
    a. decreased about nine years.
    b. increased about eight years.
    c. stayed the same.
    d. is unknown.

5. All of the following services are included in CAM, EXCEPT
    a. massage therapy.
    b. hypnosis.
    c. laparoscopic surgery.
    d. acupuncture.

6. Which of the following health care professionals is typically the first to attend to a patient in a health care crisis outside of a hospital?
    a. Registered nurse
    b. Thoracic surgeon
    c. Pharmacist
    d. Paramedic

7. Noninvasive diagnostics have been enhanced by the transition to
    a. new medications.
    b. digital imaging.
    c. laparoscopic surgery.
    d. vaccinations.

8. Infant mortality has _____ from 1960 to 2009.
    a. increased
    b. decreased
    c. stayed the same
    d. not been accurately measured

9. Health care administrators are needed in
    a. large hospital corporations.
    b. nursing homes and assisted living facilities.
    c. small physician group practices.
    d. all of the above

10. Health care administrators are required to
    a. perform risk assessments.
    b. design crisis management plans.
    c. implement performance improvement activities.
    d. all of the above

FILL-IN-THE-BLANK

Fill in the blank with the accurate answer.

11. As of 2011, 25% of the population of the United States is _____.

12. Technology has a big impact on health care finances, especially with the implementation of electronic claim creation and submission, as well as _____.

13. The way individuals use the resources of the health care industry is known as health care _____.

14. The life expectancy in the United States has increased from 69.77 years in 1960 to _____ years in 2009.

15. A flu shot and a colonoscopy are examples of _____ health care services.

16. According to the National Center for Health Statistics, CAM stands for _____.

17. According to the CDC, from 1990 to 2000, the largest number of health care services were provided during _____.

18. Fluoroscopy, ultrasound, and nuclear medicine are all types of noninvasive _____ procedures.

19. The group who rely, and will rely, on your organization for health care services is known as your _____.

20. The responsibility to ensure that everyone within the organization is following the applicable laws and regulations is known as _____.

TRUE/FALSE

Indicate whether each of the following statements is true or false.

21. In 2010, more adults eighteen years of age and over were in excellent or very good health than in previous years. _____

22. In 2010, more than three-quarters of adults eighteen years of age and over maintained their excellent or very good health from the prior year. _____

23. It is recommended that children age six and over be screened for hepatitis B. _____

24. Administrators oversee the health of patients, and clinicians oversee the health of the facility. _____

25. CAM stands for computerized advanced medicine. _____

26. As mentioned in the section of this chapter on CAM, more than half of all adults surveyed used some type of alternative medicine. _____

27. Preventive medicine and screening for early diagnosis has been found to cause more illness. _____

28. A vaccine is currently available to prevent HPV, a known cause of cervical cancer. _____

29. Some medications can prevent illness, while others can treat illness. _____

30. A successful health care administrator needs to have managerial understanding of every aspect of the facility. _____

WHEN YOU ARE THE ADMINISTRATOR . . .

Critical Thinking and Analysis

Case Study #1

Better Service to Current Patient Population

You are the administrator of a 250-bed hospital. A recent report from the county tells you that the population within a 25-mile radius of your facility is getting younger—the median age in the area has decreased from 35 years of age to 29 years of age. This was an expected impact of the opening of a new state university campus about five miles away.

a. What do you need to review and analyze in order to ensure that you can provide the services required by this changing population in your area?

b. Are there any departments in your hospital that may need to be added or expanded? If so, specifically, which services?

c. Are there any departments you might be able to reduce or eliminate? If so, specifically, which services?

d. What details about clinical staff and administrative staff do you need to take into consideration for any of these changes?

Case Study #2

Proposal for New Program or Service

Figure 1-10 ■ is information taken directly from the report "Health, United States, 2010," published by the National Center for Health Statistics, Centers for Disease Control and Prevention, U.S. Department of Health and Human Services regarding adults who are overweight or obese. **Review the statistics and details presented in this report and create a proposal for a new program or service your facility could provide to help these patients improve their health.**

(Continued)

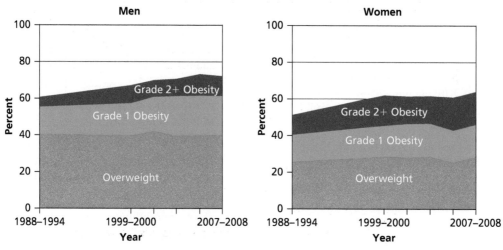

FIGURE 1-10 Health, United States, 2010.

Source: New Health, United States, 2010.

Case Study #3

Expanded Services Presentation

Figure 1-11 ■ is a chart from the National Health Statistics Reports, December 10, 2008, on the use of complementary alternative medicine by adults and children.

Analyze the data included and create a PowerPoint presentation to propose that your facility should expand the services provided to your patient population to include some form of CAM.

Case Study #4

Strategic Planning for a Nursing Home

Evaluate the data presented in Figure 1-12 ■ concerning the age distribution of nursing home residents, along with the data presented in Table 1-1 concerning population by age.

As the health care administrator of a nursing home, how can you use these specifics to begin creating a strategic plan for the future of this facility? Be specific. Are there any changes or expansions you might consider, based on this information? What can you estimate will be the age of the population of the nursing home ten years from now? Twenty years from now?

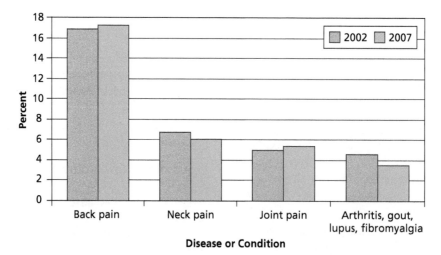

FIGURE 1-11 Use of complementary alternative medicine services.

Source: CDC/NCHS, National Health Interview Survey, 2002 and 2007.

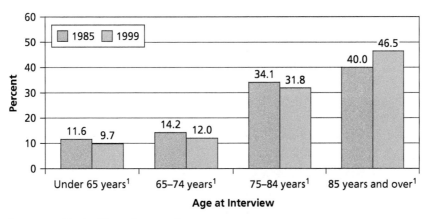

[1]Time trend is significant ($p < 0.05$).

FIGURE 1-12   Age distribution of nursing home residents: United States, 1985 and 1999.

Source: Centers for Disease Control and Prevention, National Center for Health Statistics, National Nursing Home Survey (NNHS).

INTERNET CONNECTIONS

Healthfinder

Healthfinder connects you with a range of health-related resources. Discover these resources at
www.healthfinder.gov/.
The same service is available in Spanish at:
www.healthfinder.gov/espanol/

National Health Information Center

The U.S. Federal Government maintains several health clearinghouses and information centers that connect you to various credible resources on specific topics. This makes searching for information easier and brings you to trusted, credible sites. To see what's out there, visit:
http://www.health.gov/nhic/pubs/2010clearinghouses/clearinghouses.htm

National Center for Complementary and Alternative Medicine

The National Center for Complementary and Alternative Medicine (NCCAM) Information Clearinghouse provides great information about the various types of health care services categorized as complementary medicine and alternative medicine. Discover them here at:
http://nccam.nih.gov/

CHAPTER 1 ENDNOTES

1. World Bank, World Development Indicators. Last updated: Feb 10, 2012. Retrieved from http://www.google.com/publicdata
2. *USPSTF A and B Recommendations*. August 2010. U.S. Preventive Services Task Force. http://www.uspreventiveservicestaskforce.org/uspstf/uspsabrecs.htm
3. Barnes, P. M., Powell-Griner, E., McFann, K. Nahin, R. L. Complementary and alternative medicine use among adults: United States, 2002. Advance data from vital and health statistics; no. 343. Hyattsville, MD: U.S. Department of Health and Human Services, CDC, National Center for Health Statistics; 2004. Available at http://www.cdc.gov/nchs/data/ad/ad343.pdf

CHAPTER 2

TYPES OF FACILITIES AND SERVICES

KEY TERMS

acute care hospital
ambulatory surgical center
  (ASC)
assisted living facility
board-certified physician
certified nurse midwife (CNM)
certified registered nurse
  anesthetist (CRNA)
clinic
demographics
dietetic technician, registered
  (DTR)
domiciliary
economics
home health agency
hospice
inpatient facility
not-for-profit (nonprofit)
  facility
nurse practitioner (NP)
outpatient facility
physicians' office
proprietary facility
rehabilitation center
registered dietitian (RD)
skilled nursing facility (SNF)

LEARNING OBJECTIVES

Upon completion of this chapter, you should be able to:

- Define commonly used terms, abbreviations, and acronyms.
- Identify the different types of health care facilities.
- Enumerate the various types of services offered.
- Compare the types of services provided to various segments of the population.
- Describe the types of services offered in different types of facilities.
- Evaluate the personnel requirements for the different types of services.

WHEN YOU ARE THE ADMINISTRATOR . . .

As a health care administrator, you will need to be able to:

- Assess and identify specific services, equipment, and personnel needed to address the current and future health care needs of the community and the funding required to provide such services.
- Research, analyze data, and determine recommendations for the addition, expansion, or reduction of specialized services currently provided by the organization.

INTRODUCTION

A perfectly balanced health care industry ensures that providers have appropriate state-of-the-art services available for each and every patient, as required when needed. This means that doing the job of a health care administrator necessitates the ability to predict the health care requirements of the population that surrounds the facility. Don't misunderstand. No single facility has to expertly provide all services. As with any other team of specialists, the industry as a whole should be able to provide the solution to each patient's health care concern. Therefore, each administrator must evaluate the goals and capabilities of their individual facility and determine the scope of services that this facility needs to provide in order to maintain its own financial health.

TYPES OF FACILITIES

The official type of facility is directly aligned with the types of health care services that the entity provides. Of course, there are facilities that provide multiple types of services.

The administrative or business aspect of health care facilities will fall under one of two categories: proprietary or not-for-profit.

- *Proprietary facilities* are owned and run by corporations with shareholders.
- *Not-for-profit (nonprofit) facilities* might be owned and run by the public (a public entity such as the federal or state government, or an agency of the government, such as a military hospital) or a specialized group, such as a religious organization or community association.

Generally speaking, a health care facility is categorized as either an inpatient or outpatient facility. Note that there are acute care facilities that provide both types of services, in separate departments, under one roof.

- *Inpatient facilities* are those that provide health care treatments and procedures, along with room, nourishment, and ancillary services, to a patient who requires medically supervised care twenty-four hours a day, for at least twenty-four to forty-eight hours (Figure 2-1 ■).

proprietary facility
an organization owned and operated by a for-profit corporation.

not-for-profit (nonprofit) facility
an organization with a tax status that is designated to reinvest excess revenue into the organization for the betterment of its patients (customers).

inpatient facility
a facility providing room and meals in addition to health care services on a continuous basis.

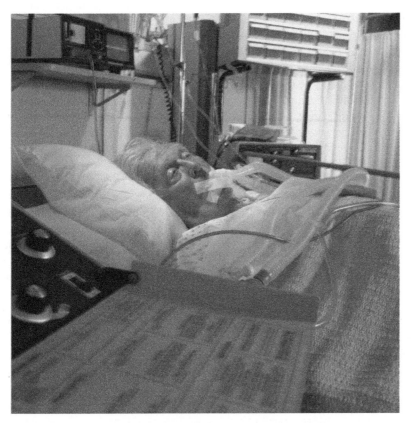

FIGURE 2-1   Inpatient facilities help patients who require "round the clock" medical support.
Photo credit: Ken Tannenbaum/Shutterstock.

outpatient facility
a facility that provides health care services alone, without room and board.

- *Outpatient facilities* provide only health care services, generally without an overnight stay. There are occasions when a patient will stay in the facility overnight, but generally not longer than twenty-four hours.

NOTE: In health care, there is a specific difference between *date of service* and *twenty-four hours.*

A *date of service* is a calendar day—12:01 A.M. to 11:59 P.M.—while twenty-four hours is exactly as it sounds—twenty-four consecutive hours. In some cases, a patient may be kept in the facility for twenty-four hours and this actually represents two *dates of service.*

For example: After his surgery, Dr. Lennox decides to keep Roger Johnson for twenty-four hours. It is now 3:30 P.M. Tuesday. The next day (Wednesday), Dr. Lennox reviews Roger's test results, the nursing notes from overnight and this morning, and decides to discharge Roger. Discharge notes state: 3:15 P.M. Roger was in the facility for twenty-four hours, but he received care on two dates of service: Tuesday and Wednesday.

Within these two general categories, there are subsets of facilities that are typically described by the types of health care (medical) services they provide.

acute care hospital
a facility providing medical care in an inpatient setting to diagnose and treat an injury or illness for a limited duration of time.

- *Acute care, or general, hospitals* provide immediate and short-term care in an inpatient environment for the purposes of diagnostic and therapeutic care. Inpatient medical and surgical services may be administered for conditions, diseases, and injuries that need various types of care around the clock (twenty-four hours a day).
- *Emergency or trauma centers* are health care facilities that are open 24 hours a day/365 days a year to provide services to those who require immediate (unscheduled) medical attention based on a single situation or circumstance. For example: trauma care (e.g., injuries from a car accident; fall); acute medical conditions (e.g., heart attack, labor and delivery); psychiatric emergency (e.g., emotional crisis, severe shock); and so on. These facilities will often employ physicians and staff specially trained in emergency medicine or trauma medicine. Independent facilities may be known as *urgent care centers.* On the other hand, *emergency departments* (ED) are more often a part of an acute care hospital.
- *Community or regional hospitals*, as their name implies, are focused on providing services identified as important to those in their patient population. Whether large or small (measured by the number of beds), this facility will be licensed as an "acute care hospital," and it will virtually always include an emergency department.
- *Critical access hospitals (CAH)* are specifically designated as such by participating in a federal program designed to assure that facilities based in rural areas will not lose the ability to provide quality health care services to the community within which the facility is located. This classification helps to keep them financially stable by enhancing reimbursement for the procedures, services, and treatments they provide. CAH are protected by the *State Medicare Rural Hospital Flexibility Program* (Flex), developed as a part of the Balanced Budget Act (BBA) of 1997.
- *Specialty (acute care) hospitals* narrow the scope of services provided, either by specific medical specialty (e.g., MD Anderson Cancer Centers, Resnick Neuropsychiatric Hospital at UCLA) or a narrow portion of the patient population (e.g., Boston Children's Hospital, Winnie Palmer Hospital for Women and Babies). This category will be discussed further in the next section of this chapter.
- *Teaching hospitals* are acute care facilities with a specific accreditation to provide medical education and training to the health care professionals of the future. Those with this formal designation are affiliated with an accredited medical school and are integrally involved with the approved curriculum for these students.
- *Veterans Affairs (VA) hospitals* provide a full scope of health care and medical services to veterans (those individuals honorable discharged from military service). These facilities are all encompassing, meaning they will offer inpatient and outpatient services, extended (long-term) care, rehabilitation care, and more.
- *Research hospitals* may be separate, free-standing organizations, or they may be a department or division within a teaching hospital. These facilities care for the future patient by studying methodologies for new vaccinations, new procedures or treatments, new surgical techniques, or new pharmaceuticals that may cure conditions that plague individuals today.

ambulatory surgical center (ASC)
facility that provides surgical procedures on an outpatient basis.

- *Ambulatory Surgical Centers (ASC)* are free-standing facilities that provide surgical procedures on an outpatient basis only. ASCs are also known as same day surgery centers.

- *Clinics*, also known as walk-in clinics, free clinics, or urgent care centers, are outpatient facilities that accept overall responsibility for an individual's health care and provide a limited scope of services.
- *Physicians' offices* are outpatient facilities that exist in a various number of sizes: solo practice, small group practice, or large group practice. Physicians' offices may offer general services or specialized health care services, such as an endocrinologist, orthopedist, or urologist.
- *Home health agencies* organize clinicians, typically physicians, registered nurses, and licensed practical nurses to provide health care services in the patient's residence.
- *Rehabilitation hospitals/centers* provide care to patients who have suffered some type of disability, either mental or physical, with the intent of supporting their recovery to a level of function and independence. These facilities will typically offer a variety of physical therapy, occupational therapy, and speech therapy services on either an inpatient or outpatient basis. A rehabilitation center may be affiliated with an acute care hospital, teaching hospital, or a skilled nursing facility.
- *Domiciliaries* provide patients who are independent with a place to live and supervised, limited health care support (such as medication management). The participants may be provided with a room in a group home or an individual apartment. They are commonly known as halfway houses. Domiciliaries are a part of VA services, psychiatric residential programs, and other patient population-focused services.
- *Skilled nursing facilities (SNF)* furnish short-term and long-term inpatient care services, twenty-four hours a day, seven days a week, and include both health care and personal services.
- *Assisted living facilities* supply long-term, residential services to patients who have some independence yet need assistance with medication administration, activities of daily living (ADL), and medical services (Figure 2-2 ■).
- *Intermediate care facilities for individuals with mental retardation (ICF/MR*)* are optional benefits offered by all fifty state Medicaid programs. ICF/MR are designed to provide both health care and rehabilitation services to individuals with an intellectual disability (ID) in

clinic
a health care facility providing a limited range of services on an outpatient basis.

physicians' office
a private facility in which a licensed health care professional can provide outpatient services.

home health agency
an organization that provides health care services to a patient in their own home.

rehabilitation center
a health care facility providing services and therapies designed to restore an individual to an optimal level of physical, mental, and/or vocational health and independence.

domiciliary
a place of residence for independent individuals requiring supervision, e.g. halfway house.

skilled nursing facility (SNF)
an inpatient facility providing twenty-four hour continuous health care services provided by health care professionals, including registered nurses.

assisted living facility
an inpatient facility providing long-term care for individuals requiring help with the activities of daily living (ADL) and requiring limited medical services.

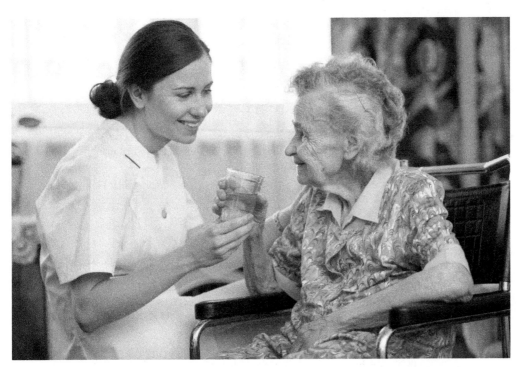

FIGURE 2-2 Assisted living facilities provide assistance with ADLs, medication management, and other non-nursing care.
Photo credit: Alexander Raths/Fotolia.

**CMS prefers using the term* intellectual disability (ID) *as a replacement for the term* mental retardation (MR). *However, the acronym ICF/MR has become a standard part of the nomenclature, so this continues to be the accepted phrase.*

hospice

an organization that provides health care services, most often palliative care to those who are terminally ill.

order to promote the individual's functional status and independence. The facilities in this program are a good alternative to home and community-based services.

• *Hospice* is a facility that delivers end-of-life care (also known as palliative care) to termi-nally ill patients in their own homes or in an inpatient hospice facility. These patients are expected to die within six months (a Medicare limitation that is accepted industry-wide).

Medicare has a specific list of every type of health care organization or provider, each iden-tified by a two-digit code. These codes are used, most often, in relation to reimbursement from Medicare, on each claim to report the type of facility in which the services were provided to the patient, as you can see in Table 2-1 ■. This list gives you some additional insights to the various types of facilities that provide health care services.

TABLE 2-1   **Place of Service (POS) Codes for Professional Claims Database (updated November 1, 2012)**

Place of Service (POS) Code(s)	Place of Service (POS) Name	Place of Service Description
01	Pharmacy	A facility or location where drugs and other medically related items and services are sold, dispensed, or otherwise provided directly to patients.
02	Unassigned	
03	School	A facility whose primary purpose is education
04	Homeless Shelter	A facility or location whose primary purpose is to provide temporary housing to homeless individuals (e.g., emergency shelters, individual or family shelters).
05	Indian Health Service Free-standing Facility	A facility, or location, owned and operated by the Indian Health Service, which provides diag-nostic, therapeutic (surgical and nonsurgical), and rehabilitation services to American Indians and Alaska natives who do not require hospitalization.
06	Indian Health Service Provider-based Facility	A facility or location, owned and operated by the Indian Health Service, which provides diag-nostic, therapeutic (surgical and nonsurgical), and rehabilitation services rendered by, or under the supervision of, physicians to American Indians and Alaska natives admitted as inpatients or outpatients.
07	Tribal 628 Free-standing Facility	A facility or location owned and operated by a federally recognized American Indian or Alaska native tribe or tribal organization under a 638 agreement, which provides diagnostic, therapeutic (surgical and nonsurgical), and rehabilitation services to tribal members who do not require hospitalization.
08	Tribal 638 Provider-based Facility	A facility or location owned and operated by a federally recognized American Indian or Alaska native tribe or tribal organization under a 638 agreement, which provides diagnostic, therapeutic (surgical and nonsurgical), and rehabilitation services to tribal members who do not require hospitalization.
09	Prison/Correctional Facility	A prison, jail, reformatory, work farm, detention center, or any other similar facility main-tained by either federal, state or local authorities for the purpose of confinement or rehabilita-tion of adult or juvenile criminal offenders.
10	Unassigned	
11	Office	Location, other than a hospital, skilled nursing facility (SNF), military treatment facility, com-munity health center, state or local public health clinic, or intermediate care facility (ICF), where the health professional routinely provides health examinations, diagnosis, and treatment of illness or injury on an ambulatory basis.
12	Home	Location, other than a hospital or other facility, where the patient receives care in a private residence.
13	Assisted Living Facility	Congregate residential facility with self-contained living units providing assessment of each resident's needs and on-site support twenty-four hours a day, seven days a week, with the capacity to deliver or arrange for services including some health care and other services.
14	Group Home	A residence, with shared living areas, where clients receive supervision and other services such as social or behavioral services, custodial service, and minimal services (e.g., medication administration).
15	Mobile Unit	A facility/unit that moves from place to place equipped to provide preventive, screening, diag-nostic, or treatment services.

TABLE 2-1 *(Continued)*

Place of Service (POS) Code(s)	Place of Service (POS) Name	Place of Service Description
16	Temporary Lodging	A short-term accommodation such as a hotel, camp ground, hostel, cruise ship or resort where the patient receives care, and which is not identified by any other POS code.
17	Walk-in Retail Health Clinic	A walk-in health clinic, other than an office, urgent care facility, pharmacy or independent clinic and not described by any other POS code, that is located within a retail operation and provides, on an ambulatory basis, preventive and primary care services.
18	Place of Employment—Worksite	A location, not described by any other POS code, owned or operated by a public or private entity where the patient is employed, and where a health professional provides ongoing or episodic occupational medical, therapeutic or rehabilitative services to the individual.
19	Unassigned	
20	Urgent Care Facility	Location, distinct from a hospital emergency room, an office, or a clinic, whose purpose is to diagnose and treat illness or injury for unscheduled, ambulatory patients seeking immediate medical attention.
21	Inpatient Hospital	A facility, other than psychiatric, which primarily provides diagnostic, therapeutic (both surgical and nonsurgical), and rehabilitation services by, or under, the supervision of physicians to patients admitted for a variety of medical conditions.
22	Outpatient Hospital	A portion of a hospital, which provides diagnostic, therapeutic (both surgical and nonsurgical), and rehabilitation services to sick or injured persons who do not require hospitalization or institutionalization.
23	Emergency Room—Hospital	A portion of a hospital where emergency diagnosis and treatment of illness or injury is provided.
24	Ambulatory Surgical Center	A freestanding facility, other than a physician's office, where surgical and diagnostic services are provided on an ambulatory basis.
25	Birthing Center	A facility, other than a hospital's maternity facilities or a physician's office, which provides a setting for labor, delivery, and immediate postpartum care as well as immediate care of newborn infants.
26	Military Treatment Facility	A medical facility operated by one or more of the Uniformed Services. Military Treatment Facility (MTF) also refers to certain former U.S. Public Health Service (USPHS) facilities now designated as Uniformed Service Treatment Facilities (USTF).
27–30	Unassigned	
31	Skilled Nursing Facility	A facility that primarily provides inpatient skilled nursing care and related services to patients who require medical, nursing, or rehabilitative services but does not provide the level of care or treatment available in a hospital.
32	Nursing Facility	A facility which primarily provides to residents skilled nursing care and related services for the rehabilitation of injured, disabled, or sick persons, or, on a regular basis, health-related care services above the level of custodial care to other than mentally retarded individuals.
33	Custodial Care Facility	A facility which provides room, board and other personal assistance services, generally on a long-term basis, and which does not include a medical component.
34	Hospice	A facility, other than a patient's home, in which palliative and supportive care for terminally ill patients and their families are provided.
35–40	Unassigned	
41	Ambulance—Land	A land vehicle specifically designed, equipped, and staffed for lifesaving and transporting the sick or injured.
42	Ambulance—Air or Water	An air or water vehicle specifically designed, equipped and staffed for lifesaving and transporting the sick or injured.
43–48	Unassigned	
49	Independent Clinic	A location, not part of a hospital and not described by any other POS code, that is organized and operated to provide preventive, diagnostic, therapeutic, rehabilitative, or palliative services to outpatients only.
50	Federally Qualified Health Center	A facility located in a medically underserved area that provides Medicare beneficiaries preventive primary medical care under the general direction of a physician.

(Continued)

TABLE 2-1   (Continued)

Place of Service (POS) Code(s)	Place of Service (POS) Name	Place of Service Description
51	Inpatient Psychiatric Facility	A facility that provides inpatient psychiatric services for the diagnosis and treatment of mental illness on a twenty-four-hour basis, by or under the supervision of a physician.
52	Psychiatric Facility— Partial Hospitalization	A facility for the diagnosis and treatment of mental illness that provides a planned therapeutic program for patients who do not require full time hospitalization, but who need broader programs than are possible from outpatient visits to a hospital-based or hospital-affiliated facility.
53	Community Mental Health Center	A facility that provides the following services: outpatient services, including specialized outpatient services for children, the elderly, individuals who are chronically ill, and residents of the CMHC's mental health services area who have been discharged from inpatient treatment at a mental health facility; twenty-four hour a day emergency care services; day treatment, other partial hospitalization services, or psychosocial rehabilitation services; screening for patients being considered for admission to state mental health facilities to determine the appropriateness of such admission; and consultation and education services.
54	Intermediate Care Facility/Mentally Retarded	A facility which primarily provides health-related care and services above the level of custodial care to mentally retarded individuals but does not provide the level of care or treatment available in a hospital or SNF.
55	Residential Substance Abuse Treatment Facility	A facility that provides treatment for substance (alcohol and drug) abuse to live-in residents who do not require acute medical care. Services include individual and group therapy and counseling, family counseling, laboratory tests, drugs and supplies, psychological testing, and room and board.
56	Psychiatric Residential Treatment Center	A facility or distinct part of a facility for psychiatric care, which provides a total twenty-four-hour therapeutically planned and professionally staffed group living and learning environment.
57	Nonresidential Substance Abuse Treatment Facility	A location that provides treatment for substance (alcohol and drug) abuse on an ambulatory basis. Services include individual and group therapy and counseling, family counseling, laboratory tests, drugs and supplies, and psychological testing.
58–59	Unassigned	
60	Mass Immunization Center	A location where providers administer pneumococcal pneumonia and influenza virus vaccinations and submit these services as electronic media claims, paper claims, or using the roster billing method. This generally takes place in a mass immunization setting, such as, a public health center, pharmacy, or mall but may include a physician office setting.
61	Comprehensive Inpatient Rehabilitation Facility	A facility that provides comprehensive rehabilitation services under the supervision of a physician to inpatients with physical disabilities. Services include physical therapy, occupational therapy, speech pathology, social or psychological services, and orthotics and prosthetics services.
62	Comprehensive Outpatient Rehabilitation Facility	A facility that provides comprehensive rehabilitation services under the supervision of a physician to outpatients with physical disabilities. Services include physical therapy, occupational therapy, and speech pathology services.
63–64	Unassigned	
65	End-Stage Renal Disease Treatment Facility	A facility other than a hospital that provides dialysis treatment, maintenance, or training to patients or caregivers on an ambulatory or home-care basis.
66–70	Unassigned	
71	Public Health Clinic	A facility, maintained by either state or local health departments, that provides ambulatory primary medical care under the general direction of a physician.
72	Rural Health Clinic	A certified facility, which is located in a rural medically, underserved area that provides ambulatory primary medical care under the general direction of a physician.
73–80	Unassigned	
81	Independent Laboratory	A laboratory certified to perform diagnostic or clinical tests independent of an institution or a physician's office.
82–98	Unassigned	
99	Other Place of Service	Other place of service not identified above.

Source: Centers for Medicare and Medicaid Services.

TYPES OF SERVICES

The various types of services you provide in your facility will require staff members with specialized training and credentials as well as specific equipment and materials. Specialization is a directed focus of advanced education and provision of care, and it indicates a level of expertise in the specific discipline. Therefore, administrators want to ensure that the individual professing knowledge and skill in a specialized area of health care has the credentials to support the provision of services.

Medicare has indicators to identify the specific category of a type of service provided to one of its beneficiaries. You can see, in Table 2-2 ■, how they classify this data.

Facility Specializations

Health care facilities can focus on narrow areas of services to provide to their patients by assembling personnel with specialized certifications (knowledge and skill), along with equipment and supplies that provide a heightened level of care for those patients with a particular diagnosis.

Acute care specialty hospitals are becoming more widespread around the country. Some are quite well known throughout the United States, such as the Shriner's Hospitals, which provide

TABLE 2-2   Type of Service Indicators

"TYPE OF SERVICE" INDICATORS	
0	Whole Blood
1	Medical Care
2	Surgery
3	Consultation
4	Diagnostic Radiology
5	Diagnostic Laboratory
6	Therapeutic Radiology
7	Anesthesia
8	Assistant at Surgery
9	Other Medical Items or Services
A	Used DME
B	High Risk Screening Mammography
C	Low Risk Screening Mammography
D	Ambulance
E	Enteral/Parenteral Nutrients/Supplies
F	Ambulatory Surgical Center (Facility Usage for Surgical Services)
G	Immunosuppressive Drugs
H	Hospice
J	Diabetic Shoes
K	Hearing Items and Services
L	ESRD Supplies
M	Monthly Capitation Payment for Dialysis
N	Kidney Donor
P	Lump Sum Purchase of DME, Prosthetics, Orthotics
Q	Vision Items or Services
R	Rental of DME
S	Surgical Dressings or Other Medical Supplies
T	Outpatient Mental Health Treatment Limitation
U	Occupational Therapy
V	Pneumococcal/Flu Vaccine
W	Physical Therapy

Source: Medicare Claims Processing Manual Chapter 26—Completing and Processing Form CMS-1500 Data Set Table of Contents (Rev. 2516, 08-10-12) (Rev. 2598, 11-23-12).

specialty care to both orthopedic and burn patients; St. Jude's Children's Research Hospital, which provides expert care to children with cancer; and MD Anderson Cancer Center, which has oncology specialists for adults with a variety of affected anatomical sites. In addition, you may know of the Arnold Palmer Hospital for Children or the Winnie Palmer Hospital for Women and Babies, or you may have a specialty hospital in your area of the country.

Some general acute care hospitals provide specialty areas within their facility. As you become more involved in the industry, you may become aware of a local hospital that has the best reputation for trauma care in their emergency department, specialty clinics such as those for diabetic care, or a center within the general hospital that specializes in cardiac care.

Short-term care rehabilitation specializations are becoming quite common, especially with their frequent mention in the news for treating celebrities. These include alcohol rehabilitation centers, drug rehabilitation centers, mental health facilities, as well as therapeutic centers that focus on post-CVA (stroke), post-orthopedic surgery, and/or speech therapy. You might remember the short-term care facilities for sex addiction that were mentioned during recent celebrity scandals.

Home health agencies are becoming more prevalent around the country as older individuals choose to stay in their homes rather than go to a group or institutional setting. While some agencies may provide general care, such as medication management or assistance with activities of daily living (ADL), others provide specialized services such as intravenous (IV)/intramuscular (IM) hydration and therapeutic administration, stoma maintenance, pre/post-natal care, mechanical ventilation care, respiratory therapy care, catheter care and maintenance, hemodialysis, nutrition assessment and intervention services, along with self-care and home management training.

Clinician Specializations

board-certified physician
a credential signifying the completion of additional education in a specific area of health care, as authenticated by the passing of an exam administered by an authorized association.

Once accredited education and assessment has been completed successfully, the American Board of Medical Specialties (ABMS) awards physicians certification deeming them **board-certified physicians** in that specific specialty or subspecialty. The required education is focused on a specialized area of health care (such as cardiology, neonatology, or pediatric oncology) and is above and beyond that required for graduation from medical school and licensing. The many different board specialties and sub-specialties available for physicians are listed in Table 2-3 ■. Visit www.ambs.org for the most current version, as this information may change from time to time.

TABLE 2-3   Approved Specialty and Subspecialty Certificates in which the ABMS Member Boards Can Offer Certification

General Certificate(s)	Subspecialty Certificates
American Board of Allergy and Immunology	
Allergy and Immunology	No Subspecialties
American Board of Anesthesiology	
Anesthesiology	Critical Care Medicine
	Hospice and Palliative Medicine
	Pain Medicine
	Pediatric Anesthesiology[1]
	Sleep Medicine
American Board of Colon and Rectal Surgery	
Colon and Rectal Surgery	No Subspecialties
American Board of Dermatology	
Dermatology	Dermatopathology
	Pediatric Dermatology
American Board of Emergency Medicine	
Emergency Medicine	Emergency Medical Services[2]
	Hospice and Palliative Medicine
	Internal Medicine-Critical Care Medicine
	Medical Toxicology
	Pediatric Emergency Medicine
	Sports Medicine
	Undersea and Hyperbaric Medicine

TABLE 2-3   (Continued)

General Certificate(s)	Subspecialty Certificates
American Board of Family Medicine	
Family Medicine	Adolescent Medicine
	Geriatric Medicine
	Hospice and Palliative Medicine
	Sleep Medicine
	Sports Medicine
American Board of Internal Medicine	
Internal Medicine	Adolescent Medicine
	Adult Congenital Heart Disease[3]
	Advanced Heart Failure and Transplant
	Cardiology
	Cardiovascular Disease
	Clinical Cardiac Electrophysiology
	Critical Care Medicine
	Endocrinology, Diabetes and Metabolism
	Gastroenterology
	Geriatric Medicine
	Hematology
	Hospice and Palliative Medicine
	Infectious Disease
	Interventional Cardiology
	Medical Oncology
	Nephrology
	Pulmonary Disease
	Rheumatology
	Sleep Medicine
	Sports Medicine
	Transplant Hepatology
American Board of Medical Genetics	
Clinical Biochemical Genetics*	Medical Biochemical Genetics
Clinical Cytogenetics*	Molecular Genetic Pathology
Clinical Genetics (MD)*	
Clinical Molecular Genetics*	
American Board of Neurological Surgery	
Neurological Surgery	No Subspecialties
American Board of Nuclear Medicine	
Nuclear Medicine	No Subspecialties
American Board of Obstetrics and Gynecology	
Obstetrics and Gynecology	Critical Care Medicine
	Female Pelvic Medicine and Reconstructive . . . Surgery[1]
	Gynecologic Oncology
	Hospice and Palliative Medicine
	Maternal and Fetal Medicine
	Reproductive Endocrinology/Infertility
American Board of Ophthalmology	
Ophthalmology	No Subspecialties
American Board of Orthopaedic Surgery	
Orthopaedic Surgery	Orthopaedic Sports Medicine
	Surgery of the Hand

(Continued)

TABLE 2-3   *(Continued)*

General Certificate(s)	Subspecialty Certificates
American Board of Otolaryngology	
Otolaryngology	Neurotology
	Pediatric Otolaryngology
	Plastic Surgery Within the Head and Neck
	Sleep Medicine
American Board of Pathology	
Pathology—Anatomic/Pathology-Clinical*	Blood Banking/Transfusion Medicine
Pathology—Anatomic*	Clinical Informatics[1]
Pathology—Clinical*	Cytopathology
	Dermatopathology
	Neuropathology
	Pathology—Chemical
	Pathology—Forensic
	Pathology—Hematology
	Pathology—Medical Microbiology
	Pathology—Molecular Genetic
	Pathology—Pediatric
American Board of Pediatrics	
Pediatrics	Adolescent Medicine
	Child Abuse Pediatrics
	Developmental-Behavioral Pediatrics
	Hospice and Palliative Medicine
	Medical Toxicology
	Neonatal-Perinatal Medicine
	Neurodevelopmental Disabilities
	Pediatric Cardiology
	Pediatric Critical Care Medicine Pediatric Emergency Medicine
	Pediatric Endocrinology
	Pediatric Gastroenterology
	Pediatric Hematology-Oncology
	Pediatric Infectious Diseases
	Pediatric Nephrology
	Pediatric Pulmonology
	Pediatric Rheumatology
	Pediatric Transplant Hepatology
	Sleep Medicine
	Sports Medicine
American Board of Physical Medicine and Rehabilitation	
Physical Medicine and Rehabilitation	Brain Injury Medicine[4]
	Hospice and Palliative Medicine
	Neuromuscular Medicine
	Pain Medicine
	Pediatric Rehabilitation Medicine
	Spinal Cord Injury Medicine
	Sports Medicine
American Board of Plastic Surgery	
Plastic Surgery	Plastic Surgery Within the Head and Neck
	Surgery of the Hand

TABLE 2-3   *(Continued)*

General Certificate(s)	Subspecialty Certificates
American Board of Preventive Medicine	
Aerospace Medicine*	Clinical Informatics[1]
Occupational Medicine*	Medical Toxicology
Public Health and General Preventive . . . Medicine*	Undersea and Hyperbaric Medicine
American Board of Psychiatry and Neurology	
Psychiatry*	Addiction Psychiatry
Neurology*	Brain Injury Medicine[4]
Neurology with Special Qualification in Child Neurology*	Child and Adolescent Psychiatry
	Clinical Neurophysiology
	Epilepsy[2]
	Forensic Psychiatry
	Geriatric Psychiatry
	Hospice and Palliative Medicine
	Neurodevelopmental Disabilities
	Neuromuscular Medicine
	Pain Medicine
	Psychosomatic Medicine
	Sleep Medicine
	Vascular Neurology
American Board of Radiology	
Diagnostic Radiology*	Hospice and Palliative Medicine
Interventional Radiology and Diagnostic . . . Radiology*[3]	Neuroradiology
Radiation Oncology*	Nuclear Radiology
Medical Physics*	Pediatric Radiology
	Vascular and Interventional Radiology
American Board of Surgery	
Surgery*	Complex General Surgical Oncology[4]
Vascular Surgery*	Hospice and Palliative Medicine
	Pediatric Surgery
	Surgery of the Hand
	Surgical Critical Care
American Board of Thoracic Surgery	
Thoracic and Cardiac Surgery	Congenital Cardiac Surgery
American Board of Urology	
Urology	Female Pelvic Medicine and Reconstructive Surgery[1]
	Pediatric Urology

*Specific disciplines within the specialty where certification is offered.

[1]Approved 2011; first issue 2013. [2]Approved 2010; first issue 2013. [3]Approved 2012; first issue to be determined. [4]Approved 2011, first issue to be determined.

Source: American Board of Medical Specialties: www.abms.org. Reprinted with permission.

Nurses also earn specialty certifications, such as:

- *Nurse practitioner (NP)* is a registered nurse (RN) with advanced education and clinical training. These professionals can provide both general and acute-care services.
- *Certified Nurse Midwife (CNM)* is a nationally certified professional after successfully completing advanced education (many with master's degrees) on a wide range of services beyond just the birthing process. These professionals most often work alongside obstetricians (OB).

nurse practitioner (NP)
a credential signifying the successful completion of additional, specialized training, authorizing a registered nurse (RN) to provide basic health care services to patients including determining diagnosis and treatment plan for common acute injuries and illnesses.

certified nurse midwife (CNM)
a credential signifying the successful completion of additional, specialized training in assisting the delivery of a neonate.

certified registered nurse anesthetist (CRNA)

a credential signifying the successful completion of additional, specialized training in the administration of anesthesia.

registered dietitian (RD)

a credential signifying the successful completion of additional, specialized training in nutrition.

dietetic technician, registered (DTR)

a credential signifying the successful completion of additional, specialized training in nutrition.

- *Certified Registered Nurse Anesthetist (CRNA)* is a qualified, advance-practice registered nurse with specialized education and board certification in anesthesia.
- *Registered Dietitian (RD) or a Dietetic Technician, Registered (DTR)* is an individual with academic and professional qualifications in food and nutrition and has been certified by the Commission on Dietetic Registration. In addition, one might become a board certified specialist in gerontological nutrition, sports dietetics, pediatric nutrition, renal nutrition, and/or oncology nutrition.

In addition, nurses also have subspecialty certifications. These require additional training and education in a particular area of health care. See Box 2-1 ■.

| BOX 2-1 | ANCC Nursing Certifications |

Nurse Practitioners
- Acute Care NP
- Adult NP
- Adult-Gerontology Acute Care NP
- Adult-Gerontology Primary Care NP
- Adult Psychiatric–Mental Health NP
- Emergency NP
- Family NP
- Gerontological NP
- Pediatric NP
- Psychiatric–Mental Health NP

Clinical Nurse Specialists
- Adult Health CNS
- Adult-Gerontology CNS
- Adult Psychiatric–Mental Health CNS
- Child/Adolescent Psychiatric–Mental Health CNS
- Gerontological CNS
- Pediatric CNS

Specialties
- Ambulatory Care Nursing
- Cardiac-Vascular Nursing
- Forensic Nursing—Advanced
- General Nursing Practice
- Gerontological Nursing
- Informatics Nursing
- Medical-Surgical Nursing
- Nurse Executive
- Nurse Executive, Advanced
- Nursing Case Management
- Nursing Professional Development
- Pain Management Nursing
- Pediatric Nursing
- Psychiatric–Mental Health Nursing
- Public Health Nursing—Advanced

Source: American Nurses Association. Reprinted with permission.

Ancillary Clinical Specializations

In addition to physicians and nurses, other members of your clinical staff who provide specialized services for your patients may include:

Physical therapists are trained to assist patients with injuries or illnesses focused on a goal of increasing mobility and flexibility. These treatments may be needed to support healing and ultimate recovery, enable the patient to accomplish, or more easily accomplish, activities of daily living (ADL), or assist with pain management, especially for those with chronic conditions.

All fifty states require physical therapists to be licensed. Although licensing requirements vary from state to state, it is not unusual for the passing of the *National Physical Therapy Examination* (NPTE) or a similar state-administered exam to be a part of the obligations for licensure. A number of states require continuing education for physical therapists to keep their license. Physical therapists typically need a doctoral degree in physical therapy.

Occupational therapists incorporate modalities that seek to support improvement of physical, cognitive, and social behaviors into their treatment plans for patients with disabilities, those recovering from an injury or surgery, as well as those suffering from age-related physiological changes.

These therapists need to have earned a master's degree in occupational therapy, successfully passed the *National Board for Certification of Occupational Therapists* (NBCOT) and are required, in all fifty states, to be licensed. National certification is optional, however, only those who pass the certification exam are permitted to identify themselves as an *Occupational Therapist Registered* (OTR).

Speech-language pathologists work with patients who are experiencing communication disorders including cognitive-communication dysfunction, swallowing concerns, as well as other speech and language disorders.

Almost all states require a speech-language pathologist to be licensed. The licensing process typically requires a master's degree from an accredited program in conjunction with supervised clinical experience. *Certificate of Clinical Competence in Speech-Language Pathology* (CCC-SLP) offered by the American Speech–Language–Hearing Association (ASLHA), will often satisfy some or all of the requirements for licensure and may be required by employers.

GENERAL PRACTICE OR SPECIALIZED SERVICES

As a health care administrator, one of the responsibilities you hold is to determine what types of services your patient population needs, and will need, from your facility. Why is this important? You must remember that health care facilities are businesses, too. Services provided must bring in revenue so the facility has the money to support necessary expenditures such as payroll, equipment, and supplies. If your facility is not able to provide the specific type of care your patients need, your revenue opportunities will be severely limited. For example, how financially secure do you think an obstetrics and birthing center would be if the facility were situated in the middle of a retirement area where the surrounding population's average age is sixty-five? This facility would have a difficult time getting enough patients to keep it open. This is one of the reasons why you, as the administrator, must know the demographics and economics of the area around the facility.

The first step is to look at the population for the given area. Those facilities located within an urban community will typically analyze using a smaller geographical radius because individuals live tighter together and will often seek health care services close to where they live. A facility in a rural area will need to draw from a larger geographical radius due to a lower number of people per square mile. Patients in rural areas are more likely to need to travel greater distances to obtain health care services.

It is important to evaluate the makeup of the population of your facility's primary and secondary service areas—the geographical range from which the organization will attract patients. The most common definition used for a health care facility's primary service area is that geographical area from which the facility will attract 75 percent of its patients. The other 25 percent of the geographic region will define the secondary service area.

Demographics

Demographics are the statistical measures and categorization of individuals in a specific geographic area, most often sorted by age, gender, and race. These three key foci of the population can tell you a great deal about the potential health care needs of your community.

AGE   Knowing the largest percentage of the area's population as determined by age will provide insights as to what services may be needed the most. Think about the different requirements of services needed by the residents of a college town (average age twenty-six) versus a retirement community (average age sixty-five). This illustrates the fact that all individuals require different types of health care as they age—from birth to adolescence, from adulthood to seniority. This is the reason behind age-specific guidelines that have been established for annual physical exams, also known as preventive medical examinations. Review Box 2-2 ■. Notice how some of the elements for assessments, such as behavioral assessments, blood pressure screenings, and dyslipidemia screening, have different components of the evaluation based on the child's age: 0 to 11 months, 1 to 4 years, 5 to 10 years, 11 to 14 years, and 15 to 17 years. If you go to www.healthcare.gov/prevention you can see how the guidelines for preventive services vary based on the patient's age: adults, children, and seniors each have their own recommendations for screenings and assessments.

It is known by clinical professionals that certain diseases and conditions exhibit different signs and symptoms depending upon the patient's age. For example, while the presence of a fever is a typical indicator of infection in children and adults, this sign is less likely to be present in elderly patients. A well-baby check will include different milestones than a routine prenatal examination. While a general practitioner (GP) certainly could competently perform all of these exams, the reputation of your facility and the quality of care perceived by current and prospective patients would be higher at a facility with a gerontologist, a pediatrician, or an obstetrician on staff.

GENDER   Understanding the balance of gender in your area may also provide interesting insights. What could this mean to you, as an administrator?

Review the numbers shown in Table 2-4 ■ as if they were the specific county or community surrounding your organization. They can be used to support the addition or expansion of certain gender-related services. For example, evaluate this limited data set and you can observe that there are 283,997 women aged 40 to 49 who might support your facility's purchase of a mammography machine and there are 246,066 males aged 15 to 25—a fact that might support the opening of a sports medicine clinic.

Above and beyond the obvious differences between men and women with regard to genital health, there are other conditions that affect one gender greater than the other. According to the American Stroke Association, more men than women will suffer a cerebrovascular accident (CVA), also known as stroke—a fact that is consistent across virtually all age groups. Interestingly though, more women will die as a result of a stroke.

The American Cancer Society predicted that 9,840 men would be newly diagnosed with cancer of the larynx (voice box) in 2012 in comparison to 2,520 women, and more than twice as many men than women are expected to be diagnosed with cancer of the urinary system, including an estimated 55,600 new cases of urinary bladder cancer (versus 17,900 new cases for women). On the other side of the gender scale, it was estimated that 43,210 women will be diagnosed with thyroid cancer in 2012 compared to an estimated 13,250 men with that same new diagnosis.

These statistics could help hone the scope of a cancer department that provides education, support, counseling, and community outreach to gender-specific groups. Especially with such sensitive subjects, individuals often prefer to discuss these issues amongst those of the same gender because they find it less embarrassing.

CULTURE/ETHNICITY   Ethnicity can be a component of consideration with specific regard to known genetic diseases that are prevalent amongst those of certain races. According to the Centers for Disease Control, hypertension affects non-Hispanic black adults twenty years of age and older more than any other group (see Table 2-5 ■). In addition, sadly, infant mortality

BOX 2-2	Preventive Services for Children Covered Under the Affordable Care Act

1. **Alcohol and Drug Use** assessments for adolescents
2. **Autism** screening for children at 18 and 24 months
3. **Behavioral** assessments for children of all ages
   Ages: *0 to 11 months, 1 to 4 years, 5 to 10 years, 11 to 14 years, 15 to 17 years.*
4. **Blood Pressure** screening for children
   Ages: *0 to 11 months, 1 to 4 years, 5 to 10 years, 11 to 14 years, 15 to 17 years.*
5. **Cervical Dysplasia** screening for sexually active females
6. **Congenital Hypothyroidism** screening for newborns
7. **Depression** screening for adolescents
8. **Developmental** screening for children under age 3, and surveillance throughout childhood
9. **Dyslipidemia** screening for children at higher risk of lipid disorders
   Ages: *1 to 4 years, 5 to 10 years, 11 to 14 years, 15 to 17 years.*
10. **Fluoride Chemoprevention** supplements for children without fluoride in their water source
11. **Gonorrhea** preventive medication for the eyes of all newborns
12. **Hearing** screening for all newborns
13. **Height, Weight and Body Mass Index** measurements for children
    Ages: *0 to 11 months, 1 to 4 years, 5 to 10 years, 11 to 14 years, 15 to 17 years.*
14. **Hematocrit or Hemoglobin** screening for children
15. **Hemoglobinopathies** or sickle cell screening for newborns
16. **HIV** screening for adolescents at higher risk
17. **Immunization** vaccines for children from birth to age 18—doses, recommended ages, and recommended populations vary:

    • Diphtheria, Tetanus, Pertussis
    • Haemophilus influenzae type b
    • Hepatitis A
    • Hepatitis B
    • Human Papillomavirus
    • Inactivated Poliovirus
    • Influenza (Flu Shot)
    • Measles, Mumps, Rubella
    • Meningococcal
    • Pneumococcal
    • Rotavirus
    • Varicella

18. *Learn more about immunizations and see the latest vaccine schedules.*
19. **Iron** supplements for children ages 6 to 12 months at risk for anemia
20. **Lead** screening for children at risk of exposure
21. **Medical History** for all children throughout development
    Ages: *0 to 11 months, 1 to 4 years, 5 to 10 years, 11 to 14 years, 15 to 17 years.*
22. **Obesity** screening and counseling
23. **Oral Health** risk assessment for young children
    Ages: *0 to 11 months, 1 to 4 years, 5 to 10 years.*
24. **Phenylketonuria (PKU)** screening for this genetic disorder in newborns
25. **Sexually Transmitted Infection (STI)** prevention counseling and screening for adolescents at higher risk
26. **Tuberculin** testing for children at higher risk of tuberculosis
    Ages: *0 to 11 months, 1 to 4 years, 5 to 10 years, 11 to 14 years, 15 to 17 years.*
27. **Vision** screening for all children

Source: Healthcare.gov. Posted on: September 23, 2010. Last updated: September 27, 2012.

rates, consistently over the last ten years, have been highest for those born to mothers of non-Hispanic black, American Indian, Alaska Native, and Puerto Rican descent. This data can be used to promote a specialty clinic or a community outreach program.

Cultural differences are critical to an accurate health care assessment. Cultural values have an impact on the patient's decision making regarding specific health care services. In other

TABLE 2-4   **Population by Age and Gender**

AGE	NUMBER		
	Both Sexes	Male	Female
Total population	3,574,097	1,739,614	1,834,483
Under 5 years	202,106	103,475	98,631
5 to 9 years	222,571	113,763	108,808
10 to 14 years	240,265	122,924	117,341
15 to 19 years	250,834	128,949	121,885
20 to 24 years	227,898	117,117	110,781
25 to 29 years	214,145	107,986	106,159
30 to 34 years	206,232	102,038	104,194
35 to 39 years	222,401	108,637	113,764
40 to 44 years	262,037	127,555	134,482
45 to 49 years	291,272	141,757	149,515
50 to 54 years	284,325	138,961	145,364
55 to 59 years	240,157	116,699	123,458
60 to 64 years	203,295	96,939	106,356
65 to 69 years	149,281	70,258	79,023
70 to 74 years	105,663	47,331	58,332
75 to 79 years	89,252	37,908	51,344
80 to 84 years	77,465	30,369	47,096
85 to 89 years	53,759	18,651	35,108
90 years and over	31,139	8,297	22,842

Source: U.S. Census Bureau, 2010.

TABLE 2-5   **Percentage of Persons with Elevated Blood Pressure by Race/Ethnicity and Sex, 20–74 Years of Age, for Selected Years**

Race/Sex	1988–1994	1999–2002	2003–2006
African American men	30.3	28.2	26.5
White men	19.7	17.6	17.4
Mexican American men	22.2	21.5	15.3
African American women	26.4	28.8	23.9

Note: Percentages are age adjusted. Elevated blood pressure is defined as having systolic pressure of at least 140 mm Hg or diastolic pressure of at least 90 mm Hg. Those with elevated blood pressure may be taking prescribed medicine for high blood pressure.

Source: National Center for Health Statistics (2008). Table 71. Hypertension and elevated blood pressure among persons 20 years of age and over, by selected characteristics: United States, 1988–1994, 1999–2002, and 2003–2006. Health, United States, 2008. With chartbook on trends in the health of Americans. Hyattsville, MD, 312–313.

words, some cultures find certain common procedures, such as transfusion or vaccinations, unacceptable. With this knowledge, an administrator can possibly find alternatives that can provide the health benefit without violating the patient's belief system.

Language may be another barrier than can negatively affect the provision of quality health care services. Clear communication between the patient and the facility staff is mandatory and therefore, you may need to consider having a translator available. You might poll existing staff to identify those proficient in other languages. Contact your local public or university library system; many have translation lines that enable you to phone in a request for a translator.

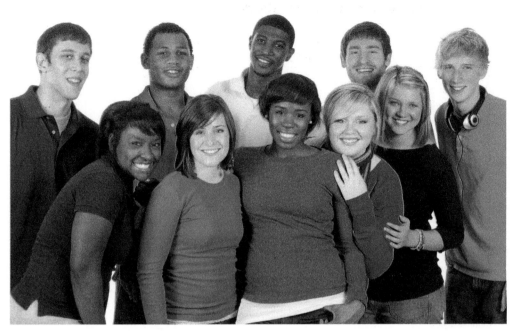

FIGURE 2-3 Diversity means respect and understanding for the various cultures and races that constitute your staff as well as your patient population.
Photo credit: Mike Flippo/Shutterstock.

Creating an environment of cultural sensitivity, thereby establishing mutual respect between your facility and the patient's heritage, can connect in a partnership of enhanced benefit to everyone involved (Figure 2-3 ■). Every individual in your facility, from the front desk receptionist through the administration staff, as well as every clinician from medical assistants to physicians, must be trained to acknowledge the cultural differences of these groups in your community, put aside their personal biases, and be willing to connect with these patients in a respectful manner— for the good of the patient and the good of the organization.

Economics

Economics is a statistical evaluation of employment and income levels in the geographic area being studied. Employment statistics can be used to cull two important pieces of data that will help you determine important aspects of your health care facility. First, you may be able to determine the percentage of the population in your community that has health insurance coverage (Table 2-6 ■). Those individuals with health care insurance will typically seek services more often, and will take advantage of preventive medicine screenings. Those without coverage are more likely to delay seeking medical care, or avoid it altogether, resulting in increased complications, greater severity of the condition, and potentially longer hospital stays. You might find that a segment of your community that is unemployed would benefit from your facility offering a free clinic once a week.

economics
the study of the production, distribution, and consumption of goods and services, often referring to the financial well-being, or lack thereof, of a group.

TABLE 2-6   Health Insurance Coverage by Source

United States	Estimate for 2010
HEALTH INSURANCE COVERAGE	
Civilian noninstitutionalized population	301,501,772
With private health insurance	67.7%
With public coverage	28.5%
No health insurance coverage	15.0%

Note: Total percentage may add to over 100% due to dual coverage (two or more policies) held by some participants.

Source: U.S. Census Bureau, 2008–2010 American Community Survey.

Reviewing data, such as that provided in Table 2-7 ■, that reports the types of businesses, or industries, in which the population is employed, may also provide some predictive insights. For example, an area with many construction workers would likely need more orthopedic services while employees at local manufacturing plants may require more respiratory support (Figure 2-4 ■).

Income levels can also reveal important information. Research shows that individuals with higher income levels often have completed higher levels of education. Several studies indicate that people with more education have a greater probability of participating in wellness programs and taking advantage of preventive services regularly.

TABLE 2-7   Employment by Industry

United States	Estimate for 2010
INDUSTRY	
Civilian employed population 16 years and over	141,848,097
Agriculture, forestry, fishing and hunting, and mining	1.9%
Construction	6.8%
Manufacturing	10.7%
Wholesale trade	2.9%
Retail trade	11.6%
Transportation and warehousing, and utilities	5.0%
Information	2.3%
Finance and insurance, and real estate and rental and leasing	6.8%
Professional, scientific, and management, and administrative and waste management services	10.5%
Educational services, and health care and social assistance	22.6%
Arts, entertainment, and recreation, and accommodation and food services	9.1%
Other services (except public administration)	4.9%
Public administration	4.9%

Source: U.S. Census Bureau, 2008–2010 American Community Survey.

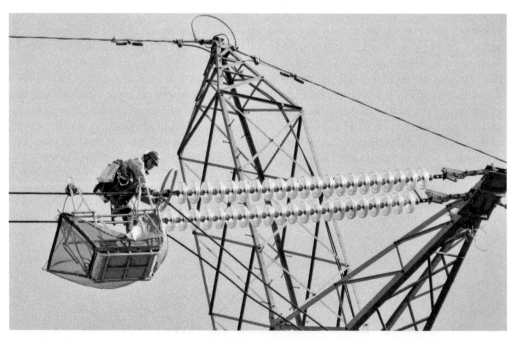

FIGURE 2-4   Those individuals working in some occupations and at certain types of workplaces have higher incidents of needing health care services.
Photo credit: © Justin Kase zninez/Alamy.

GATHERING DATA

There are many sources for gathering data about the population surrounding your facility. You will not have to go door to door or conduct any surveys yourself (although you certainly can if you want to do this and you have the budget). The federal and state governments, as well as non-profit organizations interested in health care, collect a great deal of data that you can access and use for free (most of the time). Some examples are shown in Table 2-8 ■.

You must be very careful from where you collect data, especially when you are downloading information from the Internet. Not all websites are the same with regard to quality (accuracy) of information. Therefore, you want to ensure that you evaluate the credibility of the source prior to accepting and using data from that source. There are some elements you can check rather easily:

1. *What can you tell from the URL?* The URL is the address of the website (such as http://www.pearson.com or http://www.cms.gov), and you can see this in the address bar of your browser screen. Begin by looking at the domain name—the last part of the address. You can tell a great deal from this small segment. Some of the most common domain names include:
   * .gov = U.S. government
   * .mil = U.S. military
   * .edu = post-secondary school, college, or university
   * .org = a nonprofit organization
   * .com = business/commercial

   In addition to these, also look for designations that the website might be hosted in another country. When you are pulling statistics and other elements about the population, you want to confirm whose population the numbers represent. Look for two letter designations, such as .jp = Japan, .uk = United Kingdom, .nz = New Zealand

2. *Specifically who created the site?* Once you click to the home page, you should be able to determine who created and maintains the information on the site. Look for a link to "About Us" or something similar. Is it an individual, a group, or business? Is contact information including phone numbers, street address, and e-mail addresses easily found? Are there any credentials, such as college degrees, accreditation, or certification and any validation from a third-party that this information is valid and not just someone's opinion? For example,

TABLE 2-8 Examples of Population Data Websites

Name of Agency	URL
U.S. Department of Health and Human Services, Health Resources and Services Administration, Area Resource Files	http://arf.hrsa.gov
Quick Health Data Online	http://www.healthstatus2020.com/owh/
Agency for Healthcare Research and Quality (AHRQ) Data and Surveys	www.ahrq.gov/data/
U.S. Census	http://www.census.gov
State and County Quick Facts	http://quickfacts.census.gov/qfd/index.html
Centers for Disease Control and Prevention (CDC)	http://www.cdc.gov
CDC Data and Statistics	http://www.cdc.gov/datastatistics/
National Center for Health Statistics: Healthy People 2020, DATA2010, Health Indicators Warehouse	http://www.cdc.gov/nchs/
Centers for Medicare and Medicaid Services Research, Statistics, Data and Systems	http://www.cms.gov/home/rsds.asp
Quality of Care	www.hospitalcompare.hhs.gov
Kaiser Family Foundation State Health Facts	http://www.statehealthfacts.org
American Cancer Society	http://www.cancer.org
American Heart Association	http://www.heart.org

Wikipedia is not considered a credible source because anyone can go into a page and alter the contents. The site does not require valid references, credentials, or supporting data in accepted literature to prequalify the information that is available on their site. Therefore, you cannot immediately discern whether you are reading facts supported by data and valid research or merely one person's opinion.

3. *When was the site last updated or when was the data collected?* You can typically find this at the very bottom of the home page or subsequent pages. Especially when you are dealing with health care data, only that information gathered and analyzed within the last five years is considered current. If you think about all that has been established as standard of care, all the new knowledge about various diagnoses and procedures, and the technological advancements in health care during just the last five years, you can understand why this makes sense. Confirm that the information is the latest release of data available. For example, the U.S. Census only gathers information every ten years. Often, it takes a year or two for large quantities of data to be collated, analyzed, and released. Therefore, it is not unusual for the freshest, newest data sources to be from one, two, or even three years ago.

4. *Is the data clearly labeled, organized, and cited?* Professionally trained statisticians ensure that the data is organized so that anyone can clearly understand what details the numbers in the table or graph represent (Figure 2-5 ■). Those who are trying to influence policy and public opinion with false data may attempt to confuse you by presenting the information in a way that is not easily comprehended. They hide behind the fact that some individuals who are not experts will assume it is the reader that is not sophisticated or educated enough to interpret what is there.

In addition, important data can be pulled from your own facility's electronic patient records and patient management software. Printing a patient contact list can provide patient zip codes for analysis to determine primary and secondary service areas. Practice analysis reports can provide details on the most frequent diagnoses identified and procedures performed. Another area of important data can come from an analysis of referrals made by your facility, possibly revealing some services that may be profitable for you to provide in-house in the future. Adding these services would also give your patients a great convenience—allowing them to stay in a facility

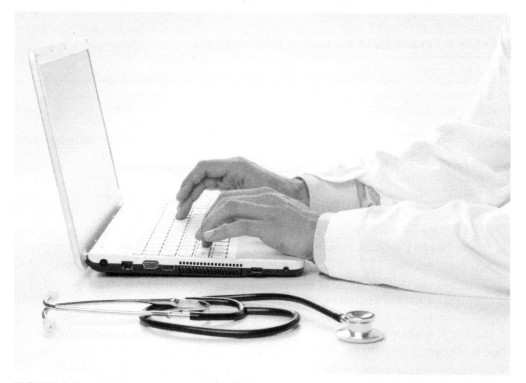

FIGURE 2-5 Computers make statistical analysis and interpretation of data more accurate and more easily accessible.
Photo credit: rangizzz/Fotolia.

where they know the physician and the support staff and don't have to travel or use unfamiliar providers.

The capability of pulling this data is available in the smallest, as well as the largest, of health care facilities. As of 2012, all health care facilities must be in the process of converting and using electronic health records.

USING THE DATA

Now that you have learned about multiple sources for gathering data, the next step is to review the various ways you can use this information to benefit your facility.

National and State Data

Consider what you, as an administrator, might do with this data to support the addition, expansion, or reduction of specific services offered in your facility. As mentioned in the previous section, you can pull a report of your facility's current patient list by zip code to identify the primary and secondary service areas. It may also reveal pockets of outlying areas that have been unrealized as potential patient regions. For example, you may find that a group of your patients live in a rural area and come to your facility because it is near their job rather than choosing a health care provider near their home. This can potentially open new patient opportunities with the employees of local businesses.

Next, the identification of all other health care providers within that same geographic scope should be done, along with a list of the types of services provided by each. You have to know what the competition is doing so you can develop a strategy to complement existing facilities. This can be done by pulling zip code information by industry (health care providers) using the business listings or the "find a provider" lists for those third-party payers (insurance companies and Medicare, for example) with whom you participate and matching this to your primary and secondary service area zip code(s).

Figure 2-6 ■ contains population data that may be used to determine what services may be good business to offer. The administrator for a health care facility in any one of these counties

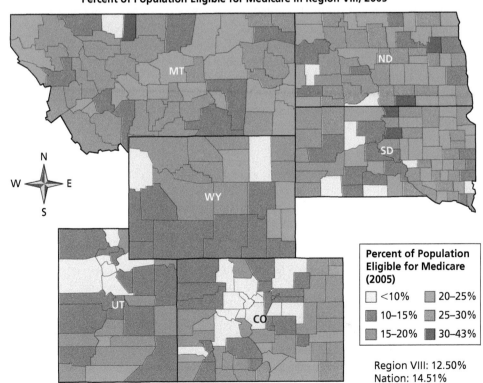

Percent of Population Eligible for Medicare in Region VIII, 2005

Percent of Population Eligible for Medicare (2005)

- <10%
- 10–15%
- 15–20%
- 20–25%
- 25–30%
- 30–43%

Region VIII: 12.50%
Nation: 14.51%

FIGURE 2-6 Medicare Eligibles Region VIII.

Source: Health Resources and Services Administration.

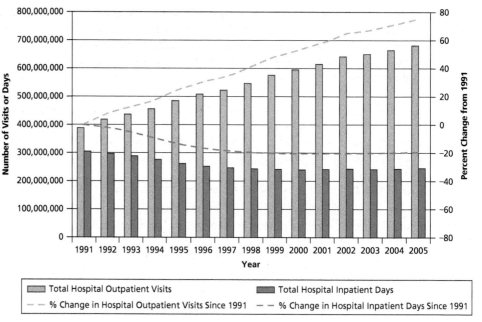

FIGURE 2-7 Change in Hospital Outpatient Visits and Inpatient Days, 1991–2005.

Source: Health Resources and Services Administration.

could use this data from the U.S. Department of Health and Human Services (Health Resources and Services Administration, Area Resource Files). You can clearly see the areas with a younger population in north central Colorado versus an older population in North Dakota. If you were located in North Dakota, you would want to make certain your facility is a participating provider with Medicare. In addition, you might ensure you have the capability to provide geriatric services, perhaps have a board-certified gerontologist or a Registered Dietician board-certified in geriatric nutrition on staff.

Over the fifteen years shown in Figure 2-7 ■, outpatient visits increased 80 percent and inpatient days decreased 20 percent. Gathering similar data for your community or region could lead you to recommend an increase in your facility's outpatient services rather than adding more inpatient beds. Ambulatory surgical centers (ASC) and clinics could look at expanding the types of services they provide, and physicians' offices in the area might consider investing in an expansion of in-office procedure rooms and appropriate personnel.

Facility Data

As mentioned earlier in this chapter, there is a great deal of useful data sitting in your facility's computers. Virtually all software programs used for electronic patient records and patient management (claims creation) programs provide certain reports with a single mouse click. If you are uncertain, contact the software manufacturer (you may want to start with the user's manual, the help module within the software, or the manufacturer's website) to discover how to pull the statistics you need.

These statistical reports can provide you with tremendous insights beyond the zip code information already discussed. Potential insights for services can be drawn from:

Diagnosis reports. Evaluate the clusters of diagnoses most often seen in your facility. These may reveal additional services that can be provided, expanding revenue opportunities while supporting patient comfort level. For example, an increased percentage of patients with hypertension could spur the development of additional services such as acupuncture or a massage therapist. Perhaps you could establish patient education classes presented by your staff registered dietician to teach patients how to adjust their diet.

Procedure reports. Over the past decade, many procedures that formerly required an operative theater (inpatient procedure at a hospital) are now approved to be performed in an outpatient facility (in a physician's office or ASC). An analysis of the most frequent procedures provided to the current patient list, performed at an outside location such as an ASC, may give you some insights about additional services that may be viable to provide within your facility.

Age reports. Find out the age ranges of your current patients and determine if they might benefit from additional services. You might make an arrangement with a durable medical equipment supplier to provide canes, wheelchairs, and the like, to a large patient population of elderly patients or orthopedic patients. Offer a late-night hotline for parents of young children to phone with a concern, manned by a nurse practitioner. Call forwarding means the nurse on call would not have to come into the office, and remote access (password protected, of course) to electronic health care records could enable a quick update on the patient's personal history so that the nurse could provide more accurate advice.

Referral reports. There are times when a patient requires more services, such as lab tests, imaging, or a specialist and must go elsewhere. This can delay treatment and be inconvenient for patients, especially those with disabilities or transportation problems. Are there enough of these referrals to warrant your facility taking on some of these services? Will there be enough opportunity to support the expense of obtaining and maintaining the equipment? Will adding this service require the hiring of additional personnel or can members of the current staff handle the tasks? The answers to these questions will guide you through an analysis that can produce some data valuable to decision making about facility services.

CHAPTER REVIEW

SUMMARY

An important step to building a successful health care organization is to begin by getting a clear picture of what type of facility it is and what services are being provided. To determine if the facility is providing the maximum selection of services as required by its patient population, statistics must be gathered and analyzed as to the demographics and economics of the primary and secondary service areas. Once the population is identified and described, you, a good administrator, can analyze the value of how best to provide care for the current and future health care needs of the community.

REVIEW QUESTIONS

MULTIPLE CHOICE

Choose the most accurate answer.

1. Acute care hospitals are also known as _____ facilities.
   a. assisted living
   b. inpatient
   c. rehabilitation
   d. ambulatory surgical

2. Hospices are health care facilities that provide
   a. same day surgical procedures.
   b. physical therapy.
   c. preventive care services.
   d. end-of-life care.

3. A CRNA is a(n)
   a. RN with special training in anesthesia.
   b. RN with training in nutrition.
   c. board-certified physician.
   d. RN with special training in obstetrics.

4. Demographics are statistics that measure all of the following factors EXCEPT
   a. age.
   b. economics.
   c. gender.
   d. ethnicity.

5. Reviewing statistics on population economics can give you the answer to which of the following questions?
   a. How many potential patients are over age sixty-five?
   b. What zip codes do my potential patients live in?
   c. How many potential patients have health insurance?
   d. How many patients are of Hispanic heritage?

6. A facility's primary service area is the geographic zone in which _____ of its patients live.
   a. 25 percent
   b. 50 percent
   c. 75 percent
   d. 100 percent

7. An ambulatory surgical center (ASC) provides
   a. preventive medical services, such as annual physicals.
   b. ongoing medical services, such as allergy shots.
   c. long-term physical therapy services.
   d. outpatient surgical procedures.

8. Facility data can be combined with _____ to support decision making for the addition, expansion, or reduction of services within a facility.
   a. county
   b. state

   c. national
   d. all of the above

9. Ethnicity can be a component of health care services with regard to
   a. contagious diseases.
   b. genetic illness.
   c. traumatic injury.
   d. industrial accidents.

10. The American Board of Medical Specialties confirms
    a. certified nurse midwives.
    b. board-certified physicians.
    c. registered dietitians.
    d. certified registered nurse anesthetists.

MATCHING

Match the facility to the procedure, service, or treatment it would provide.

11. acute care hospital
12. ambulatory surgical center
13. physician's office
14. assisted living facility
15. hospice
16. rehabilitation center
17. home health agency
18. skilled nursing facility
19. domiciliary
20. clinic

a. annual physical exam
b. palliative care
c. post-CVA speech therapy
d. continuous nursing care
e. urgent care center
f. open heart surgery
g. halfway house
h. stoma maintenance
i. cataract surgery
j. support of ADL

FILL-IN-THE-BLANK

Fill in the blank with the accurate answer.

21. A health care facility owned and operated by a corporation with shareholders is known as a _____ facility.

22. A _____ participates in a federal program designed to assure that facilities based in rural areas will not lose the ability to provide health care services.

23. A freestanding facility that provides outpatient surgical procedures only is called an _____.

24. Short-term and long-term inpatient care services, twenty-four hours a day, seven days a week, including health care and personal services, are provided by facilities known as _____.

25. The _____ awards physicians certification deeming them board-certified in a specific specialty or subspecialty.

26. Pediatric urology is a subspecialty of a general _____ board certification.

27. In the certification title "Gerontological CNS," the acronym CNS stands for _____.

28. All fifty states in the United States require physical therapists to be _____.

29. An _____ provides only health care services without an overnight stay.

30. The statistical measures and categorization of individuals in a specific geographic area is known as the _____ of that area.

WHEN YOU ARE THE ADMINISTRATOR . . .

Critical Thinking and Analysis

Case Study #1

Connecting Professional Skills with Health Care Utilization

The first part of this chapter discusses the various types of health care facilities as well as the various types of health care services a facility might provide. **Choose a type of facility and make a list of the credentials and skills that would be required from your clinical staff. Include an explanation of why you feel that each credential on your list is important.**

For example: a facility specializing in women's health would need to have a physician board-certified in obstetrics and gynecology, possibly with a subspecialty in ___?___, as well as possibly a certified nurse midwife and a nurse certified in perinatal nursing. Is there any benefit to this facility hiring an occupational therapist? If so, why? If not, why not?

Case Study #2

Compliance with Professional Licensing Regulations

Go to the website for the state in which you live. **Choose one specific type of health care facility and print out the requirements (credentials) for two of the specific clinicians you would need to hire to work in your facility.**

For example, what does your state require of a professional in order to provide midwife services to an obstetrics patient in your birthing center?

Case Study #3

Using Statistics to Support Expansion Plans

Evaluate the data from the Agency for Healthcare Research and Quality (AHRQ) Data and Surveys (www.ahrq.gov/data) shown in Figure 2-8 ■.

After reading the statistics (in the next paragraph) and referencing Figure 2-8, **determine what services you would recommend if you were the administrator of a health care facility in Illinois, to expand what is available at your facility.** Support your recommendation with specific statistics from the table.

Illinois Profile

Of the state's 6.5 million women, nearly two thirds are non-Hispanic White. Its largest minority populations are non-Hispanic Black, at 16 percent, and Hispanic, at 14 percent. It ranks in the top 15 states in its low rates of death for suicide, unintentional injuries, diabetes-related causes and chronic obstructive pulmonary diseases. It has a much poorer record in rates of death for breast cancer, coronary heart disease, influenza and pneumonia, and colorectal cancer. Not surprisingly, it ranks among the worst states in the percentage of women who have had recent colorectal cancer screening. Illinois ranks in the middle of the nation in cholesterol screening, mammograms, and Pap smears. Eighty-seven percent of its women have health insurance, with Hispanic women having the lowest rate of insurance coverage, at 68 percent.

FIGURE 2-8 Illinois Profile

	Non-Hispanic White	Non-Hispanic Black	Hispanic	American Indian/ Alaskan Native	Asian/ Pacific Islander	State Total	Healthy People 2020 National Target	State Rank
Female population (2009) (all ages)	65.4	15.5	14.3	0.4	4.7	**6,550,783**		
Major causes of death among females (rate per 100,000) ¶								
All cause	654.3	843.8	367.7	255.9	304.0	**662.5**	+	30
Heart disease	160.1	216.7	81.4	65.1	72.9	**163.9**	+	32
Coronary heart disease	106.1	154.5	55.7	51.3	55.8	**110.0**	100.8	35
Total cancer	162.8	199.8	83.0	46.0	77.7	**161.4**	160.6	40
Breast cancer	24.3	35.3	11.2	*	10.0	**24.7**	20.6	44
Colorectal cancer	15.8	23.6	8.2	*	10.5	**16.3**	14.5	49
Lung cancer	43.6	50.3	11.6	*	12.8	**41.8**	45.5	28
Stroke	42.7	56.5	28.4	*	26.9	**44.1**	33.8	31
Chronic obstructive pulmonary diseases (age 45 & over)	110.5	58.7	23.9	*	11.6	**97.9**	98.5	10
Diabetes-related	53.7	92.0	59.1	*	36.4	**58.5**	65.8	14

(Continued)

FIGURE 2-8 *(Continued)*

	Non-Hispanic White	Non-Hispanic Black	Hispanic	American Indian/ Alaskan Native	Asian/ Pacific Islander	State Total	Healthy People 2020 National Target	State Rank
Influenza and pneumonia	17.6	18.2	10.6	*	8.7	**17.5**	+	37
Unintentional injuries	21.6	22.9	10.4	*	9.0	**20.5**	36.0	12
Suicide	4.0	1.7	1.0	*	2.9	**3.3**	10.2	8
Health risk factors (percent) §								
Diagnosed high blood pressure (2007–2009)	23.8	39.8	20.0	*	22.3	**26.1**	26.9	34
Obesity (2008–2010) (age 20 & over)	23.5	43.9	32.5	*	11.7	**27.5**	30.6	34
No leisure-time physical activity (2008–2010)	24.3	36.3	37.7	30.5	27.4	**27.8**	32.6	34
Binge drinking (2008–2010)	15.2	9.9	10.3	9.1	3.4	**13.0**	24.3	44
Smoking currently (2008–2010)	16.9	19.2	13.9	19.9	2.4	**16.2**	12.0	26
No smoking during pregnancy ◊ (all ages) (2006–2008)							98.6	
Eats 5+ fruits and vegetables a day (2007–2009)	27.6	25.3	25.9	*	43.9	**27.8**	+	29
Preventive care (percent) §								
Cholesterol screening in past 5 yrs. (2007–2009)	76.6	80.1	62.2	*	73.2	**75.4**	82.1	33
Mammogram in past 2 yrs. ◊ (2008–2010) (age 50–74)	77.7	83.7	75.1	*	*	**78.4**	81.1	34
Pap smear in past 3 yrs. ◊ (2008–2010) (age 21–65)	86.6	88.9	84.0	*	74.4	**86.1**	93.0	19
Colorectal cancer screening #0 (2008–2010) (age 50–75)	58.5	58.7	41.4	*	*	**57.2**	70.5	36
Routine check-up in past 2 yrs. (2008–2010)	83.7	92.7	84.6	81.7	91.3	**85.7**	+	29
Dental visit within the past year (2008–2010)	75.0	61.7	59.2	*	62.5	**70.4**	+	31
First trimester prenatal care ◊ (2006–2008)							77.9	
Health insurance coverage (percent)								
Health insurance coverage (2008–2010) (ages 18–64)	92.0	84.5	67.8	*	86.3	**87.4**	100.0	19

¶ Estimate age-adjusted and for all ages unless noted.
§ Estimate age-adjusted and for 18 years of age and over unless noted.
* Figure does not meet standard of reliability or precision.
+ No Healthy People 2020 target associated with this health indicator.
#Blood stool test in the past year, sigmoidoscopy in the past 5 years and blood stool test in the past 3 years, or a colonoscopy in the past 10 years
◊ Definition for Healthy People 2020 Objective differs from Healthy People 2010; Data are not comparable to values presented in prior editions of the Chartbook.

Note: All data are from 2005 to 2007 unless noted.
Note: Low numerical rankings indicate better relative health status.
Note: State rank includes the 50 states, the District of Columbia, Guam, Puerto Rico and the US Virgin Islands, where data are available and reliable.
Note: Healthy People targets correspond with the Healthy People 2020 Objectives.
Note: No smoking during pregnancy and First trimester prenatal care data from states using the 2003 revision of the U.S. Standard Certificate of Live Birth. States that are blank had not yet implemented the revised certificate items corresponding to the variable(s) for at least two of the three years from 2006 to 2008.

Source: Agency for Healthcare Research and Quality (AHRQ) Data & Surveys.

INTERNET CONNECTIONS

Healthcare Facilities Accreditation Program

CMS created the Healthcare Facilities Accreditation Program (HFAP) to monitor all participating hospitals, ambulatory care/surgical facilities, mental health facilities, physical rehabilitation facilities, clinical laboratories, and critical access hospitals to ensure compliance with the Medicare Conditions of Participation and Coverage. HFAP also provides certification reviews for Primary Stroke Centers.
http://www.hfap.org/

The Joint Commission

The Joint Commission accredits and certifies health care organizations and programs in the United States and oversees their commitment to meeting certain performance standards. While Joint Commission accreditation is voluntary, many third-party payers use this status for qualification of participation.
http://www.jointcommission.org/

Types of Health Care Providers

Medline Plus, a section of the National Library of Medicine, provides complete descriptions of the various types of health care providers. Explanations are easy to understand and links are provided for more in depth learning.

- Primary Care Provider
- Nursing Care
- Drug Therapy
- Specialty Care

http://www.nlm.nih.gov/medlineplus/ency/article/001933.htm

CHAPTER 3

FINANCING THE PROVISION OF CARE

KEY TERMS

capitation plan
case mix
Centers for Medicare and
   Medicaid Services (CMS)
commercial loan
episodic care
expenditures
fee-for-service (FFS)
fixed costs
for-profit organization
grant
medical necessity
not-for-profit (nonprofit) facility
private health insurance
private investment
public health care facility
revenue
secured bonds
shares of stock
third-party payer
variable expenditures
Veterans' Administration
workers' compensation

LEARNING OBJECTIVES

Upon completion of this chapter, you should be able to:

- Define commonly used terms, abbreviations, and acronyms.
- Enumerate the differences between for-profit, not-for-profit, and public health facilities.
- Evaluate the impact of the facility's relationship with third-party payers.
- Describe the various methods of payment received from third-party payers.
- Identify the options for funding various types of facilities.
- Explain how case mix and occupancy rates can be used to balance the budget of a health care facility.

WHEN YOU ARE THE ADMINISTRATOR . . .

When managing the financing of health care, administrators need to be able to:

- Assess and identify specific services, equipment, and personnel needed to address the current and future health care needs of the community and the funding required to provide such services.
- Create a balanced budget along with strategic planning to maintain fiscal health for the organization.
- Supervise the activities of all departments, including: clinical, human resources, finance (accounts receivable and payable), operations, maintenance, housekeeping, and admissions/scheduling.

INTRODUCTION

All of the great intentions in the world to heal the sick and repair the injured cannot be fulfilled without money. The truth is that most of us are unable to work for free, so there must be money (known as revenue) coming into the organization for salaries. In addition to salaries, the facility, no matter how large or small, must also pay for expenses such as rent, utilities, and phones. There is no way around this. Even free clinics have bills to pay. This chapter will discuss various aspects of the financial facets of a health care facility; things that you, as an administrator, need to know.

◗ BUSINESS STRUCTURE

There are three types of business structures from which a health care facility may choose. For the most part, this designation affects the bookkeeping of the **revenue** coming into and out of the organization and the company's relationship with the Internal Revenue Service (IRS). However, depending upon the structure, different sources of funding will be available for growth activities.

revenue
income; monies received.

For Profit

A **for-profit organization** is set up with the intention of making a profit, similar to many other businesses. The goal is always to bring in more revenue than needed for expenditures (expenses, costs, and taxes). When these two numbers are equal, this is known as *breaking even*. Once the amount of revenue exceeds expenditures, this is called *profit*. A simple formula is used: Profit = Total Revenue minus Total Expenditures. Virtually every company, from a one-physician office to a multilocation hospital corporation, holds a goal of making a profit.

for-profit organization
an organization that is structured to share excess revenue with its shareholders.

The owners of a for-profit organization can do anything they want with this "extra" money (in accordance with the company's articles and structure). They can pay bonuses to personnel, pay dividends to stockholders (investors), or invest it back into the company to fund improvements or growth activities.

When evaluating an expansion, addition, or reduction of services, the profitability of such an action must be considered. The analysis of an activity may include questions, such as: Will there be enough patients to ensure sufficient revenue? Is the organization able to fund the upfront costs until a profit can be made? How long might it take to realize a profit?

Not-for-Profit

Not-for-profit facilities, also referred to as **nonprofit**, still care about the balance of revenue and expenditures. The difference between a nonprofit and a for-profit company is that while the for-profit facility might pay out profits to investors, a not-for-profit organization *must* reinvest the money back into the facility or into enhancing the services provided by the facility. In addition, not-for-profit corporations that are Internal Revenue Service (IRS) designated as a 501c(3) are tax-exempt (do not pay taxes). Funds coming into the company from sources other than patient services may be considered donations rather than investments. Donations to a 501c(3) are often tax-deductible for the donor. This can be an advantage for the facility to enhance its financial stability or fund an expansion. Examples of a nonprofit health organization are a clinic sponsored by United Cerebral Palsy and the Shriner's Hospital.

not-for-profit (nonprofit) facility
an organization with a tax status that is designated to reinvest excess revenue into the organization for the betterment of its patients (customers).

Public Health

Public health care facilities are owned and operated by a local, state, or federal government, such as a community-based free clinic sponsored by the state's department of health or a clinic situated within a public school. They are supported by tax dollars, so rather than having a focus on the number of dollars brought in, a greater importance is placed on how the money is used and the number of citizens served. Documentation of these statistics must support the value to tax payers. Administrators often need to interact with politicians to lobby for funds.

public health care facility
an organization, established by a government agency, to provide health care services to its citizens.

◗ THIRD-PARTY PAYERS

The term **third-party payer** describes an agency, organization, or individual that pays for health care services even though it is not directly involved in the encounter. In this regard, the physician or other provider is the first party and the patient is the second party when health care services are rendered. A government agency, such as Medicare, or a private company, such as Prudential or Aetna

third-party payer
an individual or organization who pays for a health care service yet is not either the provider or the receiver of these services.

health insurance, is the third party encompassed in this encounter. It is the third party that is paying for those services provided, making them the third-party payer. Note that not all third-party payers are health insurance companies, which is why the health care industry uses this umbrella term.

Government Agencies

The **Centers for Medicare and Medicaid Services (CMS)** is an agency of the federal government within the Department of Health and Human Services. *Medicare* provides payment for health care services to its beneficiaries. Essentially, those in the United States who are age sixty-five years or older; individuals of any age with a permanent disability, such as someone who is blind; and those of any age diagnosed with end stage renal disease (ESRD) are eligible to apply for benefits. *Medicaid* pays for health care services for those who are indigent (poor, needy) and low-income.

Federal government programs, specifically Medicare and Medicaid, are funded only in part by the federal government. The state governments pay the rest. The federal government establishes the minimum required benefits to be provided to these beneficiaries across the country. Each individual state is responsible for administering the program on a day-to-day basis. In addition to processing claims for services provided to those beneficiaries who live within its borders, each state is permitted to entitle additional benefits (cover additional services and procedures) to those mandated by the federal program. Therefore, what is a covered procedure to a Medicare beneficiary in Ohio may not be covered to a beneficiary in Arkansas. You, as an administrator, must be aware of this fact, in case your facility treats a Medicare beneficiary who lives in another state, you must be aware that your facility may not be reimbursed for nonemergency services provided.

State governments often maintain **workers' compensation** coverage. These funds are available to reimburse the costs of providing health care to an individual who becomes ill or injured while doing their job. Industrial accidents, work-related illness, and even a car accident during work-related driving are examples of cases that may be covered by workers' compensation insurance. Note that some large industrial organizations fund worker's compensation coverage themselves. This is known as being "self-insured."

The **Veterans' Administration**, another federal government agency, supports health care services for its beneficiaries. *TriCare* is a federal program that covers medical expenses for the dependents (spouse and children) of those who are currently serving in the uniformed services* (active military), retired military and their families, as well as the dependents of deceased active-duty military. *CHAMPVA* (Civilian Health and Medical Program of the Department of Veterans Affairs) provides health care benefits for dependents of those veterans who suffered a 100 percent service-connected disability and the dependents of those who died from service-connected disabilities.

In addition to the Medicaid program mentioned earlier in this chapter, in certain circumstances, there are other federal and state funds available to reimburse a health care provider for services provided to an individual who is indigent or uninsured. The process to access these funds is very similar to the reimbursement process with any other third-party payer. That is, **medical necessity** must be documented, along with other requirements.

Let's look at two examples: one from the federal government (Box 3-1 ■) and one from a state government (Box 3-2 ■).

Federal provisions under the Community Assistance Act:

For those facilities that are eligible for funds under the Hill-Burton Act, Community Services Assurance has been established under Title VI of the Public Health Service Act.

Centers for Medicare and Medicaid Services (CMS)
a federal government agency authorized to manage Medicare and Medicaid programs.

workers' compensation
an insurance plan specifically designated to pay for medical care for an individual who was injured or became ill as a result of their occupation.

Veterans' Administration
an agency of the federal government with the authority to care for members of the uniformed services.

medical necessity
determination that an individual has need for a procedure, service, or treatment based on the standards of care.

| BOX 3-1 | **Public Health Service Act Title VI** |

The Community Service Assurance under Title VI of the Public Health Service Act requires recipients of Hill-Burton funds to make services provided by the facility available to persons residing in the facility's service area without discrimination on the basis of race, color, national origin, creed, or any other ground unrelated to the individual's need for the service or the availability of the needed service in the facility.

Source: Health and Human Services, Office for Civil Rights.

The classification "uniformed services" includes: U.S. military (Navy, Army, Marines, Air Force, and Coast Guard), Public Health Service, North Atlantic Treaty Organization (NATO), and the National Oceanic and Atmospheric Administration (NOAA).

BOX 3-2	Covered Hospital Services; Review and Approval

"In-patient and out-patient hospital and physician services, when rendered in a hospital, are covered when such services are medically necessary for the treatment of a medical condition that manifested itself by symptoms of sufficient severity that the absence of immediate medical attention would probably result in:

(1) placing the person's life in jeopardy;
(2) serious impairment to bodily functions; or
(3) serious dysfunction of any bodily organ or part.

(b) A qualified resident of Indiana shall be eligible to receive assistance to pay for any part of the cost of care that is a direct consequence of the medical condition that necessitated the emergency care providing such care is rendered in the hospital. No post-hospital care shall be reimbursable under the hospital care for the indigent program.

(c) Any costs of services rendered by a physician pursuant to the hospital care for the indigent program must conform to the global or single billing concept as defined in 405 IAC 1-7-1 *[405 IAC 1-7 was repealed filed Jul 25, 1997, 4:00 P.M.: 20 IR 3365.]* and be included in the charges initially incurred by an eligible patient while hospitalized.

(d) Any emergency medical transportation costs reasonably necessary to transport an eligible patient to a hospital for the treatment of a medical condition described in subsection (a), above, shall be reimbursed to said transportation provider if said provider is properly licensed in the state of Indiana to render the transportation service for which he seeks payment. The department shall not pay more to the transportation provider than the prevailing rate in the community for similar service."

Source: From Indiana Administrative Code ARTICLE 11.1. Hospital Care For The Indigent. Material reprinted with permission of Thomson Reuters.

State provisions: Example from the state of Indiana:
In the Indiana Administrative Code, article 11.1. *Hospital Care for the Indigent* is the list of essential requirements that must be met for a hospital to request reimbursement for services provided to those who do not have the money or health insurance to pay for that health care. Note that Indiana limits this reimbursement to hospitals, as you can see in Box 3-2, first line, ". . . when rendered in a hospital . . ."

It is important to note that none of these funds are available to cover nonemergency services. The laws do not mandate any facility to provide nonemergency medical care to anyone. However, this gap is often filled by the public health services through state and federal programs.

Private Health Insurance Companies

You are probably familiar with **private health insurance** companies, such as Prudential, Aetna, Humana, and United Healthcare, which provide health insurance coverage to businesses for the benefit of their employees, members of large organizations, and individuals. These days, most health insurance policies reimburse for preventive care, such as a flu shot or a mammogram, as well as for medical care, such as surgery or applying a cast.

private health insurance
a third-party payer that is not affiliated with the federal government.

Patient Payments

Patients with health care benefits from a third-party payer will often have to make their own financial contribution to the payment for care, in addition to the premiums they pay for the policy. Typically, an insured patient may be responsible for any of three types of payments to the provider.

Co-payment: Also known as the *co-pay*, a co-payment is a fixed amount paid by the patient to the provider for each encounter regardless of what is provided during the visit. These co-pays are usually $10, $20, or $50, depending upon the policy and the location of the encounter.

Coinsurance: In some policies, the patient agrees to pay a percentage of the allowed amount, while the policy pays the rest. This cost sharing is often known as coinsurance. For example, with an 80/20 policy, the third-party payer reimburses 80 percent and the patient pays 20 percent.

Deductible: This is the amount of money, based on the allowed amounts, that a patient must pay out of pocket each year before third-party payer benefits begin. The deductible may be as small as $200 or as large as $3,000 and is stated in the policy agreement between the policyholder (the patient) and the third-party payer.

THIRD-PARTY PAYER REIMBURSEMENT

A large portion of a health care facility's revenue comes from the care provided to patients. There are several different types of reimbursement received and a financially stable organization should seek to have a balance among these various source types so as to avoid total dependence on any one system. This is known as *case mix*.

A balanced **case mix**, with regard to reimbursement sources, should be part of the financial plan of the organization (Figure 3-1 ■). This means that the facility, as a whole, needs to seek a balance of patient cases reimbursed by various third-party payers. While virtually all third-party payers have set fee schedules, you will find that not all allowed amounts (the amount of money paid for each procedure, service, or treatment provided to an insured) are the same. For example, you may discover that Medicare pays $20 for each flu shot, but Blue Cross Blue Shield pays $25, and Humana pays $22 (numbers are for illustrative purposes only). As you monitor your patient roster, it is important to review data on third-party payers so you can have your staff work toward attaining and keeping a healthy equilibrium.

There is a business philosophy that discourages businesses from becoming dependent upon one vendor or one customer. What this means is that you want to do everything possible to avoid total dependence on anyone outside of your organization or outside of your control. No single customer (in this case, no single third-party payer) should ever have control over your financial stability. If 70 percent of your patient population is covered by Aetna, then when Aetna adjusts its fee schedule, a majority of your revenue stream is affected, and there is nothing you can do.

The general rule is that no single customer should ever represent more than 30 percent of your revenue. Some health care providers consider the patient as the customer. When it comes to customer service, this is true. However, here we are discussing revenues, and because the money

case mix
a strategic plan to ensure a health care facility is caring for patients with a variety of diagnoses.

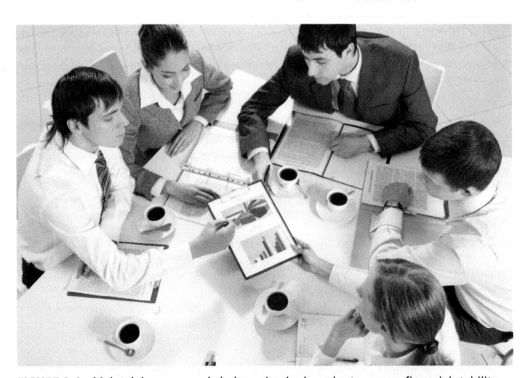

FIGURE 3-1 Maintaining a case mix balance is wise in order to ensure financial stability. *Photo credit:* Pressmaster/Shutterstock.

actually comes from the third-party payer, in this circumstance, the third-party payers are the customers. Does this mean that if Medicare beneficiaries make up 50 percent of your patient population you should tell 20 percent to go somewhere else? Not at all. It means that you need to take action that will bring in more patients who are covered by other insurers such as Aetna, Blue Cross Blue Shield, or Prudential to readjust the overall percentages.

Fee-for-Service (FFS)

A **fee-for-service (FFS)** agreement between a third-party payer and a health care provider is straightforward. For each and every covered procedure, service, and treatment that is provided to a policyholder (covered patient), a predetermined amount of money will be paid. Once a year, the third-party payer publishes a *fee schedule* itemizing the allowed amount for each individual procedure code. A participating provider (PAR) can agree by continuing the relationship or choose to dissolve the relationship with the third-party payer and become a NonPAR (nonparticipating provider).

fee-for-service (FFS)
a payment plan in which a health care provider receives reimbursement from a third-party payer based on the specific procedure, services, and treatments provided.

USUAL, CUSTOMARY, AND REASONABLE (UCR)   Many third-party payers will use a formula known as UCR (usual, customary, reasonable) to determine the allowed amount for each covered procedure, service, and treatment.

- Usual = the fee usually charged by this provider for this procedure
- Customary = the range of usual fees charged by other physicians with the same level of training and experience for this specific procedure within the same geographic area
- Reasonable = the justifiable payment for the service in the eyes of the third-party payer's medical review committee

RESOURCE-BASED RELATIVE VALUE SCALE (RBRVS)   Medicare uses a different formula to determine how much will be paid to each provider for each covered procedure, service, and treatment. This formula is known as RBRVS and uses a unit of measurement known as a relative value unit (RVU).

The first step in the formula is to determine the amount of work that the physician has devoted to providing the procedure. This is then assigned a weighted *Work RVU*. For example, you can understand that aligning a compound fracture requires more work by the physician than giving a patient a flu shot. Next, the cost of supplies, equipment, support personnel, and overhead, based on the national average, to the physician or facility to provide the procedure is assigned a weighted *Practice Expense RVU*. Lastly, an evaluation of the risk of providing the procedure is used to assess a *Malpractice RVU*. For example, brain surgery carries a higher risk of an adverse event than draining an abscess on a patient's finger. These are then added together to get the *Total RVU* value for this single procedure.

$$Work\ RVU + Practice\ expense\ RVU + Malpractice\ RVU = Total\ RVUs$$

However, an RVU is a unit of measurement, not a unit of money. Once a year, the U.S. Congress assigns a monetary value to one RVU, known as the *conversion factor*.

$$Total\ RVUs\ multiplied\ by\ the\ Conversion\ Factor = Total\ Dollars$$

There is one last step. The federal government understands that the cost of providing a procedure is not the same in all parts of the country. Certainly, you can understand that the rent of a physician's office, for example, is higher in New York City than it is in Kankakee, Illinois. Therefore, *geographical practice cost indices (GPCI)* are applied to the Total Dollars determined above to make the payments fair in all parts of the country.

$$Total\ Dollars\ multiplied\ by\ the\ geographical\ practice\ cost\ indices\ (GPCI) = Allowed\ Amount$$

Let's look at an example: A patient is admitted for a Mumford procedure (surgical shoulder arthroscopy with distal claviculectomy including distal articular surface). As you can see in Table 3-1 ■, Medicare will reimburse $677.69 for the facility hosting this procedure. On its face, it can appear that this is some crazy arbitrary figure. However, as you are learning, this is an amount that is calculated using the formulas for RBRVS.

FACILITY #1

TABLE 3-1 Medicare Reimbursement for a Mumford Procedure: GPCI =1

WORK RVU	PE RVU	MP RVU	CONV FACT	GPCI PE	FACILITY PRICE
8.98	9.16	1.77	34.0376	1	$677.69

Source: Physician Fee Schedule Look-Up. www.medicare.gov

Enter these numbers into the formulas:

Work RVU [8.98] + *Practice expense RVU* [9.16] + *Malpractice RVU* [1.77]
= *Total RVUs* [19.91]

Total RVUs [19.91] *multiplied by* the *Conversion Factor* [$34.0376]
= *Total Dollars* [$677.69]

Total Dollars [$677.69] *multiplied by* the geographical practice cost indices (GPCI) [1]
= Allowed Amount [$677.69]

Compare to this, a facility hosting the same exact procedure in two other cities, and you can see, in Tables 3-2 ■ and 3-3 ■, how the geographical practice cost indices (GPCI) will adjust the amount reimbursed depending upon where they are located physically:

FACILITY #2

TABLE 3-2 Medicare Reimbursement for a Mumford Procedure: GPCI = 0.866

WORK RVU	PE RVU	MP RVU	CONV FACT	GPCI PE	FACILITY PRICE
8.98	9.16	1.77	34.0376	0.866	$586.88

Source: Physician Fee Schedule Look-Up. www.medicare.gov

Enter these numbers into the formulas:

Work RVU [8.98] + *Practice expense RVU* [9.16] + *Malpractice RVU* [1.77]
= *Total RVUs* [19.91]

Total RVUs [19.91] *multiplied by* the *Conversion Factor* [$34.0376]
= *Total Dollars* [$677.69]

Total Dollars [$677.69] *multiplied* by the geographical practice cost indices (GPCI) [0.866] = Allowed Amount [$586.88]

FACILITY #3

TABLE 3-3 Medicare Reimbursement for a Mumford Procedure: GPCI = 1.218

WORK RVU	PE RVU	MP RVU	CONV FACT	GPCI PE	FACILITY PRICE
8.98	9.16	1.77	34.0376	1.218	$825.43

Source: Physician Fee Schedule Look-Up. www.medicare.gov

Enter these numbers into the formulas:

Work RVU [8.98] + *Practice expense RVU* [9.16] + *Malpractice RVU* [1.77] = *Total RVUs* [19.91]

Total RVUs [19.91] *multiplied by* the *Conversion Factor* [$34.0376] = *Total Dollars* [$677.69]

Total Dollars [$677.69] multiplied by the geographical practice cost indices (GPCI) [1.218] = Allowed Amount [$825.43]

Episodic Care

There are some third-party payers that strive to make things simpler. Based on the accepted standards of care, the theory is that once a confirmed diagnosis is made, the course of treatment (procedures, services, etc.) to be provided is predetermined. Therefore, under an **episodic care** payment plan, one allowed amount fee is assigned by the diagnosis to cover the entire course of care—the episode of care.

Diagnosis-related groups (DRG) is an episodic care payment plan used by Medicare to reimburse acute care hospitals for services provided to inpatient Medicare beneficiaries. DRG categorizes patient care by the principal diagnosis and takes into consideration any comorbidities and complications (additional diagnoses) as well as the patient's age and gender. Additional factors that will be included in this analysis are:

episodic care
a method of paying a provider with one lump sum based on the standard of care for a specific diagnosis.

- Severity of illness, including current complications and comorbidities (CC). CCs are further classified as: non-CC or minor; moderate or major (MCC); or catastrophic CC.
- Risk of mortality (death)
- Resource utilization, including the quantity and types of diagnostic and/or therapeutic services, inpatient room/bed services

There are 579 DRGs into which each Medicare beneficiary's diagnoses will be sorted and calculated into the amount of reimbursement that will be remitted to the acute care provider. The first level is determined by the principal diagnosis–as one of the major diagnostic categories (MDC) (Box 3-3 ■).

The DRG system has several variations within it, including:

- Medicare Severity DRG (MS-DRG) includes a geographic location adjustment (similar to the GFCI in the RBRVS formula), and uses an larger pool of major diagnostic categories (745 MS-DRGs versus 579 DRGs)
- All Patient DRGs (AP-DRG) include non-Medicare patients as well as Medicare patients.
- All Patient Refined DRGs (APR-DRG) add severity, mortality, and utilization into the calculation based on the AP-DRG.

BOX 3-3	**Major Diagnostic Categories (MDC)**

1. Diseases and Disorders of the Nervous System
2. Diseases and Disorders of the Eye
3. Ear, Nose, Mouth, Throat, and Craniofacial Diseases and Disorders
4. Diseases and Disorders of the Respiratory System
5. Diseases and Disorders of the Circulatory System
6. Diseases and Disorders of the Digestive System
7. Diseases and Disorders of the Hepatobiliary System and Pancreas
8. Diseases and Disorders of the Musculoskeletal System and Connective Tissue
9. Diseases and Disorders of the Skin, Subcutaneous Tissue, and Breast
10. Endocrine, Nutritional, and Metabolic Diseases and Disorders
11. Diseases and Disorders of the Kidney and Urinary Tract
12. Diseases and Disorders of the Male Reproductive System
13. Diseases and Disorders of the Female Reproductive System
14. Pregnancy, Childbirth, and the Puerperium
15. Newborns and Other Neonates with Conditions Originating in the Perinatal Period
16. Diseases and Disorders of Blood, Blood Forming Organs, and Immunological Disorders
17. Lymphatic, Hematopoietic, Other Malignancies, Chemotherapy, and Radiotherapy
18. Infectious and Parasitic Diseases, Systemic or Unspecified Sites
19. Mental Diseases and Disorders
20. Alcohol/Drug Use and Alcohol/Drug Induced Organic Mental Disorders
21. Poisonings, Toxic Effects, Other Injuries, and Other Complications of Treatment
22. Burns
23. Rehabilitation, Aftercare, Other Factors Influencing Health Status and Other Health Service Contacts
24. Human Immunodeficiency Virus (HIV) Infections
25. Multiple Significant Trauma

Source: Centers for Medicare and Medicaid Services.

Capitation Plans

capitation plan

a payment plan in which a primary care physician receives a monthly stipend for ongoing care of a managed care beneficiary.

Patients covered by a managed care plan, such as a health maintenance organization (HMO), are required to choose a primary care physician (PCP). The PCP is responsible for overall care and coordination of the patient's health. To reimburse the physician for this broad scope of responsibility, a **capitation plan** is often put into place. From this point forth, as long as that physician is documented as the PCP for that policyholder, the third-party payer will pay a fixed amount each and every month, for each and every insured, to the PCP whether any care is provided or not to that individual patient. This is called a per-member-per-month (PMPM) case management payment. Think of a cap on the head of each patient. The monthly payment is for the PCP's care for each 'Cap'—*cap*itation payment. Any care provided above and beyond what is included in the monthly stipend is separately documented and reported, resulting in additional reimbursement.

Bonus and Incentive Programs

There are many incentive programs and bonus opportunities related to health care. Here are two examples from the federal government. Your state and/or your private third-party payers may have an opportunity for your organization to get extra money for services rendered.

PHYSICIAN QUALITY REPORTING SYSTEM (PQRS) CMS must gather data about the care provided to its beneficiaries to continually work to improve coverage and services. These details, submitted on claim forms using category II codes (HCPCS Level I, category II codes) report elements of service provided by an eligible professional (Box 3-4 ■) that would not otherwise be specifically reported:

- Clinical basics (such as assessing a patient's level of activity, screening a patient for depression, or documenting a patient's body mass index (BMI);
- Lab and imaging test follow-up (such as noting that screening mammogram results were documented and reviewed or negative microalbuminuria test results were documented and reviewed); and

---

BOX 3-4 | **Health Care Professionals Eligible to Participate in PQRS**

1. Medicare physicians
   - Doctor of Medicine
   - Doctor of Osteopathy
   - Doctor of Podiatric Medicine
   - Doctor of Optometry
   - Doctor of Oral Surgery
   - Doctor of Dental Medicine
   - Doctor of Chiropractic
2. Practitioners
   - Physician Assistant
   - Nurse Practitioner
   - Clinical Nurse Specialist
   - Certified Registered Nurse Anesthetist (and Anesthesiologist Assistant)
   - Certified Nurse Midwife
   - Clinical Social Worker
   - Clinical Psychologist
   - Registered Dietician
   - Nutrition Professional
   - Audiologists
3. Therapists
   - Physical Therapist
   - Occupational Therapist
   - Qualified Speech-Language Therapist

Source: Centers for Medicare and Medicaid Services.

- Patient education provided (such as performing written/oral education appropriate for patients with heart failure; counseling regarding contraception provided to the patient prior to initiation of antiviral treatment; or instruction in therapeutic exercise with follow-up provided to patients during an episode of back pain lasting longer than 12 weeks).

Those eligible professionals who participate in PQRS will receive a bonus payment once each year.

PRIMARY CARE INCENTIVE PAYMENT PROGRAM (PCIP)   The Primary Care Incentive Payment Program (PCIP) was created by the Affordable Care Act to enhance payments for services provided by primary care professionals. Those participating health care professionals with a Medicare designation as: family medicine, geriatric medicine, pediatric medicine, internal medicine, nurse practitioner, clinical nurse specialist, and physician assistants may qualify for these incentive funds, which will be paid out through 2015.

In the first year of the program (2011), more than $560 million, equal to 10 percent of the total amount paid that year by Medicare to providers for primary care services, was meted out to those who participated.

SOURCES OF FUNDING

Some health care facilities may benefit from additional sources of monies beyond just third-party reimbursement for procedures, treatments, and services provided to patients (Figure 3-2 ■). Capital expenses, such as purchasing a magnetic resonance imaging (MRI) unit for the creation or expansion of the imaging department or the remodeling of a surgical suite, can be a huge

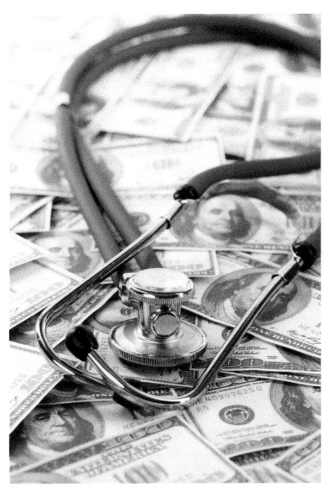

FIGURE 3-2   Health care can be funded in several different ways.
Photo credit: Zadorozhynyi Vicktor/Shutterstock.

Small Business Innovation Research Grant (SBIR: R43/R44)

Small Business Technology Transfer Grant (STTR: R41/R42)

SBIR and STTR grants are made to eligible domestic for-profit small business concerns conducting innovative research that has the potential for commercialization. SBIR/STTR awards are intended to stimulate technological innovation, use small business to meet federal research and development needs, increase private sector commercialization of innovations derived from federal research and development, and foster and encourage participation by minority and disadvantaged persons in technological innovation.

FIGURE 3-3 AHRQ small business grants.

financial concern similar to the purchase of a new house. Outside financing will be required, and there are several options for securing funds.

Grants

grant
monies provided under very specific terms.

A **grant** might be available from government and/or private sources seeking to support health care under certain terms. These sources of funding may be given with no recourse (monies do not have to be paid back) or with recourse (monies do have to be paid back). This type of funding is not often available to for-profit facilities; however some may be found—for example, Figure 3-3 ■. In addition, grants are not exclusively for large organizations. Opportunities for grant money will typically be offered across the board, based on the community's need for the service or facility. Figure 3-3 shows an example of a small business grant offering from the Agency for Healthcare Research and Quality (AHRQ)).

Grant applications are very much like business plans; they are extensive documents that will explain in specific detail why the service or equipment is needed, what portion of the population will benefit most, and precisely how the money will be used. Failure to use grant monies in the manner and time frame accepted in the grant application may be considered fraud and may subject the individuals and facility to criminal investigation and possibly prosecution. When grant monies are pursued, most often the organization will hire a professional grant writer to handle the creation of the proposal, using their knowledge of the formatting required and the technicalities involved.

Again, as an example, Box 3-5 ■ presents basic instructions for completing a grant application, from the AHRQ.

BOX 3-5   **Overview of the (AHRQ Grant) Application Process**

1. AHRQ receives most new application types three times a year: February 1, June 1, and October 1. There are set AHRQ grant receipt dates for all grant mechanisms that AHRQ accepts.
2. After AHRQ receives your application, it is logged in, given a unique Application ID number, and then it is assigned to a peer review group (study section committee) or to a special emphasis panel.
3. You will receive written notification indicating your review assignment within six weeks. CSR mails application to reviewers to read and asks them to streamline the list of applications.
4. Your application will undergo initial peer review at AHRQ.
5. After the application review has been conducted, you will receive a summary statement with the review results within three months.
6. AHRQ decides which applications to fund based on scientific and technical merit. Agency research priorities and availability of grant funds.
7. If your application is approved for funding, an AHRQ Grants Management staff member will contact the applicant institution to negotiate the terms of the grant award. A Notice of Grant Award will then be sent electronically to the applicant institution, usually within six weeks of the funding decision.
8. If your application did not get funded, you may contact your Project Officer to discuss options for revising and resubmitting the application.

Source: Agency for Healthcare Research and Quality (AHRQ).

Government Programs

There are some government programs that have been created to help physicians and hospitals with the cost of providing state-of-the-art services. For example, as of March 2012, CMS's *electronic health record (EHR) program* paid a $4.5 billion in incentive payments to more than 76,500 physicians and hospitals. In addition, the Health Information Technology for Economic and Clinical Health (HITECH) Act, signed into law in 2009, has expanded the number of funding opportunities to assist health care facilities of all sizes to implement technology to improve the provision of health care services throughout the United States.

More government programs are available. Earlier in this chapter, we looked at the incentive programs PQRS and PCIP. Take a look at the snippet of information from this Healthy People 2020 Request for Proposal (RFP) from small organizations shown in Box 3-6 ■. When searching for grant opportunities, it is important to keep an open mind. While we may be involved in health care, federal government grants may be available through various government agencies. Take a look at the list shown in Table 3-4 ■. You may not have known that some of these agencies even existed and yet, they have money to share for health care projects.

Commercial Loans

A standard **commercial loan** may be available for those facilities that maintain good relationships with banks and other lending institutions. Along the same lines as a car loan or a mortgage to purchase a house, this enables the facility to borrow the money necessary to accomplish the expansion or purchase of equipment and then pay it back with interest according to a predetermined schedule.

commercial loan
a loan provided by a bank.

Private Investments and Endowments

There are very wealthy individuals throughout the world who desire to make a **private investment** in small- and medium-size companies. These investors are known as *angels*, and they

private investment
an individual endowing money to an individual or organization.

BOX 3-6   **Healthy People 2020 Community Innovations Project Purpose**

This Request for Proposal (RFP) is to solicit community-level projects that use Healthy People 2020 overarching goals, topic areas, and objectives to promote improved heath at a community level. Funding is intended to support activities above and beyond general operations. Using the projects funded through this RFP, the Office of Disease Prevention and Health Promotion (ODPHP) intends to evaluate how the Healthy People 2020 overarching goals, topic areas, and objectives are being used to improve the health of communities.

Funding Information
- This is a one-time funding opportunity.
- Awards will range from $5,000 to $10,000.
- Up to 170 projects will be funded.
- Multiple submissions representing a single eligible entity will *not* be reviewed. (Please see "Who Can Apply" section for eligibility criteria).
- Awardees will be chosen to represent a variety of themes, activities, and regions.

Who Can Apply?
Nonprofit, community-based organizations with budgets less than $750,000 can apply for these funds.

Types of Projects to be Funded
Healthy People 2020 has four overarching goals, covers 42 topics, and has over 600 objectives, encompassing 1200 measures. In order to be eligible for consideration, proposed projects must address at least **one** of the Healthy People 2020 topics and incorporate at least **one** of the following priorities that are linked to the Healthy People 2020 overarching goals. Please click on the referenced links for more information about each priority:

- Environmental justice: *supporting the rights of all people to live in a healthy environment.* http://www.epa.gov/environmentaljustice/
- Health equity: *dealing with issues that cause some groups of people to have worse health than others.* http://minorityhealth.hhs.gov/npa
- Healthy behaviors across all life stages: *activities to improve the opportunities for people of all ages to make healthy choices.* http://www.cdc.gov/healthyliving

TABLE 3-4 Government Grant Opportunities

Opportunity Title	Agency
The Eldercare Locator	Administration for Community Living
Bureau of Democracy, Human Rights and Labor (DRL)–Request for Proposals for International Labor Rights Programs in Cameroon and Pakistan	Bureau of Democracy, Human Rights and Labor
USSOCOM BAA (U.S. Special Operations Command–Broad Agency Announcement)	Department of the Army–USAMRAA
Rural Health Information Technology (HIT) Workforce Program	Health Resources and Services Administration
Disaster Preparedness for Effective Response (PREPARE)	Philippines USAID–Manila
Electronic Data Methods (EDM) Forum: Second Phase (U18)	Agency for Health Care Research and Quality
Land Use Change and Disease Emergence	Thailand USAID–Bangkok
Rapid Hepatitis C Virus Screening and Referral	Substance Abuse and Mental Health Services Administration
STD Surveillance Network (SSuN)	Centers for Disease Control and Prevention
Enhancing Opioid Treatment Program Patient Continuity of Care through Data Interoperability	Substance Abuse and Mental Health Services Administration
Rapid Response to Pakistanis Affected by Disasters–Phase Two (RAPID II)	Agency for International Development
Dental Reimbursement Program	Health Resources and Services Administration
Agriculture and Food Research Initiative–Childhood Obesity Prevention	National Institute of Food and Agriculture
MCH (Maternal and Child Health) Navigator Program	Health Resources and Services Administration
National Farmworker Jobs Program Grants	Employment and Training Administration
MCH Knowledge to Practice Program	Health Resources and Services Administration
Health Promotion and Disease Prevention Research Centers: Special Interest Project Competitive Supplements (SIPS)	Centers for Disease Control and Prevention
FY14 Farm to School Grant Program	Food and Nutrition Service
Maternal and Child Health (MCH) Nutrition Training Program	Health Resources and Services Administration

Source: Grants.gov.

prefer to find an organization that has great potential for growth. In some cases, their motivation for donating is to support a personal cause that they believe in or gratitude for excellent care. Health care, being an industry of economic growth, innovations, and bright futures, is a very popular target for these individuals.

Health care facilities structured as nonprofit might also decide to seek out wealthy individuals to request a donation for the support of the good works of the organization. Certainly this can be a one-time gift; however, a larger version of a donation can be made in a manner that will provide funds now and in the future. One type of perpetual donation is known as an endowment.

Typically, the initial donation or endowment is invested so that the gift itself (the principal) remains intact over the years and the money generated by the investment (interest, for example) can be used by the facility. If you have ever been to a hospital with an area or department named after an individual, such as the Henry Harris Cardiac Care Center or the Renee Radon Imaging Annex, there is a good chance that Henry and Renee made an endowment to the facility, monies from which support the ongoing operations of these areas.

An example: In his last will and testament, Arnold Unger left an endowment of $1 million to Community General Hospital. Accordingly, when Mr. Unger passed away, his estate made the gift to Community General. The money was invested and the structure of the investment produced

5 percent per year. Each year, the investment vehicle issued $50,000 to Community General Hospital, allowing them to purchase equipment, add staff members—whatever was needed.

Shares of Stock

Both private (held by the owners) and public (sold on the stock market) for-profit companies may issue **shares of stock**. A share of stock essentially represents a small percentage of the company. Individuals and other organizations can purchase shares of stock in a company, thereby owning a portion of that company. This ownership entitles them to benefit from the profits (paid as dividends to stockholders) or suffer loss when the company loses money (evidenced by the drop in value of each share of stock). Purchasing shares of stock in a company is an unsecured investment. If the management of the company does not succeed using the money to make a profit, the company can go out of business, and its stock becomes worthless.

shares of stock
percentage of ownership of a company.

Selling more shares of stock can provide a facility with the opportunity to bring in additional investment dollars. However, before people will invest in a company, they will typically want to know details about the business including what major debt may already be obligated.

Secured Bonds

Secured bonds are bonds that are backed with some type of asset (something of value). This might be a parcel of land or a revenue stream that the project for which the bond is raising capital (money) is expected to generate. Typically, a bond issuance is used to raise millions of dollars for the organization to expand, to build a new hospital building, or a medical center. There are unsecured bonds, called *debentures*, which are not supported by anything that currently has value. Investors purchase bonds through a broker, in a similar fashion to purchasing stock shares. However, rather than representing a percentage of ownership in a company, bonds have a set interest rate and maturity date. Often, a government or municipal bond will mature within a three- to ten-year range. During this time, the organization can use the money raised to implement the project and, hopefully, have it begin earning a profit—money that can then be used to repay the bond investors.

secured bonds
an investment vehicle backed by another asset.

Compare these forms of raising capital (money) to business transactions with which you are familiar. For example, suppose you want to purchase a car, and you get several of your friends to chip in and loan you the money to buy the car. You agree to pay them back with interest in one year. This is similar to a secured bond. If you do not pay the loan back as agreed, they can take your asset—the car. The value of the car will, in part, give them back some of the money they invested in you.

In another scenario, you love to paint and want to enter a contest, whose prize is $10,000. But you need $500 for the entry fee plus another $250 for the canvas, paints, brushes, and other supplies. You tell your friends that if they lend you the $750, you will pay them back 10 percent of your winnings ($1,000 – the principal [$750] + interest [$250]). Your investors can get more than 30 percent return on their money (profit); however, if your painting does not win the contest, they lose it all. This would be similar to a debenture, an unsecured bond, because there is nothing of value to support the repayment of the investment.

BUDGETING

Your facility must maintain economic stability to ensure that you can financially support your staff and your patients (Figure 3-4 ■). For all of us—whether it be an individual household or a mega-hospital corporation—financial stability is all about the balance of the same two things: revenue and expenditures. The quantity of money coming in and being paid out. As a health care administrator, part of your responsibilities will be to oversee the financial well-being of your organization.

Revenues

In any health care facility, revenue, also known as receivables (money that is owed to your facility and that the facility will be receiving), comes primarily from payment for services provided to patients. The types of services offered determine the scope of the facility's revenue, and the gross amount (before taxes) is determined by the quantity of patients served. As you have learned, one

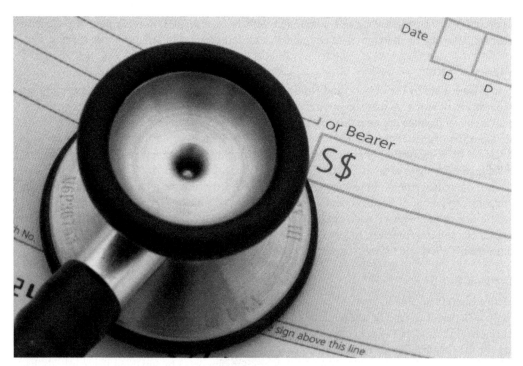

FIGURE 3-4 Money is required to provide health care services.
Photo credit: IRP/Shutterstock.

of your responsibilities as an administrator is to analyze ways to increase revenue while controlling expenditures. You have two ways to do this:

1. Grow the business horizontally by increasing the types of services your facility provides so the same people can benefit from, and pay for, more services, thereby increasing revenue.
2. Grow the business vertically by increasing the number of patients to whom your facility can provide the same services.

Some may think that you, as the administrator, could simply increase the charges for services provided. Because a large portion of every health care facility's revenue is received from third-party payers, such as Medicare, Medicaid, Aetna, Prudential, and the like, pay rates cannot be changed because the fee for each procedure, service, and treatment provided is set by the payers, not by the facility itself.

Expenditures

expenditures
money spent or paid out.

fixed costs
expenses that remain the same, month after month.

variable expenditures
expenses or debt that changes month to month.

Expenditures, also known as payables (the money that the health care facility owes and must pay to others) are, again, similar to what you and I must pay out of our personal budgets. Items such as rent or mortgage payments, utilities, and telephones are known as **fixed costs**. This type of expenditure is consistent—the same every month—and is absolutely necessary to keep the business functioning. These costs can be reduced slightly by, for example, moving to a smaller building. But, for the most part, these are bills that must be paid to enable the facility to stay in business, no matter how many patients are treated that month.

Variable expenditures are those that increase or decrease based on the actual number of patients served. Examples of these may be gauze bandages, rolls of paper that cover exam room tables, and syringes. If you have no patients with wounds, no packages of gauze bandages will be used, and therefore, you will not need to purchase more. When the economy gets rocky and the number of patients being treated decreases, these are the items that will be most affected by cutbacks.

Salaries fall into this category as well. While the facility must have some staff, the number of individuals required will be based on the number of patients for which the facility is providing care. For example, a nursing home with 100 beds may desire to have a 1:10 ratio of nurses-to-residents (one nurse for every ten patients). This means that if all beds are occupied, the facility must hire ten nurses. However, if half of the beds are empty, only five nurses are required to support that same level of care. In some states, the law controls the ratio of nurses-to-patients for inpatient facilities. For example, Florida Statutes (2012, Title XXIX, Chapter 400.23), "*A facility may not staff below one certified nursing assistant per 20 residents . . . A facility may not staff below one licensed nurse per 40 residents.*" Variations on these staffing requirements are typically determined by the severity of the patients' conditions. For example, California (R-37-01, Section 70217 Nursing Service Staff) requires, "*the licensed nurse-to-patient ratio in an emergency department shall be 1:4 or fewer at all times that patients are receiving treatment.*" Salaries, payroll taxes, employee benefits, plus equipment and supplies all require the dispersing of funds.

Every health care provider also has an ethical obligation to provide care and medical services to a patient whose life is in peril without concern for getting paid or reimbursed. There is also a legal obligation to do this, to an extent, as required by laws such as the Emergency Medical Treatment and Active Labor Act (EMTALA), the Good Samaritan Law, Physician Duty to Care, and the Hill-Burton Act.

There is some recourse for a health care provider to seek reimbursement for medical treatment afforded to an individual who does not have the ability to pay for those services. Many states have budgets to reimburse within limitations. The Hill-Burton Act allots federal funds to financially assist hospitals, nursing homes, public health centers, and rehabilitation facilities expressly for the provision of services to these individuals.

There are several industry terms used for this category of care: charity care, uncompensated care, free care, and indigent/uninsured care. As an efficient and effective health care administrator, you must include an allotment in all financial discussions and planning for the expenses of services to those individuals for whom there will be no reimbursement received.

Creating a Budget

It can be overwhelming to create a budget for yourself and your family. Imagine creating a budget for an organization, such as a physician practice or a 200-bed hospital. As with any other large project, one way to tackle this task is to break it up into several smaller steps.

Essentially, the budget has two sections: revenue (income) and expenses. In each of these two sections, the organization is likely to have both fixed and variable aspects. For example, existing endowments are fixed revenues, while utilities payments (gas, electric, water, telephone) are fixed expenditures. In addition, there are variable revenue streams, such as third-party payer reimbursements. These monies are variable because the facility will not have an identical number of patients to treat with the exact same types of procedures every month, so the income will vary from month to month. Due to this fact, your facility's expenditures for medical supplies will vary as well. When creating a budget, you need to predict what services will be provided in the future. This can be quite a challenge. However, even without a crystal ball, there are ways to figure this out sufficiently so you and your staff can properly prepare.

For a company that is currently in business, the place to begin is with a review of past years' accounting records to give you insights about these numbers. When reviewing, it is best to look for trends so that you can use this historical perspective as a foundation for the future. Whenever possible, pulling the statistics for the last five years will provide enough data to support predictive decision making.

In those cases where the existing facility has not been around long enough to be able to provide five-year data, or if the budget is being created for a brand new facility, you can seek out financial data for a similar type of facility in a similar geographic region. Looking at existing budgets will give you some insights as to all of the line items that must be taken into consideration when preparing a budget. For example, it is not enough to include the monthly payment for the copy machine. You must also include the funds to pay for the paper, toner, and maintenance contract. You must include not only the gross salaries for your personnel but also the cost of benefits (health insurance, dental insurance, sick pay, paid time off (PTO), pension or 401K contributions, taxes, and more). You must include everything including the money to purchase toilet paper for the bathrooms, landscape professionals to ensure the outside of the building is maintained, window washers for the outside surfaces of the windows, security equipment and personnel, and more. In addition to paying the rent or mortgage for the building, you must include property and liability insurance. A percentage of the budget will need to be allotted for replacements of furniture and equipment, revenue that goes uncollected (known as bad debt), marketing, expansion plans, disaster recovery (after a hurricane or earthquake, for example). Yes, there is a lot to consider, and a dollar amount can be determined for each.

Balancing the Budget

As we have been discussing, every organization strives for financial stability. This means that you, as the administrator, must be able to keep revenue and expenditures in harmony. There are elements over which you will have no control, such as the tax rate or the allowed amount from Medicare for a hip replacement procedure. However, there are also many elements over which you can take control that can have a positive impact on the financial health of your facility. Somehow, no one ever has difficulty in spending money. So let's look at some methods that can be used to firm up the facility's revenue stream.

FINANCIAL LEAKS   In every business, there is the potential for financial leakage—the small amounts of money that get wasted. Large organizations, at times, might lose respect for the single dollar. However, as we all know, these single dollars can add up quickly and result in the institution paying out thousands of dollars for rent payments for equipment that is no longer used, and consulting retainers for services no longer needed. If the shuttle bus service has been eliminated because patients were not using it, and the drivers have been reassigned to other duties, then the money paying for the bus itself, the insurance, and the maintenance of a bus that is not being used is wasted money.

Another money hole, especially in physician's practices, lies in the piles of rejected and denied claims that have not been corrected and resubmitted or researched and appealed for reconsideration. Some practices have been found to be losing $20,000 to $30,000 a month or more because everyone is too busy to deal with this rather simple process. Sometimes, the notice is *not* a rejection or denial, but a request for more information before the third party will pay. Connected to this money leak is that some facilities do not learn from their mistakes. In other words, when an error is found, especially when it is discovered that the same error is made month after month, this correction should be brought to the attention of the billing and coding staff. This may present itself as a wonderful opportunity for retraining so this doesn't happen again.

While rejected and denied claims are financial leaks occurring in the health information management department, your clinical staff may have their behaviors cost your facility thousands or hundreds of thousand dollars, as well with the occurrence of hospital-acquired conditions (HAC).

Starting with hospital discharges on or after October 1, 2008, reimbursement is adjusted down, allowing no additional reimbursement for the care of the HAC. This means, of course, that the hospital itself must pay to treat the issue—an expense that should be, for the most part, preventable with proper training of the staff.

Some of the non-reimbursable conditions are:

• Foreign object retained after surgery (left in the patient)
• Air embolism
• Blood incompatibility (giving a patient blood of the wrong type)
• Pressure ulcers—stages III and IV
• Falls and trauma, including fractures, dislocations, intracranial injuries, burns, and the like
• Catheter-associated urinary tract infection (UTI)
• Vascular catheter-associated infection
• Surgical site infections

Consider the following example of a non-reimbursable HAC: John Madison was in the hospital for knee surgery. After taking a nap, he awoke and felt the need to go to the bathroom. The bed rails were down, so John attempted to get out of bed by himself. His knee was not strong enough to support his body weight and he fell and fractured his wrist. Patient safety protocol requires bed rails to be up, in position, whenever the patient is in the bed for the express purpose of preventing accidents just like this. Now, the hospital will have to pay for the x-rays, the casting, the physician's time for additional care, the nurse's time for additional care, pain medication, medical supplies, physical therapy (if necessary), and so on. In addition, the facility must hope that the patient doesn't sue. One seemingly small failure to act (not putting up the bed rails) resulted in a cost to the hospital of thousands of dollars—not to mention the pain and suffering of the patient.

CASE MIX   The industry term 'case mix' actually has two references. The first use of this term refers to ensuring a balanced mix of patient diagnostic cases. Of course, some conditions will cost the facility more money to achieve a positive outcome for the patient than others. You want to monitor the active patient roster to track current diagnoses being treated. To promote better balance, you can actively promote the facility services for other diagnoses. For example, as discussed earlier in this chapter, you might grow the facility's case mix horizontally by offering specialized services to those with diabetes or establishing a childhood obesity clinic.

The other reference is to seek a balanced mix of patient cases covered by various third-party payers. You learned about this type of case mix earlier in this chapter.

Occupancy Rate

The formula for calculating the bed occupancy rate is used frequently by inpatient facility administrators. Remember the example discussed earlier about a nursing home with 100 beds used to determine how many nurses needed to be on staff. Whether this is an empty patient room in a hospital or an unused examination room in a physician's office, this data may alert you to the fact that your facility is not working to its full potential and revenue is being lost. On occasion, this is not a significant factor. However, when this happens on a regular basis, your facility is losing a substantial amount of money. What can you do?

Remember that we discussed your options earlier:

1. Increase the types of services you provide so the same people can benefit from, and pay for, more services, thereby increasing revenue.
2. Increase the number of patients to whom you can provide the same services.

In situations such as this, you, the administrator, need to evaluate the facility as a whole and determine the opportunities that are the most reasonable to pursue. Community outreach can enrich the relationship between your facility and the residents. Perhaps converting an examination room into a casting room to apply fracture care will make more profitable use of the space. Inpatient facilities might host an open house or other interactive event to increase referrals from local health care professionals to you.

CHAPTER REVIEW

SUMMARY

The financial health of an organization is critical to its ability to continue to exist. The greatest physician on earth still
needs equipment and supplies to properly care for a patient.
The revenue (money coming in) is required for the purchase
of these materials and other obligations such as salaries and
taxes. Remember, a free clinic is only free to the patients.
Various types of facilities have multiple ways to find additional
revenue sources, beyond that which comes from third-party
payers. Third-party payers provide reimbursement in various
methodologies. In addition, there are federal and state grants,
government programs, private investors, and bonds issuance,
to name a few, that may provide a health care facility with the
money it needs to expand or enhance the services it provides to
the community.

REVIEW QUESTIONS

MULTIPLE CHOICE

Choose the most accurate answer.

1. Revenue is the term used to identify money that is
   a. owed to others.
   b. coming into the organization.
   c. paid by patients to third-party payers.
   d. a financial obligation.

2. A health care facility may be structured as a
   a. for-profit organization.
   b. nonprofit organization.
   c. public health organization.
   d. all of the above

3. IRS designation 501c(3) indicates that the facility
   a. does have to pay taxes.
   b. has to pay taxes in advance.
   c. does not have to pay taxes.
   d. has third-party payers who pay taxes for them.

4. Which type of business structure can pay dividends to
   stockholders when there is profit?
   a. For-profit organization
   b. Nonprofit organization
   c. Public health organization
   d. All of the above

5. Unsecured bonds are also known as
   a. tax-exempt investments.
   b. angel investments.
   c. debentures.
   d. commercial loans.

6. Which entity may be known as a third-party payer?
   a. Physician
   b. Patient
   c. Internal Revenue Service
   d. Health insurance company

7. All of the following are government third-party payers
   EXCEPT
   a. Humana.
   b. Medicare.
   c. workers' compensation.
   d. Veterans' Administration.

8. Which of the following is a type of payment that would
   come to the facility from a patient?
   a. Fee-for-service
   b. RBRVS
   c. Capitation
   d. Coinsurance

9. DRGs are a type of _____ paid by Medicare to acute
   care hospitals.
   a. fee-for-service
   b. episodic care
   c. capitation
   d. coinsurance

10. *Breaking even* means that the facility has
    a. revenues exceeding expenditures.
    b. expenditures exceeding revenues.
    c. revenues and expenditures that are equal.
    d. no expenditures at all.

11. Analysis of the facility's case mix means that the administrator is evaluating
    a. the percentage of revenue coming from each third-party payer.
    b. the percentage of all patients by diagnosis.
    c. the percentage of beds or exam rooms that are not used.
    d. Both a and b

12. Evaluation of the facility's occupancy rate may reveal that
    a. the facility is not working to its full potential and revenue is being lost.
    b. too much revenue is coming from a single third-party payer.
    c. patients are not paying their fair share of costs.
    d. the facility is a nonprofit organization.

13. Medicare beneficiaries may
    a. be sixty-five years of age and older.
    b. be diagnosed with ESRD.
    c. have a permanent disability.
    d. all of the above

14. Which statement is true about Medicaid?
    a. This program is funded and run exclusively by each state.
    b. This program covers health care costs for those who are indigent.
    c. This program is funded by secured bonds.
    d. This program is only available for services at for-profit hospitals.

15. The general business rule is that no single customer should ever provide _____ of the facility's revenue.
    a. less than 10 percent
    b. more than 30 percent

c. less than 50 percent
d. more than 75 percent

16. Which of the following is an example of a variable expenditure?
    a. Rent
    b. Telephone
    c. Salaries
    d. Utilities

17. Which of the following is an example of a fixed expenditure?
    a. X-ray film
    b. Bandages
    c. Aspirin tablets
    d. Furniture

18. Which of the following is the formula for the definition of profit?
    a. Profit = total expenditures minus total revenues
    b. Profit = total taxes owed minus total taxes paid
    c. Profit = total revenues minus total expenditures
    d. Profit = total expenditures minus dividends paid

19. A grant or commercial loan may be used to fund
    a. the purchase of a CT scanner.
    b. a new building.
    c. the creation of a new operating suite.
    d. all of the above

20. A facility might increase revenue by
    a. increasing the fee charged for each procedure or service.
    b. increasing the number of services provided.
    c. increasing the number of patients for whom they care.
    d. both B and C

FILL-IN-THE-BLANK

Fill in the blank with the accurate answer.

21. For a health care facility to grow its revenue _____, it would increase the types of services it provides to its current patient population.

22. Diagnosis-related groups (DRG) is an example of a(n) _____ care payment plan.

23. A community hospital and a state health department clinic are examples of a(n) _____ care facility.

24. The Shriner's Hospital and a United Cerebral Palsy clinic are examples of a(n) _____ health care facility.

25. Each year, Dr. Jebber's office receives a list of how much this third-party payer will reimburse him for each and every procedure, service, and treatment provided to one of their insureds. Dr. Jebber is being paid under a(n) _____ agreement.

26. A(n) _____ is a fixed amount paid by the patient to the provider, regardless of what is provided during this visit.

27. You, as the administrator, instruct your staff to keep an eye on the third-party payers from whom the facility receives reimbursement so that no single payer represents more than 30 percent of the total revenue stream. This concept is known as _____.

28. The three parts of the RBRVS formula for total RVU calculation is: physician work, practice expense, and _____.

29. Unreimbursed indigent care, staff salaries, and medical supplies are known as _____.

30. A bond that is backed with some type of asset is called a _____.

WHEN YOU ARE THE ADMINISTRATOR . . .

Critical Thinking and Analysis

Case Study #1

Case Mix Stability

Evaluate the data in Figure 3-5 ■. **If you were the administrator of this health care facility, what actions would you recommend to ensure your organization maintains financial good health?** Support your recommendations with specific statistics from the table.

Note: Numbers included on this table have been created only for this assignment.

Case Study #2

Determining Opportunities to Increase Revenues

Evaluate the data available in Figure 3-6 ■, which is from the Health, United States, 2010 report from the U.S. Department of Health and Human Services. If you were the administrator of a health care facility, **what actions would you recommend to ensure your organization can increase revenues?** Support your recommendations with specific statistics from Figure 3-6.

Case Study #3

The Cost of Providing Care

The Office of Civil Rights, an agency within the U.S. Department of Health and Human Services, is involved in investigating health care providers, amongst others, to ensure they are compliant with federal law. In response to complaints, the case shown in Box 3-7 ■ was investigated and eventually resolved.

The ability for an infirmed individual to be able to stay in their own home, rather than be relocated into an assisted living facility or a nursing home, is an endeavor that has become sanctioned by government agencies over the past decade. Medicare has expanded its coverage for home health services to accommodate the provision of the medical services so that patients can get what they need in the environment that they desire.

The case discussed in Box 3-7 describes a situation in which a woman, who needed specialized health care, was able to negotiate with the state of Colorado so she could have the quality of life she needs in her own home without being forced to move.

Read through the allegation and the disposition of this case. From the point of view of the state of Colorado, **create a list of pros and cons** for paying for the services this woman needs to stay in her own home. **How much money would you need to add to the budget to provide these services for one year?**

Take into consideration:

- The average salary for a certified nursing assistant (CNA) in Fort Collins, Colorado (city picked randomly for purposes of this exercise), is $27,039, or roughly $104 per eight-hour shift day.

- Typically, those in the National Guard must complete duty of one weekend a month and two weeks during the summer.

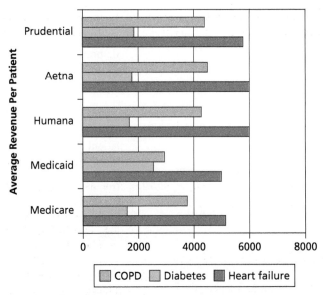

FIGURE 3-5 Average revenue per patient by diagnosis and by third-party payer.

(Continued)

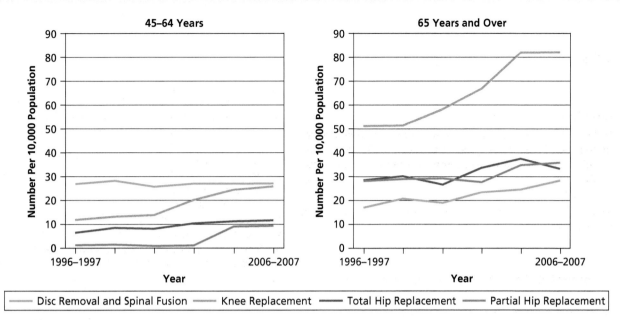

FIGURE 3-6 Health Care Utilization: Total Knee Replacements Procedures.

Source: Health, United States, 2010: Health Care Utilization.

BOX 3-7 **Colorado State Department of Health Care Policy and Financing**

Allegation: This complaint was filed on behalf of a woman with multiple sclerosis. The complainant, who lives at home, alleged that the state's policies put her at risk of unnecessary institutionalization because she could not obtain the daily and overnight care she needed to continue living in her home when the complainant's husband was carrying out responsibilities related to his National Guard service.

Disposition: Office for Civil Rights (OCR) worked with the state and the complainant to resolve the issues in this matter. The complainant began receiving two additional certified nursing assistant (CNA) visits a day when her husband is away for National Guard duty. The complainant found this level of care adequate for her needs. The state also provided information as to the complainant's options should she believe that the level of home health care services she receives is inadequate. The complainant continues to receive Medicaid waiver services, including cleaning, meal preparation, and the use of certain medical equipment.

 INTERNET CONNECTIONS

Healthcare Finance News

This is an online publication focused on the financial issues related to the business of health care and the various organizations involved with the provision of care.

http://www.healthcarefinancenews.com/

Healthcare Financial Management Association (HFMA)

The Healthcare Financial Management Association (HFMA) is a national organization for health care financial management executives and leaders from all aspects of the health care industry. Its website features many news articles and discussion spots covering virtually every aspect of financing the provision of care.

http://www.hfma.org/

Joint Committee on Health Care Financing

The Commonwealth of Massachusetts

This site, from the state of Massachusetts, provides interesting insight into one state's handling of the direct funding of health care programs and any other Medicaid or public health assistance matters, fiscal matters relating to health care policy, Medicaid, MassHealth, and the Uncompensated Care Pool.

http://www.malegislature.gov/committees/joint/j24

CHAPTER 4

QUALITY OF CARE

KEY TERMS

acute myocardial infarction (AMI)
credentials
evidence-based medicine (EBM)
heart failure (HF)
hospital acquired conditions (HAC)
medical necessity
patient-related encounter
patient safety practice
quality improvement strategies
quality indicators (QI)
socio-demographic
Surgical Care Improvement Project (SCIP)
true need

LEARNING OBJECTIVES

Upon completion of this chapter, you should be able to:

- Define commonly used terms, abbreviations, and acronyms.
- Identify the methods available to perform due diligence on clinicians.
- Interpret clinical practice guidelines for implementation.
- Evaluate the impact of outdated equipment and supplies.
- Comprehend the regulatory mandates with regard to quality of care.

WHEN YOU ARE THE ADMINISTRATOR . . .

When you are the administrator overseeing a health care facility, you must take into account your responsibility to:

- Structure and execute a cohesive strategic plan designed to ensure the effective and efficient delivery of services.
- Promote clinical excellence using evidence-based health care principles.
- Verify clinical practice guidelines and quality indicators to ensure patient safety and quality of care.
- Oversee and confirm professional and staff development.

INTRODUCTION

There can be no argument that everyone wants a health care industry that provides quality care. An administrator must be diligent to ensure that the facility is able to provide the best possible care while maintaining financial health and complying with state and federal laws. This may seem like an impossible feat but you can find a way to have these elements work together and augment efforts throughout the organization.

QUALITY STAFF

When a physician wants privileges to care for patients in your facility or a nurse applies for an opening stating he or she is qualified, sadly, you cannot simply take them at their word. You must confirm their identity and their credentials. If this person is lying or even just exaggerating, this can endanger not only your patients, but also everyone who works in your facility, due to the liability.

Of course, this process is the responsibility of the human resources (HR) department. However, as the administrator, you must establish the policies by which the HR staff must abide. In a smaller facility, this may be a part of your job as the administrator. Here is a checklist you can use to verify a physician's clinical **credentials**:

credentials
documentation of knowledge and skills as confirmed by an authorized association or agency.

1. Meet with the individual face-to-face and place a copy of photo identification (such as a driver's license) in the file. (Figure 4-1 ■)
2. While you will certainly require documentation of state licensure for your files, it is recommended that you check with your state's medical licensing board to confirm this individual has a license to practice medicine in your state. Another state in the United States will not do because each has its own requirements. Medicare and Medicaid require participating providers to monitor the quality of care provided to patients in several ways, including credentialing of medical staff. See Box 4-1 ■ for an example of what may happen without this confirmation.
3. Confirm any claim for specialty board certifications with the American Board of Medical Specialties (www.abms.org).
4. If the individual is a physician, check his or her National Provider Identifier (NPI) and ensure that information provided by the individual matches this record (https://nppes.cms.hhs.gov/NPPES/NPIRegistryHome.do).

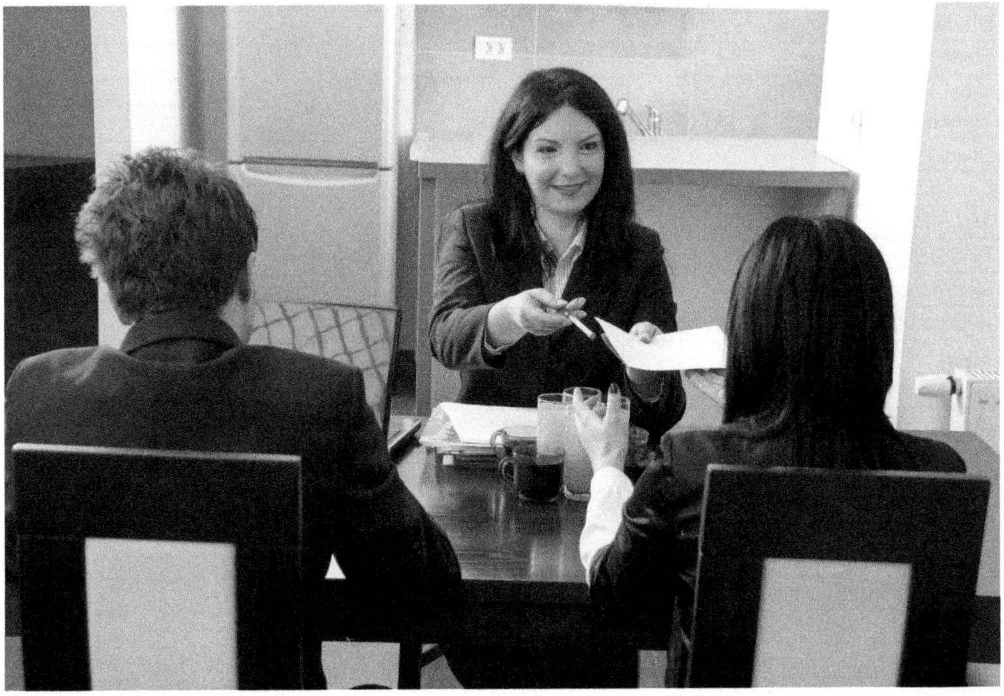

FIGURE 4-1   A face-to-face interview is an important part of the hiring process.
Photo credit: Blaj Gabriel/Shutterstock.

BOX 4-1	Michigan Man Arrested on Health Care Fraud Charge

BUFFALO, N.Y.–U.S. Attorney William J. Hochul Jr. announced today that Fitzgerald Anthony Hudson, 51, of Dearborn Heights, Michigan, was arrested and charged by Criminal Complaint with health care fraud. The charge carries a maximum penalty of 10 years imprisonment, and a fine of $250,000.

Assistant U.S. Attorney Aaron J. Mango, who is handling the case, stated that according to the Criminal Complaint, in October 2007, the defendant obtained a New York State medical license. Thereafter, from August of 2008 to August of 2010, Hudson provided medical care in the Western District of New York at Jones Memorial Hospital in Wellsville, N.Y. and the Nicholas H. Noyes Memorial Hospital in Dansville, N.Y. The defendant allegedly obtained his medical license by listing on his New York State application that he graduated from York University-Facility of Science, North York, Ontario, Canada, when in fact, he had not. In addition, Hudson failed to list that he had been dismissed from the Warren Hospital Family Practice residency program in July 2003.

As a result of his fraudulently obtained medical license, the defendant was improperly reimbursed approximately $200,000 under the Medicare Part-B and Part-D programs. Hudson was arrested today in Michigan, and an initial appearance on the charge has been scheduled for March 29, 2012 at 3 P.M. before United States Magistrate Judge H. Kenneth Schroeder Jr.

The arrest is the culmination of an investigation on the part of Special Agents of the Federal Bureau of Investigation, under the direction of Christopher M. Piehota, Special Agent in Charge and Special Agents of the U.S. Department of Health and Human Services, Office of Inspector General, Office of Investigations under the direction of Thomas O'Donnell, Special Agent in Charge.

Source: The United States Department of Justice.

Privileging and Credentialing Checklist			
Provider Name	**Provider Type**	**Date Last Performed/ Expiration Date/Period**	**Status/Comment**
CREDENTIALING			
Governement Issued Picture I.D. (e.g. Drivers License, State I.D., etc.)			
State License			
DEA License			
NPDB Query			
Undergraduate Degree			
AMA Profile			
Graduate School Degree			
Medical School Degree			
Other Relevant Education, Training or Experience			
Board Certification			
Curriculum Vitae			
ACLS/BCLS			
FTCA/Malpractice Ins.			
Health Fitness Verfication			
Hepatitis B			
TB/PPD			
Job Description			
Employment Agreement			
CMEs			
Performance Evaluation			
Board Approval of Credentials			
PRIVILEGING			
Health Center Privileges			
Hospital Admitting Privileges			
Board Approval of Privileges			
Other			

FIGURE 4-2 Privileging and Credentialing Checklist.

Source: Primary Care: The Health Center Program, U.S. Health Resources and Services Administration.

5. Check the applicant physician's information on the National Practitioner Data Bank (NPDB) and the Healthcare Integrity and Protection Data Bank (HIPDB) (http://www. npdb-hipdb.hrsa.gov). Now that they are together on one website, you will be able to obtain data on physicians, health care practitioners, providers (such as facilities), and suppliers, based on reports filed as required by federal law. The NPDB will enable you to check licensure information in all fifty states, professional memberships, medical malpractice history, and details of clinical privileges. The HIPDB will provide information regarding any fraud or abuse activities.

6. Run a criminal background check on *all* potential staff members, both intrastate (within your state) and nationwide. You can't take a chance that your new pediatrician might be a known sex offender or the new gynecologist is a convicted rapist. The federal law HIPAA (Health Insurance Portability and Accountability Act) Security Rule requires that your organization perform criminal background checks on *all potential* staff members, no matter what job they will perform.

Your staff is the heart of your organization. In reality, they are your product. You must do everything possible to ensure that only qualified, honest health care professionals are on your roster. Figure 4-2 ■ is a checklist created by the U.S. Health Resources and Services Administration to provide a foundation for this process. It is the legal thing to do; it is the moral thing to do; it is the right thing to do.

QUALITY INITIATIVES

Quality care initiatives guide health care professionals in all areas to provide better, more effective care to patients. These initiatives and policies come from the federal government as well as supporting agencies and organizations such as the Joint Commission and the Agency for Healthcare Research and Quality (AHRQ).

AHRQ has created a wide variety of materials that clinicians can use as they work to make important decisions regarding the care of each patient. Of course, administrators can use these same **quality indicators (QI)** to aid in the development of internal policies as well as budget making. AHRQ produces four types of QI documents available on their Quality Indicators website:

quality indicators (QI)
specific standard measures of benefit provided.

- Prevention quality indicators (PQI);
- Inpatient quality indicators (IQI);
- Patient safety indicators (PSI); and
- Pediatric quality indicators.

Let's take a look at a portion of a PQI as an example so you can get an idea of how you might use this data to improve quality in your facility:

"Summary of Evidence

Hospital admission for diabetes short-term complications is a PQI that would be of most interest to comprehensive health care delivery systems. Short-term diabetic emergencies arise from the imbalance of glucose and insulin, which can result from deviations in proper care, misadministration of insulin, or failure to follow a proper diet.

Although risk adjustment with age and sex does not impact the relative or absolute performance of areas, this indicator should be risk-adjusted. Some areas may have higher rates of diabetes as a result of racial composition and systematic differences in other risk factors.

Areas with high rates of diabetic emergencies may want to examine education practices, access to care, and other potential causes of non-compliance when interpreting this indicator. Also, areas may consider examining the rates of hyperglycemic versus hypoglycemic events when interpreting this indicator." *

Whether you are an administrator at a hospital or a physician's office with patients diagnosed with diabetes, you can find recommendations for actions your facility can take to improve patient outcomes and reduce the number of health crises experienced by your patients. Let's analyze this together using this PQI as a point of discussion.

---

*AHRQ Quality Indicators.

1. *"Short-term diabetic emergencies arise from the imbalance of glucose and insulin, which can result from deviations in proper care, misadministration of insulin, or failure to follow a proper diet."* From this single sentence you can pick up several opportunities to add policies in your facility, such as directing nurses and physicians to be certain to discuss diet restrictions for diabetics. You can create a handout listing the titles of diabetic cookbooks that patients may want to purchase for guidance, or you might look into offering a series of diabetes workshops for patients to provide tips on proper diet, the proper administration of insulin, and how to use a blood glucose monitor to test their levels.

2. *"Some areas may have higher rates of diabetes as a result of racial composition and systematic differences in other risk factors."* There are known specific racial and risk factors that increase the probability for a patient to develop diabetes. Risk factors for developing type 2 diabetes include obesity, a personal history of gestational diabetes, little-to-no physical activity, current hypertension, and having dyslipidemia (an abnormal lipoprotein metabolism). Research shows that those of African American, Latino, or Native American ancestry have an inherited increased probability of developing type 2 diabetes. Understanding these factors can help you, as an administrator, evaluate the racial components of your community and determine policies and services that may increase the quality of care. These statistics are usually available from the U.S. Census Bureau or your local Chamber of Commerce.

3. *"Also, areas may consider examining the rates of hyperglycemic versus hypoglycemic events when interpreting this indicator."* Additionally, the quality indicator provides you with tips on how you might use this information. This is an important detail; hyperglycemic (too much glucose in the blood) versus hypoglycemic (too little glucose in the blood) may lead to some insights about what specific problems your diabetic patients may have. You can easily do this analysis by referring to a report in your facility on current patient diagnosis codes, comparing, for example, ICD-9-CM code 790.29 hyperglycemia *with* ICD-9-CM code 250.3x diabetic hypoglycemia. The same comparison can be done with ICD-10-CM codes E10.65 Type 1 diabetes with hyperglycemia/E11.65 type 2 diabetes with hyperglycemia *with* E10.649 type 1 diabetes with hypoglycemia without coma/ E11.649 type 2 diabetes with hypoglycemia without coma.

As a great tool for any health care administrator in any size facility, AHRQ created the following list of nine **quality improvement strategies**. Researchers studied these strategies with the intent of identifying policies or internal practices that support and promote the highest possible level of quality care that could be provided during routine encounters with patients. These have been identified as best practices, ready for implementation in your facility:

quality improvement strategies
a group of plans designed to raise the level of benefit derived from the organization.

1. Physician reminder systems (such as notes in paper charts or computer-based alerts)
2. Improved delivery of clinical patient data, such as lab reports and documentation from other providers, to the physician
3. Internal audits with feedback including physician performance evaluations, implementation of quality indicators, and so on
4. Continuing education for clinicians including supporting attendance at workshops and professional conferences, distribution of educational materials, and so on
5. Providing patient education including seminars, brochures, one-on-one, and the like
6. Encouraging patient self-management by offering workshops, providing materials such as reminder cards, blood pressure clinics, or glucose monitoring devices for use at home
7. Patient reminder systems such as e-mails, telephone calls, or postcards from the facility or the physicians to their patients
8. Top down organizational improvement programs, such as Total Quality Management (TQM), Continuous Quality Improvement (CQI) programs, improved interdepartmental communication processes, and creating a culture of quality throughout the organization
9. Financial rewards including performance-based bonuses, alternative reimbursement systems for physicians, and the like

In addition to the Quality Indicators, AHRQ also hosts the National Quality Measures Clearinghouse (NQMC) [http://www.qualitymeasures.ahrq.gov/]. The information you can get from this website applies to the clinical side of health care as well as the administrative side. In addition to hundreds of quality measures categorized by disease/condition and treatment/intervention, the NQMC offers a great deal of guidance, including this list of options:

Health Services Administration

Analytical, Diagnostic, and Therapeutic Techniques and Equipment
Phenomena and Processes
Disciplines and Occupations
Anthropology, Education, Sociology, and Social Phenomena
Information Science
Named Groups
Health Care
Publication Characteristics

For example, the following is included under Health Services Administration > Health Care > Health Care Quality, Access, and Evaluation:

Ambulatory care: summary of utilization of ambulatory care in the following categories: outpatient visits and emergency department visits. National Committee for Quality Assurance–Health Care Accreditation Organization.

CDC/Healthy People 2020

The Centers for Disease Control (CDC) and Prevention have collected science-based data that includes goals and objectives created to promote good health and disease prevention. *Healthy People 2020*, a project of the CDC, includes more than a thousand good health objectives covering more than forty topics, such as "health-related quality of life and well-being" and "determinants of health." Healthy People 2020 presents ten-year targets intended to influence national, state, and local health education projects as well as disease prevention programs with the expectation that this will lead to improved health of all people in the United States. Table 4-1 ■ exhibits an example of this information: twenty-six leading health indicators in twelve topic areas as determined by *Healthy People 2020*. This list presents objectives for health care providers and patients alike. Several items on this list can ignite a program or an initiative for any size health care organization to implement and help their patients take one step closer to good health—the purpose of the health care industry as a whole.

The CDC brings together the most current data available for analysis, including **socio-demographic** details about the population categorized by age, gender, income, race, geographic location, education level, and more. The data is currently available online at these sites: http://www.healthindicators.gov/ and http://www.healthypeople.gov/2020/.

socio-demographic *A* a collection of specific data related to an individual's age, gender, education, income level, occupation, and other details.

Centers for Medicare and Medicaid Services (CMS) Quality Initiatives

The Centers for Medicare and Medicaid Services (CMS), an agency within the Department of Health and Human Services (HHS), has been publishing quality initiatives since 2001 with the intent of supporting quality health care through public disclosure as well as accountability. These initiatives are presented for:

- Inpatient rehabilitation facilities (IRF)
- Home health organizations
- Acute care hospitals
- Nursing homes (SNF)
- Physicians
- Providers specializing in patients with ESRD

QUALITY IMPROVEMENT ORGANIZATIONS (QIO)   CMS identifies one private organization, most often a nonprofit organization, in each state, District of Columbia, U.S. Virgin Islands, and Puerto Rico to review the provision of health care services, respond to Medicare beneficiaries who have filed complaints, and to take action by implementing quality of care improvements, as necessary. The goal, as specified in the contractual agreement between CMS and the organization, is to:

- Improve quality of care for Medicare and Medicaid beneficiaries in their designated area
- Ensure CMS pays only for services and items that are shown to be medically necessary, reasonable, and provided in the most appropriate setting

TABLE 4-1 Leading Health Indicators

12 TOPIC AREAS	26 LEADING HEALTH INDICATORS
Access to Health Services	• Persons with medical insurance • Persons with a usual primary care provider
Clinical Preventive Services	• Adults who receive a colorectal cancer screening based on the most recent guidelines • Adults with hypertension whose blood pressure is under control • Adult diabetic population with an A1c value greater than 9 percent • Children aged 19 to 35 months who receive the recommended doses of diphtheria, tetanus, and pertussis (DTaP); polio; measles, mumps, and rubella (MMR); Haemophilus influenza type b (Hib); hepatitis B; varicella; and pneumococcal conjugate (PCV) vaccines
Environmental Quality	• Air Quality Index (AQI) exceeding 100 • Children aged 3 to 11 years exposed to secondhand smoke
Injury and Violence	• Fatal injuries • Homicides
Maternal, Infant, and Child Health	• Infant deaths • Preterm births
Mental Health	• Suicides • Adolescents who experience major depressive episodes (MDEs)
Nutrition, Physical Activity, and Obesity	• Adults who meet current federal physical activity guidelines for aerobic physical activity and muscle-strengthening activity • Adults who are obese • Children and adolescents who are considered obese • Total vegetable intake for persons aged 2 years and older
Oral Health	• Persons aged 2 years and older who used the oral health care system in the past 12 months
Reproductive and Sexual Health	• Sexually active females aged 15–44 years who received reproductive health services in the past 12 months • Persons living with HIV who know their serostatus
Social Determinants	• Students who graduate with a regular diploma 4 years after starting ninth grade
Substance Abuse	• Adolescents using alcohol or any illicit drugs during the past 30 days • Adults engaging in binge drinking during the past 30 days
Tobacco	• Adults who are current cigarette smokers • Adolescents who smoked cigarettes in the past 30 days

Source: U.S. Office of Disease Prevention and Health Promotion.

- Respond to all beneficiary complaints, provider-based notice appeals, as well as violations of any applicable laws, including EMTALA
- Any and all other related responsibilities as cited in the QIO-related regulations

HOSPITAL COMPARE   CMS created *Hospital Compare* in collaboration with several organizations that represent consumers, hospitals, doctors, employers, accrediting organizations, and other federal agencies. This database is a part of the *Hospital Quality Initiative*, a tool-kit designed to encourage improvement of the quality of care provided by hospitals. *Hospital Compare* is a website available for use by the general public intended to enable any individual to review the quality of care at a particular hospital, as determined by data that is collected, analyzed, and presented for quality measures as identified in Box 4-2 ■. The website also enables comparisons of the quality of care available at thousands of Medicare-certified hospitals around the United States. For example, in Orlando, Florida, a patient or patient's family can visit the *Hospital Compare* website and compare Orlando Regional Medical Center with Florida Hospital so a decision can be made at which local hospital to have a certain procedure done. Just as the competitive advantage has helped consumers in other industries, now patients—the consumers of health care—can benefit, too.

BOX 4-2   **Quality Measures Collected for Hospital Compare**

- Timely and Effective Care (Process of Care Measures)

  - Heart Attack (**Acute myocardial infarction [AMI]**)
  - **Heart Failure (HF)**
  - Pneumonia
  - Surgery (**Surgical Care Improvement Project—SCIP**)
  - Emergency Department Care
  - Preventive Care
  - Children's Asthma Care

- Readmissions, Complications, and Deaths (Outcome of Care Measures)

  - 30-day death (mortality) rates and 30-day readmission rates
  - Serious complications–AHRQ Patient Safety Indicators (PSIs)
  - Hospital-acquired conditions
  - Health care-associated infections

- Use of Medical Imaging (Outpatient Imaging Efficiency Measures)
- Survey of Patients' Hospital Experiences [HCAHPS (Hospital Consumer Assessment of Healthcare Providers and Systems)]
- Number of Medicare patients
- Spending per hospital patient with Medicare

Source: Medicare.gov.

acute myocardial infarction (AMI)
an area of dead tissue within the heart, the result of an embolus or thrombus blocking sufficient blood flow; commonly known as a heart attack.

heart failure (HF)
a cardiac condition where the heart cannot pump enough to provide proper blood for circulation.

Surgical Care Improvement Project (SCIP)
a standard of measure used by Hospital Compare to determine the level of effort used to enhance surgical outcomes.

Of course, when an emergency occurs, patients will go, or be taken, to the nearest hospital. However, there are many circumstances under which patients can plan ahead, discuss the data with their health care provider, and make an informed decision as to which hospital will best meet their health care needs and support a greater confidence in the expected quality of care.

The focus on this competitive aspect of quality of care asks a great deal of any hospital. Even for those facilities that are not acute care hospitals and, therefore, not included in the collection of data for *Hospital Compare*, there are so many areas upon which to focus continuous quality improvements. Certainly, any individual or any group could feel overwhelmed or ill equipped (regarding finances or staff resources) to go beyond what can be done to ensure that every department and every service strives for excellence. Where does one begin? How might these statistics translate to the daily processes of running a health care facility?

Review the information in Table 4-2 ■. You can see that, for example, 8.4 percent of the patient population (the second largest group) comes into an outpatient department for conditions related to their respiratory system. There are two quality measures listed in Table 4-2 directly related to the respiratory system: pneumonia and children's asthma care. Starting a quality of care initiative with a focus on this specific department would bring benefit to potentially the largest number of people. Using statistics such as these available from the federal government, can help you, as the administrator, create a plan for improvement using a logical, step-by-step strategic plan.

HOSPITAL VALUE-BASED PURCHASING PROGRAM (HVBP)   The Hospital Value-Based Purchasing Program (HVBP) was implemented for fiscal year 2013 affecting payments for hospital discharges on or after October 1, 2012. (Note that CMS's fiscal year runs October 1 through September 30.)

The terms of the HVBP provide for incentive payments to be made by CMS to a hospital determined by the level of performance on specific quality measures during a specified period of time. Logically, the higher the hospital's total performance score (TPS), or the greater the measured improvement over the previous year, the higher the incentive payment would be. The TPS consists of the hospital's score for their Clinical Process of Care domain, which represents 70 percent of the TPS, and the Patient Experience of Care, representing 30 percent of the TPS.

The formula for determining the level of performance on the quality measures identified includes the facility's score on "achievement" and "improvement." As you can see in Box 4-3 ■,

TABLE 4-2 Primary Diagnosis at Outpatient Department Visits, by Major Disease Category: United States, 2010

Major Disease Category	ICD-9-CM Code Range/ ICD-10-CM Code Range	Number of visits in thousands	Standard error in thousands	Percent distribution	Standard error of percent
All visits	....	100,742	(9,565)	100.0	(0.0)
Infectious and parasitic diseases	001-139/A00-B99	3,176	(647)	3.2	(0.6)
Neoplasms	140-239/C00-D49	5,345	(1,157)	5.3	(1.0)
Endocrine, nutritional, and metabolic diseases	240-279/E00-E89	8,225	(1,631)	8.2	(1.2)
Mental disorders	290-319/F01-F99	6,712	(904)	6.7	(0.8)
Diseases of the nervous system and sense organs	320-389/G00-H99	6,640	(839)	6.6	(0.6)
Diseases of the circulatory system	390-459/I00-I99	7,781	(1,403)	7.7	(1.1)
Diseases of the respiratory system	460-519/J00-J99	8,413	(1,009)	8.4	(0.8)
Diseases of the digestive system	520-579/K00-K95	3,791	(633)	3.8	(0.5)
Diseases of the genitourinary system	580-629/N00-N99	4,178	(555)	4.1	(0.3)
Diseases of the skin and subcutaneous tissue	680-709/L00-L99	4,190	(658)	4.2	(0.6)
Diseases of the musculoskeletal and connective tissue	710-739/M00-M99	6,970	(828)	6.9	(0.6)
Symptoms, signs, and ill-defined conditions	780-799/R00-R99	6,683	(748)	6.6	(0.4)
Injury and poisoning	800-999/S00-T88	5,171	(829)	5.1	(0.7)
Supplementary classification	V01-V86/Z00-Z99	18,210	(1,990)	18.1	(1.2)
All other diagnoses	....	3,867	(622)	3.8	(0.4)
Unknown	....	1,391	(374)	1.4	(0.3)

Note: CMS also offers *Nursing Home Compare, Physician Compare, Home Health Compare*, and *Dialysis Facility Compare.* This means that you, as the administrator, can benefit from statistical data to improve the quality of care provided by your organization, in whichever category.

Source: CDC/NCHS, National Hospital Ambulatory Medical Care Survey.

achievement points are based on the hospital's performance as compared to all other hospitals, while the improvement points are based on the hospital's performance compared to itself in a previous measured period (the base period).

The Clinical Process of Care domain consists of twelve specific actions taken by the facility's staff as specified in Box 4-4 ■. As you can see, not all of these procedures are appropriate for all patients. The Patient Experience of Care domain components are discussed in the next section.

HOSPITAL CONSUMER ASSESSMENT OF HEALTHCARE PROVIDERS AND SYSTEMS (HCAHPS) As mentioned in the previous section, one component of the formula for the HVBP incentive payment is the Patient Experience of Care domain, accounting for 30 percent of the TPS. The Patient Experience of Care score is determined by the results of the specific hospital's *Hospital Consumer Assessment of Healthcare Providers and Systems* (HCAHPS—pronounced "H-Caps"). The percentage of the patients from each hospital that choose the highest response on the survey—most positive or "top-box"—is the number used to calculate the Patient Experience of Care score for that hospital's TPS. The same calculations of "achievement" and "improvement" are used for this portion, as they are for the HVBP mentioned earlier (Box 4-3).

> **BOX 4-3**   **Scoring for HVBP Incentive Payments**
>
> Achievement points are awarded by comparing an individual hospital's rates during the performance period with all hospitals' rates from the baseline period:
>
> * Hospital rate at or above benchmark: 10 achievement points
> * Hospital rate below the achievement threshold: 0 achievement points
> * If the rate is equal to or greater than the achievement threshold and less than the benchmark:
>   * 1–9 achievement points
>
> Improvement points are awarded by comparing a hospital's rates during the performance period to that same hospital's rates from the baseline period:
>
> * Hospital rate at or above benchmark: 9 improvement points
> * Hospital rate at or below baseline period rate: 0 improvement points
> * If the hospital's rate is between the baseline period rate and the benchmark:
>   * 0–9 improvement points
>
> *Source: CMS Hospital Value-Based Purchasing Program Fact Sheet.*

The survey includes twenty-seven questions to enable CMS to collect data on each patient's perception of their hospital experience. The data collected relate back to composite measures. Each facility must offer the survey to every Medicare beneficiary patient at discharge, and they are permitted to add any additional questions about their patients' satisfaction, but may not omit any of the original twenty-seven.

The HCAHPS composite measures are:

* Communication with Nurses
* Communication with Doctors
* Staff Responsiveness
* Pain Management
* Communication about Medicines
* Discharge Information
* Hospital Cleanliness and Quietness
* Overall Rating of Hospital

> **BOX 4-4**   **Clinical Process of Care Measures**
>
> 1. AMI-7a—Fibrinolytic Therapy Received within 30 Minutes of Hospital Arrival
> 2. AMI-8—Primary PCI Received within 90 Minutes of Hospital Arrival
> 3. HF-1—Discharge Instructions
> 4. PN-3b—Blood Cultures Performed in the Emergency Department (ED) Prior to Initial Antibiotic Received in Hospital
> 5. PN-6—Initial Antibiotic Selection for Community Acquired Pneumonia (CAP) in Immunocompetent Patients
> 6. SCIP Inf -1—Prophylactic Antibiotic Received within One Hour Prior to Surgical Incision
> 7. SCIP-Inf -2—Prophylactic Antibiotic Selection for Surgical Patients
> 8. SCIP-Inf -3—Prophylactic Antibiotics Discontinued within 24 Hours After Surgery
> 9. SCIP-Inf -4—Cardiac Surgery Patients with Controlled 6:00 A.M. Post-operative Serum Glucose
> 10. SCIP-Card-2—Surgery Patients on a Beta Blocker Prior to Arrival Who Received a Beta Blocker During the Perioperative Period
> 11. SCIP-VTE-1—Surgery Patients with Recommended Venous Thromboembolism Prophylaxis Ordered
> 12. SCIP-VTE-2—Surgery Patients Who Received Appropriate Venous Thromboembolism Prophylaxis within 24 Hours
>
> *Source: CMS Hospital Value-Based Purchasing Program Fact Sheet.*

Evidence-Based Medicine

Research studies can provide statistical evidence as to what services, procedures, treatments, and policies work best. This is known in our industry as evidence-based clinical practice or **evidence-based medicine (EBM)**.

A clinician's treatment plan for a patient's condition or illness can be supported by EBM that shares proven results from credible sources. No single treatment is best for every patient with the same diagnosis. However, knowing what treatment works best for a majority of patients, as well as alternative treatments, may provide some insight to physicians, as a part of the medical decision-making process, to be weighted along with risks and benefits, costs, equipment and supplies availability, in additional to personal factors about this patient when they make the professional recommendations for treatment.

The National Guideline Clearinghouse (NGC) of the AHRQ serves as an excellent resource for evidenced-based clinical procedures, services, and treatments. These documents represent information provided from health care organizations and providers all over the world for the purposes of sharing procedures and their outcomes with the expectation that their experiences can help others. Its searchable database makes finding the applicable information a less stressful task. For example, an entry of "hypothyroidism" in the search box yields seventy-one documents originated by: the American Thyroid Association, The Endocrine Society, Children's Oncology Group, the Finnish Medical Society Duodecim, and others. The first article in the list, *"Guidelines of the American Thyroid Association for the diagnosis and management of thyroid disease during pregnancy and postpartum"* presents data and conclusions, in addition to guidance, broken out into specific categories, such as "Target Population," "Interventions and Practices Considered," and "Major Outcomes Considered."

When outcomes from the research are found to have a direct impact on specific treatment options, this data is presented in easy-to-read tables, such as the example shown in Table 4-3 ■. The determinations are indicated as "Do," "Do Not Do," or "Do Not Know," providing clear insight into those actions that have been proven to work, those that have been proven to cause harm, and those with inconclusive results.

---

evidence-based medicine (EBM)

the process of medical decision making determined by research.

TABLE 4-3   Guidelines for the Evidence-Informed Primary Care Management of Low Back Pain— Partial Summary

Recommendation: Do; Do Not Do; Do Not Know	Acute and Subacute Low Back Pain
Do	**Spinal Manipulation**
	Patients who are not improving may benefit from referral for spinal manipulation provided by a trained spinal care specialist such as a physical therapist, chiropractor, osteopathic physician, or physician who specializes in musculoskeletal medicine.
	Risk of serious complication after spinal manipulation is low (estimated risk: cauda equina syndrome, less than 1 in one million). Current guidelines contraindicate manipulation in people with severe or progressive neurological deficit.
Do	**Multidisciplinary Treatment Programs for Subacute Low Back Pain**
	For subacute low back pain (duration 4 to 8 weeks), intensive interdisciplinary rehabilitation (defined as an intervention that includes a physician consultation coordinated with a psychological, physical therapy, social, or vocational intervention) is moderately effective.
	Functional restoration with a cognitive-behavioral component reduces work absenteeism due to subacute low back pain in occupational settings.
Do Not Do	**Bed Rest**
	Do not prescribe bed rest as a treatment.
	If the patient must rest, bed rest should be limited to no more than 2 days. Prolonged bed rest for more than 4 days is not recommended for acute low back problems. Bed rest for longer than two days increases the amount of sick leave compared to early resumption of normal activity in acute low back pain.
	There is evidence that prolonged bed rest is harmful.

Source: National Guideline Clearinghouse, AHRQ, guideline.gov.

Patient Safety Practices

What health care provider would not agree that patient safety is an absolute necessity for all types of health care provider/patient interactions? This concept is in accordance with the *Hippocratic Oath* that virtually all physicians take upon entering this industry as a professional, ". . . *and I will do no harm or injustice to them*" (Hippocratic Oath, http://www.nlm.nih.gov/hmd/greek/greek_oath.html).

The Evidenced-Based Practice Center, established by AHRQ at the University of California at San Francisco and Stanford University to encourage and support a national health care quality agenda, defined the term "**patient safety practice**" as: "*A type of process or structure whose application reduces the probability of adverse events resulting from exposure to the health care system across a range of diseases and procedures.*"*

There are many sources for information on patient safety from CMS, the Joint Commission, and the Office of the Inspector General (OIG). Certainly, you can agree that all health care providers, regardless of their location or type of facility, must consistently strive to implement processes and procedures that support absolute patient safety. Humans, being prone to distractions and other events, may well present you, as the administrator, with a challenge to ensuring this safety.

Read through the article from the OIG shown in Box 4-5 ■ on this important topic. This is part of a series on various health care facility management concerns.

patient safety practice
a behavior or action performed in a manner designed to keep the patient safe.

| BOX 4-5 | **Management Issue 4: Ensuring Patient Safety and Quality of Care** |

Why This Is a Challenge

As a purchaser of health care for over 100 million Americans, the Department faces challenges in ensuring the quality of care rendered to Federal health care program beneficiaries. Despite increased attention to patient safety, quality problems persist. According to the Joint Commission, 40 wrong-site surgeries are performed in U.S. hospitals and surgicenters every week. In a 2010 report, OIG found that 13.5 percent of hospitalized Medicare beneficiaries suffered harm from adverse events (i.e., patient harm resulting from medical care) during their hospital stays. Forty-four percent of these adverse events were preventable and were caused by care failures, such as medical error, substandard care, or inadequate monitoring. OIG continues to conduct follow-up work on studying adverse events, including determining the extent to which adverse events occur in other care settings, such as nursing homes.

Other OIG work has raised concerns about overmedication with atypical antipsychotic drugs in nursing homes; more than 20 percent of atypical antipsychotic drugs claimed for Medicare patients in nursing homes violated Federal standards to protect nursing home residents from unnecessary drug use. OIG also found that nursing homes generally were not meeting all requirements for care plans and resident assessments when administering antipsychotics. OIG has also identified concerns with the licensure and qualifications of health care providers across various health care settings.

Quality of nursing home care remains a critical challenge. OIG investigations have uncovered various problems, including inadequate staffing, failure to provide adequate nutrition and hydration, patients' development of preventable or untreated pressure wounds (bedsores), inappropriate medication practices, and other serious deficiencies. Other enforcement actions target nursing homes that maximize reimbursement by rendering excessive therapy services that are medically unnecessary or even harmful to beneficiaries.

Progress in Addressing the Challenge

The Department has taken steps to improve quality of care and promote patient safety, both targeting specific populations, such as improving care coordination for Medicare beneficiaries with multiple chronic conditions, and improving care for all patients. The Department has committed up to $1 billion in ACA funding to the Partnership for Patients Initiative, a public-private partnership to keep patients from becoming injured or sicker while undergoing treatment and to help patients heal without added complication. Two specific partnership goals are to reduce hospital readmissions by 20 percent and reduce preventable harm to hospital patients by 40 percent by the end of 2013.

CMS awarded $218 million to state, regional, national, or hospital system organizations to establish Hospital Engagement Networks to make health care safer and less costly by targeting and reducing preventable injuries. Pursuant to the ACA, CMS specifically committed $500 million towards a Community Based Care Transition Program to improve patient outcomes following hospital discharge.

The Department is also testing and implementing new care delivery models in the Medicare and Medicaid programs designed to improve the quality of care by enhancing provider accountability for

*The Evidenced-based Practice Center, established by AHRQ.

quality and improving coordination of care and care transitions. The Department continues to provide incentives for improved quality of care through its value-based payment policies, including policies that link payment to quality measures and that address hospital-acquired conditions. The Department also continues to promote the adoption of electronic health records and electronic prescribing, which promise to improve quality of care, reduce medication errors, and otherwise promote patient safety. The Department established tools to help beneficiaries compare facility-specific quality indicators to better inform their decisions regarding where to seek treatment.

The Five Star Quality Rating System and Nursing Home Compare report on many important quality measures for nursing homes. Recent regulation has also targeted therapy utilization in nursing facilities. In March 2012, CMS launched a new initiative aimed at improving behavioral health and safeguarding nursing home residents from unnecessary antipsychotic drug use. A primary goal is to reduce antipsychotic drug use in nursing homes 15 percent by the end of 2012. Additionally, CMS' Nursing Home Value-Based Purchasing demonstration is currently testing ways to improve care for this population.

OIG continues to pursue enforcement actions against health care providers that render substandard care. OIG maintains corporate integrity agreements with several nursing homes, hospitals, assisted-living facilities, and dental clinics that include quality-monitoring provisions. CMS and OIG continue to work closely with law enforcement partners at the Department of Justice and through the Federal Elder Justice Interagency Working Group to promote better care for elderly persons and to prosecute providers that subject them to abuse or neglect.

What Needs To Be Done
The Department should continue to prioritize quality of care and patient safety and build upon its past efforts, including continuing to implement the quality improvement provisions of the ACA and achieving the goals set by the Partnership for Patients and the National Quality Strategy. OIG has offered recommendations that can assist the Department in this mission. For example, OIG suggested enhancements to nursing home oversight to ensure that Medicare does not pay nursing homes to overmedicate or otherwise inappropriately medicate beneficiaries. OIG also suggested enhancements to outpatient prescription drug claims that could help the Department ensure that Medicare and Medicaid beneficiaries receive only the drugs that are appropriate for their medical indications. The Department should also continue denying payments for services of such low quality that they are virtually worthless and work with OIG to exclude providers that have rendered grossly substandard care, thereby preventing additional harm to vulnerable beneficiaries.

The Department must also ensure that health care professionals working in all sites of service, such as hospitals, nursing homes, school-based facilities, and beneficiaries' homes, meet qualification and licensure requirements before they treat Federal health care program beneficiaries.

Source: Office of the Inspector General.

Medical Necessity

The performance of diagnostic testing has provoked much discussion. Do facilities perform too many tests on one patient without regard to cost? Do physicians perform too many tests on one patient in search of the most accurate diagnosis rather than making an educated guess?

Medical science has provided us with an increased number of methods to investigate the inside of the body without needing invasive procedures. The more accurate the information available about a patient, the more accurate the diagnosis and treatment plan. So, as long as there is **medical necessity** to run a test, the physician should be able to order that test and benefit from the resulting data. Doesn't that make sense?

Medical necessity encompasses those supporting factors of the patient's health issues such as signs, symptoms, and medical history that lead toward action (tests, procedures, services, or treatments) by the physician as determined by the accepted standards of care. For example, the patient has a fever (a sign). This would lead to the first action—the ordering of blood tests including a white blood cell count (WBC)—which will provide evidence, or not, of an infection in the body. Another patient complains of severe pain (a symptom) in her right wrist after falling off a ladder. This leads to the first action—ordering of an x-ray of the wrist to see if the wrist is fractured. If it is, that will lead to the second action—application of cast. If it is not, that will lead to a different second action—another test to check for muscle or nerve problems that may be causing the pain.

medical necessity
determination that an individual has need for a procedure, service, or treatment based on the standards of care.

Quality Documentation

Many within the health care industry focus on the purpose of documentation as it relates to reimbursement. Without a doubt, this is an important role for physician's notes, operative reports, imaging and pathology reports, new patient registration forms, and the like. However, health care documentation plays a critical role in the provision of continuity and quality of care.

All clinicians (physicians, nurses, etc.) are required by law to accurately document the complete details of every patient encounter and every **patient-related encounter**. Whether face to face or via telephone or e-mail, documentation must be created to include:

- Specific time and date of the encounter
- Identity of the patient as well as all others present during the encounter
- Patient medical record number (MRN) or other internal identification
- Identity of the health care professional providing the procedure, service, or treatment along with all other health care professionals involved in the encounter
- Reason for the encounter
- Details of any discussions during the encounter
- Details of physical examination, if provided
- Objective findings or conclusions
- Complete description of all procedures, services, and treatments provided at this encounter
- Follow-up orders, recommendations, instructions
- Signature (real or electronic) confirming the completeness and accuracy of the documentation

patient-related encounter
an exchange between health care professionals discussing a specific patient when the patient is not present.

It makes sense for health care professionals to understand the underlying purpose of these legal requirements. Only with knowledge of what was provided before can the next health care professional make quality medical decisions for diagnoses and treatments. Even when the same health care professional continues with care for the same patient, no one can accurately remember all of the details, especially when any length of time has passed during which the professional has cared for many other patients with many other concerns.

QUALITY EQUIPMENT AND SUPPLIES

Old equipment is not necessarily bad, and new equipment is not necessarily worth the price (Figure 4-3 ■). You probably already know this with all the electronic devices in your personal life. Purchase the newest version, and there may still be glitches that need to be worked out by the manufacturer. On the other hand, older devices will not have new features or the improved quality expected or required to provide proper care. As an administrator, it will be your job to assess the true need for new equipment and to find money in the budget to pay for it.

For example, telemedicine has become a force with great benefits to patients, as well as providers. Robotics are used to assist during surgery as well as to enable a physician to meet face to face (so to speak) with patients while being miles away. These machines have made a significant impact on the delivery of care. Video conferencing systems and digital imaging systems enable asynchronous and synchronous consultations between physicians in multiple locations—with or without patients and their families (Box 4-6 ■).

Studies continue to prove that patient outcomes are substantially improved with the increased use of various telemedicine methodologies. Robotic video visits and video conferencing have been shown to reduce the number of complications suffered by intensive care unit (ICU) patients. There is evidence of lowered mortality rates and fewer diabetic patients being hospitalized during several pilot programs. Patient-tracking software has played a meaningful role with regard to increasing physician productivity, lowering overhead costs, and enabling the earlier identification of signs, symptoms, and manifestations, thereby resulting in better patient outcomes.

The downside of this new technology is its cost. Even though units can be rented rather than purchased, the financial impact will include training and concern related to reimbursement. There is typically a lapse between adoption of new technology and approval by third-party payers to accept and reimburse for these services. One of your responsibilities, as the administrator, is to weigh the benefits with the costs and determine if this is a good investment for your facility. You don't have to do this alone, but you will have to participate in the process.

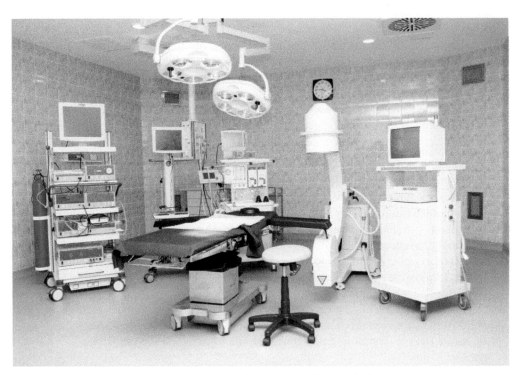

FIGURE 4-3   Hospital equipment—is replacement really needed?

Photo credit: Orkhan Aslanov/Shutterstock.

Assess the True Need

Everyone has a time in their life when new technology dazzles with the latest nifty features. This can easily lead one to confuse desire with need. Very few of us are immune to this temptation. Therefore, when an individual on your staff proposes the purchase of a new piece of equipment, your first job is to assess the **true need** and avoid being swayed by the desire.

As a non-clinician, you need to gather information from credible, objective sources about the differences between the equipment being used now and the new model being considered. During this process, you want facts rather than probabilities. Begin with the sales literature of the new model and focus on what the manufacturer is stating as the greatest benefits. Compare these with the capabilities of your current machine. Is there a difference at all? If so, is it significant?

true need

an evaluation of the level of specific requirement; differentiation between want and need.

BOX 4-6   **Real-Time Video Telehealth**

Traditionally, veterans seeking health care traveled to a Veterans Administration (VA) hospital or medical center. In order to increase veterans' access to health care, VA has so far created over 700 community-based outpatient clinics to bring VA care closer to home for veterans. However, the nearby clinics may not offer all of the specialty services and staff provided by the regional medical center. For example, if specialty care is needed from a cardiologist (heart physician), neurologist (nervous diseases specialist), surgeon for follow-up after surgery, or psychiatrist for mental health care, the clinic provider may need to refer the veteran to the VA medical center.

For many veterans, travel to the medical center can be a very complicated and sometimes arduous task, particularly if the veteran lives in a very remote or rural area, an area with sometimes severe weather, or even an urban area where congestion and traffic makes travel difficult. Some injuries, such as traumatic brain injury or spinal cord injury, further complicate travel. Travel time is time away from the veteran's work or family.

The VA is now recognized as one of the world leaders in this new area of health care. Clinical Video Telehealth (CVT) uses these telehealth technologies to make diagnoses, manage care, perform check-ups, and actually provide care.

Source: United States Department of Veterans Affairs.

Next, you can check with the trade organizations and journals. For example, if you are considering a new model of imaging equipment (x-ray, CT scanner, or MRI), check with the American College of Radiology website: *Technical Standards by Modality and Practice Guidelines* and *Technical Standards Supporting Documentation* sections. If you are considering a new surgical device, you might consult with the American College of Surgeons website: *Surgical Team Resources > Technology*.

Check with the U.S. Federal Food and Drug Administration (FDA) regarding approvals or issues with medical devices to obtain potentially important information critical to the decision-making process. In addition, the National Institute of Standards and Technology (NIST) provides up-to-date information on medical devices, diagnostics, and what it calls life sciences.

While evaluating the new model, you will also need to consider the ancillary costs. For example, if this proposal is for a new digital x-ray machine, will this require upgrades to other computer systems so the digital images can be read and shared with physicians? Will the new machine fit in the allotted space or will construction be necessary? How much time will it take for the technicians to be trained on the new equipment? How long will the facility be without service (the time in between the removal of the old equipment and the installation of the new equipment)?

Lastly, analysis of all of these facts must determine the true benefit, or lack thereof, to the facility's ability to deliver quality health care to your patients. Will the benefits to your patients justify the expense?

QUALITY REGULATIONS

It should come as no surprise that there are governmental regulations and laws with which a health care facility of any size must comply. It is important that we consider certain legal obligations while we are discussing quality of care. Although respect for a physician's knowledge and expertise is at the heart of the procedures, services, and treatments provided, you, the administrator, have your role to play in this process. It is not honorable or ethical for you to relinquish this responsibility to any other individual (such as a physician) or group of individuals (such as a third-party payer). When the entire organization works together in harmony, quality can be more confidently ensured.

Quality-of-care standards are the primary theme in a massive regulatory system on both federal and state levels. In addition, whenever possible, the maintenance of these standards, as a foundational level for assessing the quality of care provided, is tied to reimbursement and to the assessment of monetary penalties for failure to comply. CMS requires all of its participating providers to hold the clinical staff responsible for the quality of care provided to its beneficiaries.

Hospital Acquired Conditions (HAC)

Hospital acquired conditions (HAC), also known as nosocomial conditions, are those illnesses and injuries that affect a patient as a direct result of the patient's stay in the hospital. These may be caused by human error or by a lack of sterile conditions. However, they are all considered to be preventable when proper patient safety precautions are implemented. For example, if a physician forgets to change his gloves between patients, he may accidently transfer a pathogen from one patient to the other. In some cases, an HAC can be caused by a staff member's failure to comply with facility patient safety policies and procedures. For example, if a nurse forgets to put up the side rail on a patient's bed, the patient may roll over and fall out of bed, breaking his wrist.

In addition to a facility wanting to do everything possible to prevent harm from coming to patients, every administrator will want to avoid HACs because Medicare has stopped payments for the treatments of such conditions. The law specifically mandates that hospitals may *not* receive reimbursement for any treatment provided for an HAC suffered by a Medicare beneficiary, nor can that facility request payment for these treatments from the beneficiary himself or herself. There are ten categories of HACs that will not receive

hospital acquired condition (HAC)
an illness or injury that a patient contracts during a stay in an acute care hospital.

reimbursement, making the impact of causing harm to your patients a financial matter as well as an ethical one:

1. Foreign Object Retained After Surgery
2. Air Embolism
3. Blood Incompatibility
4. Stage III and IV Pressure Ulcers
5. Falls and Trauma [Fractures, Dislocations, Intracranial Injuries, Crushing Injuries, Burns, Electric Shock]
6. Manifestations of Poor Glycemic Control [Diabetic Ketoacidosis, Nonketotic Hyperosmolar Coma, Hypoglycemic Coma, Secondary Diabetes with Ketoacidosis, Secondary Diabetes with Hyperosmolarity]
7. Catheter-Associated Urinary Tract Infection (UTI)
8. Vascular Catheter-Associated Infection
9. Surgical Site Infection Following: Coronary Artery Bypass Graft (CABG)—Mediastinitis, Bariatric Surgery, Orthopedic Procedures
10. Deep Vein Thrombosis (DVT)/Pulmonary Embolism (PE)

The OIG Work Plan

The Office of the Inspector General (OIG), in collaboration with the U.S. Department of Justice, the states' Attorneys General, and health care regulatory agencies, actively investigate health care providers in all types of facilities to identify substandard care, whether perpetrated by one individual or as an institutional practice. Each October, the OIG publishes its work plan for the following calendar year, specifically identifying the foci of its upcoming or continuing investigations. Some examples from an OIG work plan are:

- *Hospital Reporting for Adverse Events:* We will review the type of information that hospitals' internal incident-reporting systems capture about adverse events and determine the extent to which hospital systems captured adverse events and reported the information to external patient-safety oversight entities. Most hospitals have incident-reporting systems that enable medical and hospital staff members to report information about patient safety incidents when they occur and to use reported information to prevent recurrence, hold staff members accountable, and notify families. We will use data collected for a 2010 OIG study examining the national incidence of adverse events among hospitalized Medicare beneficiaries. (OEI; 06-09-00091; expected issue date: FY 2012; work in progress)
- *Medicare Requirements for Quality of Care in Skilled Nursing Facilities:* We will review how SNFs have addressed certain Federal requirements related to quality of care. We will determine the extent to which SNFs developed plans of care based on assessments of beneficiaries, provided services to beneficiaries in accordance with the plans of care, and planned for beneficiaries' discharges. We will also review SNFs' use of Resident Assessment Instruments (RAI) to develop nursing home residents' plans of care. Prior OIG reports revealed that about a quarter of residents' needs for care, as identified through RAIs, were not reflected in care plans and that nursing home residents did not receive all the psychosocial services identified in care plans. Federal laws require nursing homes participating in Medicare or Medicaid to use RAIs to assess each nursing home resident's strengths and needs. (Social Security Act, §§ 1819(b)(3) and 1919(b)(3).) (OEI; 02-09-00201; expected issue date: FY 2012; work in progress)

STATISTICS TO EVALUATE QUALITY

There are several formulas that are used by hospital administrators that you can use in any size facility to identify potential problem areas when compared to national statistics. For example:

Case Fatality (percentage) = total number of patients who died due to a specific condition divided by the total number of patients who have been diagnosed with that same condition within a specified span of time.

$$\frac{\text{Total number of patients who died due to a specific condition}}{\text{Total number of patients who have been diagnosed with that same condition within a specified period of time}} = \text{Case Fatality (\%)}$$

Health care is a life and death business and, sadly and unavoidably, some patients pass away no matter how hard we try and regardless of what twenty-first century knowledge and capabilities are used. With some diagnoses, such as a stage 5 malignancy or severe sepsis, mortality (death) can be expected at a higher percentage. With other conditions, mortality is quite unusual. Greater than normal mortality rates at your facility may be a result of lack of quality care. As the facility's administrator, this is something that you must uncover and correct immediately.

Another concern often discussed throughout the health care industry is that related to readmissions. *Readmissions* is the term used to identify those patients who must be returned to inpatient status in a hospital for the same reason as the previous admission. One formula used by health care administrators to determine how their patient population stands with regard to this important measure is:

Percentage of patients who return to facility for same concern = total number of patients who unexpectedly returned to the facility for additional treatment for the same condition divided by the total number of patients who have been diagnosed with that same condition within a specified span of time.

$$\frac{\text{Total number of patients who unexpectedly returned to same facility for additional treatment for same condition}}{\text{Total number of patients who have been diagnosed with that same condition within a specified period of time}} = \text{Readmission Rate (\%)}$$

For the most part, no one is guaranteed a cure. However, there are going to be specific diagnoses that are expected to be resolved. When patients must return again and again, it may be the result of misdiagnosis or poor treatment planning. Again, as the administrator, you must look into these facts and take action to improve the provision of care.

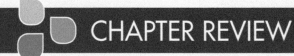

CHAPTER REVIEW

SUMMARY

The responsibility for providing quality care to your facility's patients is not just on the shoulders of the clinical staff but one that involves every member of the organization. Although respect for a physician's knowledge and expertise is at the heart of the procedures, services, and treatments provided, you, the administrator, have your role to play in this process.

Administrators should be aware of quality initiatives, such as those from the CDC and CMS, which can be used as foundations for the creation of policies and procedures in your facility. In addition to the quality of individual actions, you, as the administrator, must also evaluate the quality of the equipment and supplies with which your staff members work. All of this must be accomplished in compliance with federal and state laws. When the entire organization works in harmony, quality can be more confidently ensured.

REVIEW QUESTIONS

MULTIPLE CHOICE

Choose the most accurate answer.

1. The HIPAA Security rule requires that _____ for each potential employee; regardless of which job position they will hold in the health care facility.
   a. an embedded electronic tracking device be placed in the shoe
   b. criminal background checks, both state and federal, be performed
   c. a computer proficiency exam be administered
   d. blood tests for disease be conducted

2. The National Practitioner Data Bank can provide information on all physicians in the United States, EXCEPT
   a. physician licensure.
   b. medical malpractice history.
   c. names and addresses of immediate family members.
   d. details of clinical privileges.

3. To check if a provider or supplier has been found guilty of fraud or abuse, you should
   a. access the National Practitioner Data Bank.
   b. access the Authentication of Records systems.
   c. access the Healthcare Integrity and Protection Data Bank.
   d. perform a standard criminal background check.

4. You need to ensure that the potential staff member at the interview is actually the person he or she claims to be. Therefore, the first thing to do is
   a. talk with his or her family.
   b. contact previous employers.
   c. check photo identification such as a driver's license.
   d. ask him or her to tell you what high school he or she went to.

5. Hiring a physician office receptionist without a background check may
   a. make your office liable for any illegal actions taken.
   b. endanger your patients.
   c. save your practice money.
   d. Both A and B

6. AHRQ stands for
   a. Agency for Health Records and Quality.
   b. Agency for Healthcare Research and Quality.
   c. Association of Health Researchers and Qualifications.
   d. Association of Hospital Regulations and Qualifications.

7. AHRQ identifies all these best practices for quality improvement EXCEPT
   a. providing patient education.
   b. continuous quality improvement programs.
   c. physician alert reminders.
   d. open access for all patients to clinical patient data.

8. Statistical evidence for best clinical practices is known as
   a. evidence-based medicine.
   b. medical necessity.
   c. capital expenses.
   d. true need.

9. A facility that desires to provide the best possible care to its patients must
   a. implement the latest, newest equipment.
   b. continuously evaluate quality of care provided.
   c. hire an outside consultant.
   d. demand that physicians do things *your* way.

10. Ideas for improvement to your facility's provision of preventive care may be supported by
    a. AHRQ's prevention quality indicators.
    b. CDC's *Healthy People 2020.*
    c. Evidence-based medicine.
    d. All of the above

FILL-IN-THE-BLANK

Fill in the blank with the accurate answer.

11. A _____ is an organization contracted by CMS to review the provision of health care services in their area, respond to beneficiary complaints, and to implement quality of care improvements.

12. Heart failure, pneumonia, and children's asthma care are examples of *Hospital Compare's* _____.

13. In the calculations for a HVBP incentive payment, an _____ compares this hospital with all other hospitals.

14. The National Guideline Clearinghouse is an excellent resource for _____.

15. "*A type of process or structure whose application reduces the probability of adverse events resulting from exposure to the health care system across a range of diseases and procedures*" is a definition of _____.

16. The law specifically mandates that hospitals may not receive reimbursement for any treatment provided for a(n) _____ suffered by a Medicare beneficiary.

17. HVBP program was implemented and began affecting payments for hospital discharges on or after _____.

18. Two parts of the HVBP formula are Clinical Process of Care and _____.

19. Communication with nurses, communication with doctors, and staff responsiveness are a few of the composite measures of the _____ survey.

20. OIG suggested enhancements to _____ oversight to ensure that Medicare does not pay them to overmedicate beneficiaries.

TRUE/FALSE

Determine if each of the following statements is true or false.

21. PQI stands for prevention quality indicators.

22. AHRQ does not consider performing internal audits with physician performance evaluations to contribute to quality of care.

23. Socio-demographic data categorizes a population by health insurance coverage.

24. Nursing Home Compare and Hospital Compare are only accessible to licensed physicians.

25. The higher a hospital's TPS is, the higher the incentive payment will be.

26. Evidence-based medicine is the broad term that means that quality documentation of a patient encounter was completed and placed in the patient's chart.

27. "Do," "Do Not Do," and "Do Not Know" are determinations that may be shared in evidence-based documents that are shared on the NGC.

28. New technology, as it relates to the provision of health care, has no downside.

29. An air embolism and a catheter-associated urinary tract infection are examples of HAC.

30. Administrators have no control over the quality of care provided by the clinicians in their facility.

WHEN YOU ARE THE ADMINISTRATOR . . .

Critical Thinking and Analysis

Evaluate the research findings published by the Agency for Healthcare Research and Quality (AHRQ) shown in Case Study 1 and Case Study 2. **If you were the administrator of a heath care facility, what actions would you recommend to ensure that your facility provides the best of care for your patients? Support your recommendations with specific details from the research findings.**

Case Study #1

Good Treatments Are Available for People at Risk for Sudden Cardiac Death

Drug treatment for sudden cardiac death has improved over the years. Deaths from sudden cardiac death can be lowered by preventing the specific heart rhythm disturbances (ventricular arrhythmias) associated with it. The type I antiarrhythmic drugs (sodium channel blockers) often used in the past are no longer considered helpful. In fact, in one study, they were associated with a 21 percent increase in death rates among people at risk for sudden cardiac death.

However, some type III antiarrhythmic drugs (potassium channel blockers), including amiodarone and sotalol, are effective. In a systematic review of methods of preventing sudden cardiac death, amiodarone was identified as the most effective medication, decreasing mortality by 13 to 19 percent compared to a placebo.

Implantable cardiac defibrillators are effective and their use has expanded markedly. Surgically implanting an ICD to monitor and correct the heart rate can offer additional help. In the same review of treatments to prevent sudden cardiac death, researchers found that when ICDs were combined with other therapy (most often amiodarone), the ICDs reduced mortality by an additional 24 percent. ICDs appeared to be most effective for patients who had an episode of sustained ventricular tachycardia or ventricular fibrillation. The evidence is less strong for patients who had an earlier myocardial infarction and a low ejection fraction.

In another study, researchers examined Medicare data for 1987–95 and California hospital discharge data for 1991–95 to study trends in the use and outcomes of ICDs. During the study period, ICD use increased more than tenfold. Mortality rates fell from 6.0 percent to 1.9 percent for the first 30 days after device implantation and from 19.3 percent to 11.4 percent for the year following implantation. It could not be determined whether these better outcomes were the result of improved effectiveness of the device or improved patient selection. Over the study period, the need for device revision or replacement and overall costs remained stable.

In another study, it was found that ICD patients had higher overall costs than patients treated only with medication because of the upfront costs of the device, but their follow-up costs were lower.

Quality of life for these patients may be improving. ICDs and antiarrhythmic medications to prevent sudden cardiac death are effective in reducing deaths, but their impact on quality of life (QOL) is less clear. In a study that followed 264 patients with new cases of life-threatening ventricular arrhythmias, QOL decreased at first but gradually improved with time. The overall improvements in QOL were greater for patients with ICDs than for patients treated only with amiodarone. These findings, which contrast with previous research, may reflect advances in ICD technology and differences in study populations.

Source: AHRQ Publication No. 03-P022.

Case Study #2

Vitamin D Levels Are a Concern for Mother and Child

Breastfeeding among black women in North Carolina has risen dramatically in the past few years. Breast milk is the ideal form of nutrition for infants, but the amount of vitamin D in breast milk depends on the vitamin D status of the mother. Dark-skinned mothers need more exposure to sunlight than light-skinned mothers to produce the same amount of vitamin D. The same is true of darker skinned babies. Unless they receive vitamin supplements, breast-fed dark-skinned infants are at risk for rickets.

The amount of sun exposure an infant needs to prevent rickets depends on skin pigmentation, the amount of clothing worn, latitude, time of day, season of the year, amount of smog, and so on. Moreover, many parents do not want to expose their babies to too much sun for fear of skin cancer.

Maternal vitamin D status also plays a role in this vitamin deficiency, but it is impractical to test nursing mothers. Although there is no national reporting system for rickets that can give statistics on this condition nationwide, indications are that rickets is on the rise throughout the United States. Increasingly, it appears that vitamin supplementation for all breast-fed infants is a safe, low-cost, and reasonable option.

Source: AHRQ Publication No. 02-P001.

Case Study #3

Discuss this concept of using standard business quality initiatives and the logic of adopting them to use in health care. Choose one of the practices identified in paragraph 2, research it, summarize it, and include how you might apply this concept in your health care facility.

"Researchers now believe that most medical errors cannot be prevented by perfecting the technical work of individual doctors, nurses, or pharmacists. Improving patient safety often involves the coordinated efforts of multiple members of the health care team, who may adopt strategies from outside health care."

"The report reviews several practices whose evidence came from the domains of commercial aviation, nuclear safety, and aerospace, and the disciplines of human factors, engineering and organizational theory. Such practices include root cause analysis, computerized physician order entry and decision support, automated medication dispensing systems, bar coding technology, aviation-style preoperative checklists, promoting a 'culture of safety,' crew resource management, the use of simulators in training, and integrating human factors theory into the design of medical devices and alarms."

Source: Making Health Care Safer: A Critical Analysis of Patient Safety Practices.

INTERNET CONNECTIONS

Medicare's Hospital Compare

Hospital Compare has information about the quality of care at over 4,000 Medicare-certified hospitals across the country. You can use Hospital Compare to find hospitals and compare the quality of their care.
http://medicare.gov/hospitalcompare/

Hospital Care Quality Information from the Consumer Perspective

The HCAHPS survey seeks to collect data on patient perspectives about their health care and asks patients to rate items covering eight key topics related to recently received care from a health care facility.
http://www.hcahpsonline.org/home.aspx

Putting Evidence into Practice

This edition of *Health Affairs*, sponsored by the Agency for Healthcare Research and Quality (AHRQ), provides a variety of perspectives on the challenges and potential rewards of building and using a stronger evidence base for health care decisions.

Articles in this edition review the history and context of evidence-based decision making; they describe the challenges of developing the most relevant evidence for different clinical and policy decisions. They discuss obstacles and opportunities for practitioners and policymakers seeking to implement evidence-based decisions.
http://www.ahrq.gov/clinic/healthaff.htm

CHAPTER 5

WORKPLACE SAFETY

KEY TERMS

bloodborne pathogens
exposure control plan
(ECP)
facility maintenance
heating ventilation air
conditioning (HVAC)
other potentially infectious
materials (OPIM)
workforce health promotion
(WHP)

LEARNING OBJECTIVES

Upon completion of this chapter, you should be able to:

- Define commonly used terms, abbreviations, and acronyms.
- Identify actions that can reduce the opportunity for workplace violence and workplace illness.
- Understand the responsibilities of the maintenance and housekeeping departments.
- Evaluate the benefits of a corporate wellness program.
- Determine the costs to the organization for failure to comply with safety and health guidelines and recommendations.
- Develop plans for promoting workplace safety.

WHEN YOU ARE THE ADMINISTRATOR . . .

When you are the administrator overseeing a health care facility, you must take into account your responsibility to:

- Assess and identify specific services, facilities, equipment, and personnel needed to address the current and future health care needs of the community and the funding required to provide such services.
- Supervise the activities of all departments including: clinical, human resources, finance (including accounts receivable and payable), operations, maintenance, housekeeping, and admissions/scheduling.

INTRODUCTION

As a professional working in health care, you know how important it is to ensure that all patients are kept safe. There are so many programs, initiatives, and laws that provide administrators, like you will be, with the direction and plans to keep them safe. The fact is, you also have an obligation to keep your staff members safe, and there are laws that support your effort do this as well.

When a physician agrees to take on the responsibility for caring for a patient, this is legally known as accepting the "duty to care." Similarly, when your organization hires an individual to work for them or with them (whether paid or not), there is also an obligation for you to adopt a "duty to care"—both morally and legally. Keeping all of your people safe will take teamwork in order to plan, develop, and implement programs to avoid or minimize hazards. As the administrator, you should build your team with representatives from every department within your organization: management, union, human resources, safety and health, security, medical/psychology, legal, communications, and worker assistance, in order to ensure that all perspectives are covered.

WORKPLACE SAFETY

Dangers lurk everywhere, especially in the health care industry. We all think of health care facilities as places of healing. Yet, health care organizations frequently confront dangers that can potentially harm staff members. The administrator's job is to do everything possible to protect his or her staff.

Workplace Violence

The Center for Disease Control and Prevention, National Institute for Occupational Safety and Health (NIOSH) defines workplace violence as the occurrence of violent acts (i.e., physical assaults, threats of assaults, battery) directed toward an individual or group of individuals at work or on duty.

TYPES OF WORKPLACE VIOLENCE PERPETRATORS   Everyone in the country becomes aware of workplace violence when an incident, such as a school shooting, fills the news. In reality, none of us ever think such a thing could happen where we work. Sadly, it is not as rare an occurrence as we would all like to think. The Occupational Safety and Health Administration (OSHA) has identified health care as a "high-incidence industry" for workplace violence—regardless of the specific type of location (i.e., hospitals, clinics, physician offices, etc.). According to OSHA, workplace violence has been one of the top four causes of employment-related deaths over the last fifteen years. These incidents not only affect staff members, but family and friends, as well as the community as a whole. Think about it. How would you feel admitting your spouse into a hospital that has just had a nurse shot by a former patient?

In a way, it makes sense that health care workers are at a higher risk than those working in other industries. Emotions run high when a person or family member is ill, in pain, or passes away. Depending upon your facility, you may be more likely to deal with patients suffering from a mental illness with a greater propensity for violence or an overly excited reaction that may be misunderstood. In addition, where health care services are provided, drugs are typically present, increasing the likelihood of criminals targeting your location as well as the possibility of staff members, themselves, becoming addicts and thereby endangering those around them.

OSHA classifies workplace violence perpetrators into one of four groups:

Type 1: *Criminal Intent*   This classification of individuals comes to the workplace with the intention of committing a crime. For example, an individual might enter a physician's office or clinic with the intention of stealing drugs, and harm anyone who got in his or her way.

Type 2: *Customer/Client/Patient*   This category includes individuals who have a complaint about service that was provided or those upset with an outcome. For example, an individual may be unhappy with the results of a procedure performed on his or her family member and blame the staff. As depicted in the movie "*John Q*," where a father took over the emergency room at gunpoint because his son was refused a heart transplant when the family did not have the money to pay for the procedure, this may be someone unhappy with the facility's refusal of service.

Type 3: *Co-Worker*   This category includes individuals who are unhappy about the way they are treated at work; perhaps they have been denied a promotion or laid off due to an economic downturn. This category may also include an individual who has perceived a slight from a fellow staff member and decided to lash out at the person they blame for the event.

Type 4: *Personal*   These are cases when the individual who perpetrates the violence at the office is actually targeting someone with whom he or she has a personal relationship. Essentially, the violent act has nothing to do with the organization as a whole or any of the services provided by the staff. This is a coincidence of location—the place where the pursued individual happens to be. Sadly, it is not unusual for others to suffer the consequences as well.

CREATING A WORKPLACE VIOLENCE PREVENTION PROGRAM   As an administrator, it is within your realm of responsibilities to develop and implement a "Workplace Violence Prevention Program." It is always in the best interests of the organization as a whole to keep your people safe. Solid data proves that prevention programs are successful at reducing incidents of workplace violence. Whatever the cost of new locks or photo identification badges, it is much more expensive to enable criminal activity and endanger your staff. Based on recommendations from OSHA, here are some steps to follow when creating such a program:

1. Perform a security evaluation of the physical property—inside and outside—to create a list of specific hazards or risk factors. It is suggested that the committee assigned to perform the evaluation include both men and women. Women may be at risk from a situation in which a man will not, so it is critical to ensure your assessment includes all potential hazards.

2. Determine which physical hazards might be dramatically reduced or eliminated with adjustments, such as:
    a. Installation of locking mechanisms requiring identification or password to enter. Repair any broken locks immediately.
    b. Enable alarms or other security devices at entryways.
    c. Provide panic buttons, handheld alarms, or other manners of alerting when a risk is perceived to be imminent or possible and arrange for response systems when an alert is activated.
    d. Install and maintain bright lighting inside and outside, especially in high-risk areas such as stairwells. Ensure that burned-out lights are replaced promptly.
    e. Place curved mirrors at intersections or around corners to prevent staff members from walking into a blind spot.
    f. Enable closed-circuit recording, twenty-four hours a day, seven days a week, especially at high risk locations.
    g. If the facility is located in a high-risk area, consider installing metal detectors or other security feature to detect guns, knives, and other weapons and prevent them from being carried onto the property.
    h. Provide "quiet rooms" for patients, family members, or staff members that may be approaching an "explosion" point or acting out.
    i. Establish "safe spots"—locked areas into which staff may go to separate them from a violent episode and await security personnel or police.
    j. Arrange furniture to prevent a staff member or other innocent from becoming trapped and unable to access an exit or summon help.
    k. Limit furnishings and other accessories that may be used as an impromptu weapon.
    l. If valid, install shatterproof glass or plexiglass dividers between the public and receptionist, at nurses' stations, and other triage areas.

3. Establish policies and procedures created to align staff behaviors that keep them safe.
    a. Design work schedules so no employee is working alone, especially in an unsecured location, such as a home health visit or a parking lot at night.
    b. Provide all authorized personnel with photo identification badges to ensure access only to those individuals.

c.   Create a reporting system so staff members can identify any safety concerns and potential danger points (i.e., aggressive patient, family member, visitor, or staff member, etc.). Ensure that every report is taken seriously and addressed effectively.

d.   Include discussions in case management meetings about anyone that may be a danger currently or cause of concern in the future.

4.   Develop a mandatory training program to educate staff on protocols that will guide them as to how to address any risks that cannot be eliminated or predicted.

a.   Teach all staff members how to recognize the earliest stages of a possible assault.

b.   Ensure staff members know how to avoid or diminish potential violent encounters. Have them learn specific phrases in key languages: English, Spanish, French, and the like (determined by the community), that may be used to possibly de-escalate an assault and increase the possibility of getting help.

c.   Provide directions for seeking a safe place and contacting help if violence appears imminent.

d.   Educate all staff members on the proper use of restraints as well as release techniques.

5.   Coordinate with local law enforcement to have officers on site or on regular patrol, as well as to identify safe words or emergency signals when help is needed immediately and the staff member cannot dial 911.

6.   Map out potential places of safety and shelter at each work location—on the property and in the community.

Whether the result of a random inspection or an investigation prompted by reports of employee endangerment, OSHA will assess the facility and the preventive actions the organization employed to keep everyone safe. Box 5-1 ■ shows you what the results of a post-event inspection may reveal.

Workplace Illness

In addition to the dangers that lurk in dark stairwells and vacant parking lots, dangers to your staff lurk in the office, the examination room, the lab, and the operating room. Workers in the health care industry are, given the nature of their work, susceptible to many things that can harm them (Box 5-2 ■). You, as the administrator, must do everything you can to protect them from these perils.

The most obvious danger to health care workers is the spread of disease. Exposure to **bloodborne pathogens**—bacteria and viruses that are only contracted by exposure to infected blood or **other potentially infectious materials (OPIM)**—can be prevented by the creation and implementation of an **exposure control plan (ECP)**. An ECP includes internal policies and procedures mandating the use of personal protective equipment (PPE), including gloves, masks, gowns, and other protective clothing and equipment whenever caring for a patient who is ill. Take a look

bloodborne pathogens
bacteria and viruses that are transmitted via bodily fluids.

other potentially infectious materials (OPIM)
those materials other than bloodborne pathogens that may cause illness.

exposure control plan (ECP)
a set of policies and procedures designed to protect staff from harmful effects.

BOX 5-1   **Type 2 Workplace Violence Offender**

A patient in the psychiatric ward attacks a nurse at a local hospital.

• Known risk factor – YES

  • Working with unstable or volatile persons in health care.

• Industry or Employer Recognition – YES

  • Large body of studies on the existence of potential workplace violence in these types of health care settings. Previous incidents reported to employer.

• Existence of feasible means of abatement – YES

  • Large body of work on feasible means of abatement available to address workplace violence in these types of health care settings (e.g., having two or more employees present when unstable clients are at the facility).

Source: OSHA Instruction. Directive number: CPL 02-02-052, Enforcement Procedures for Investigating or Inspecting Workplace Violence Incidents.

| BOX 5-2 | **Health care industry has highest rate of work-related injuries and illnesses** |

More workers are injured in the health care and social assistance industry sector than any other. This industry has one of the highest rates of work related injuries and illnesses. In 2010, the health care and social assistance industry reported more injury and illness cases than any other private industry sector—653,900 cases. That is 152,000 more cases than the next industry sector: manufacturing. In 2010, the incidence rate for work related nonfatal injuries and illnesses in health care and social assistance was 139.9; the incidence rate for nonfatal injury and illnesses in all private industry was 107.7.

Nursing aides, orderlies, and attendants had the highest rates of musculoskeletal disorders of all occupations in 2010. The incidence rate of work related musculoskeletal disorders for these occupations was 249 per 10,000 workers. This compares to the average rate for all workers in 2010 of 34.

In addition to the medical staff, large health care facilities employ a wide variety of trades associated with health and safety hazards. These include mechanical maintenance, medical equipment maintenance, housekeeping, food service, building and grounds maintenance, laundry, and administrative staff.

Source: OSHA.

at Figure 5-1 ■, and you will see familiar examples of PPE. Governmental regulations require employers to provide appropriate gloves to all staff members who have even the slightest potential of being exposed to blood or OPIM. Ensure that you provide the correct size for a proper fit. Alterative materials (such as nitrile or vinyl instead of latex) must also be made available for use by those with a latex allergy or working with a patient who has a latex allergy.

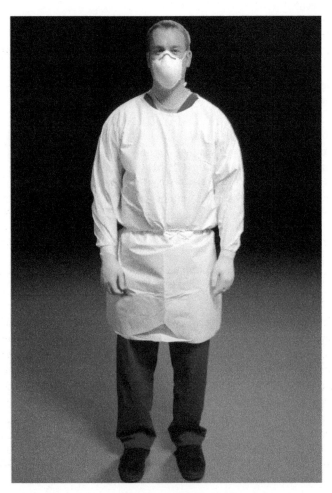

FIGURE 5-1   A staff member in personal protective equipment.

Photo credit: CDC/James Gathany.

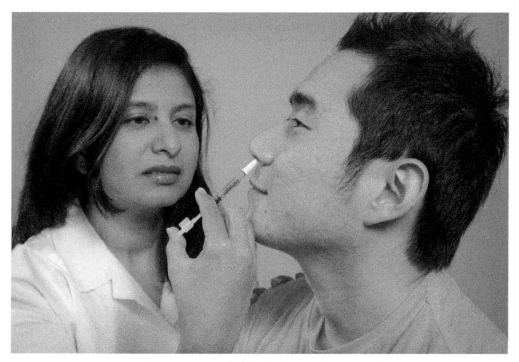

FIGURE 5-2 Administration of intranasal vaccine.

Photo credit: CDC/Dr. Bill Atkinson/James Gathany.

A needlestick and other sharps*-related injury prevention plan, and the implementation of safe medical devices, including shielded needle devices, plastic capillary tubes, and devices that do not require needles at all should be included in the ECP. Exposure to HIV-infected blood can occur by accident, involved with the performance of one's job, such as via a needlestick accident, a splash into the eyes, nose, or mouth, or contact with skin that is compromised by a cut (laceration).

Vaccination and immunization schedules must be implemented and maintained, without exception (Figure 5-2 ▬). OSHA research has found that workplace infection of hepatitis B virus (HBV) dropped 95 percent since the hepatitis B vaccination became available in 1982. Hepatitis B, influenza, MMR (measles, mumps, rubella), varicella, Tdap (tetanus, diphtheria, pertussis), and meningococcal vaccines are recommended for all health care personnel prior to beginning work. Take a look at the CDC recommendations for immunization practices for health care personnel in Box 5-3 ▬.

Of course, all the prevention plans and equipment in the world cannot prevent all accidents from happening. Specific protocols must be in place and should be followed in those situations when a staff member experiences an exposure or possible exposure. Take a look at the needle-stick post-exposure protocol in Box 5-4 ▬.

Housekeeping staff members are important combatants in the effort to keeping employees and patients safe from pathogens. OSHA requires that only EPA-approved disinfectants, used in accordance with manufacturer's directions, be used to clean all work surfaces to prevent transference of contaminants. Warnings should be strictly followed to pick up broken glass using a brush and dustpan or tongs but never with one's hand, even a gloved hand. Easily contaminated equipment, such as IV poles and reusable containers (i.e., bins, pails, cans, etc.) must be cleaned with soap and water solution prior to the use of antimicrobial cleaners and then covered with plastic wrap or foil, when possible.

As with any type of facility, the floors must be cleaned. Warning signs should be used to cordon off wet floors to prevent falls and slips. Staff should be instructed to clean one side of a hallway or other pathway at a time, so personnel can still do their jobs while the floor is drying. Mats should be in place, as appropriate, and cleaned thoroughly, as the anti-slip treads can harbor dangerous pathogens.

Don't forget that these staff members must be protected, too. Housekeeping employees should be reminded that laundry can also carry pathogens and precautions should be taken to

---

*"Other sharps" within a health care environment may include anything that is sharp enough to penetrate the skin and establish an opportunity for pathogens to get into the bloodstream. These items include: broken glass, scalpels, and dental wires.

BOX 5-3   **Immunization of Health Care Personnel (HCP)**

Hepatitis B

- HCP and trainees in certain populations at high risk for chronic hepatitis B (e.g., those born in countries with high and intermediate endemicity) should be tested for HBsAg and anti-HBc/anti-HBs to determine infection status.

Influenza

- Emphasis that all HCP, not just those with direct patient care duties, should receive an annual influenza vaccination.
- Comprehensive programs to increase vaccine coverage among HCP are needed; influenza vaccination rates among HCP within facilities should be measured and reported regularly.

Measles, mumps, and rubella (MMR)

- History of disease is no longer considered adequate presumptive evidence of measles or mumps immunity for HCP; laboratory confirmation of disease was added as acceptable presumptive evidence of immunity. History of disease has never been considered adequate evidence of immunity for rubella.
- The footnotes have been changed regarding the recommendations for personnel born before 1957 in routine and outbreak contexts. Specifically, guidance is provided for 2 doses of MMR for measles and mumps protection and 1 dose of MMR for rubella protection.

Pertussis

- HCP, regardless of age, should receive a single dose of Tdap as soon as feasible if they have not previously received Tdap.
- The minimal interval was removed, and Tdap can now be administered regardless of interval since the last tetanus or diphtheria-containing vaccine.
- Hospitals and ambulatory-care facilities should provide Tdap for HCP and use approaches that maximize vaccination rates.

Varicella

Criteria for evidence of immunity to varicella were established. For HCP they include:

- written documentation with 2 doses of vaccine
- laboratory evidence of immunity or laboratory confirmation of disease
- diagnosis of history of varicella disease by health-care provider, or diagnosis of history of herpes zoster by health-care provider.

Meningococcal

- HCP with anatomic or functional asplenia or persistent complement component deficiencies should now receive a 2-dose series of meningococcal conjugate vaccine. HCP with HIV infection who are vaccinated should also receive a 2 dose series.
- Those HCP who remain in groups at high risk are recommended to be re-vaccinated every 5 years.

Abbreviations: HBsAg = Hepatitis B surface antigen; anti-HBc = hepatitis B core antibody; anti-HBs = hepatitis B surface antibody; Tdap = tetanus toxoid, reduced diphtheria toxoid and acellular pertussis vaccine; HIV = human immunodeficiency virus.

* Updated recommendations made since publication of the 1997 summary of recommendations (CDC Immunization of health-care workers: recommendations of the Advisory Committee)

Source: CDC: Morbidity and Mortality Weekly Report, Vol. 60 No. 7, November 25, 2011.

---

avoid transference. The handling of hazardous chemicals for cleaning and laundering should follow a written protocol to ensure workers are protected from exposure that may cause harm.

One of the most important things that you, as the administrator, can do is to ensure that the culture of the organization encourages compliance. Frequently, employee attitudes about compliance with policies and procedures relating to safety come from the top—the administration—of the organization. The federal government mandates that these policies and procedures exist. However, it is the administration's own attitudes about compliance with these rules that will make the difference. When you treat compliance as crucial, so will employees.

| BOX 5-4 | Needlestick Post-exposure Procedures |

The National Institute for Occupational Safety and Health (NIOSH) recommends that if an employee experiences a needlestick/sharps injury or is exposed to blood or other body fluid during the course of work that the following steps be taken immediately:

- Wash needlestick and cuts with soap and water.
- Flush splashes to the nose, mouth, or skin with water.
- Irrigate eyes with clean water, saline, or sterile irrigates.
- Report the incident to your supervisor.
- Seek medical treatment immediately.

Source: National Institute for Occupational Safety and Health (NIOSH).

FACILITY MAINTENANCE

The physical environment of your facility needs attention to ensure that it does what it is designed to do—protect your staff as well as your patients. The building that houses your facility—whether it is just a suite in a professional office complex or a large freestanding building—is often taken for granted. Think about it. Until something goes wrong, how frequently are you aware of a building's walls, ceiling, floor, electricity, water, and temperature control (heating and air conditioning)? Certainly, it is very noticeable when the water is not working or the power is out. In a retail store or regular office building, these problems are inconvenient. In a health care facility, these problems can be life-threatening.

As the administrator, you will need to oversee **facility maintenance**. In addition to ensuring that all systems and equipment are working properly, emergency backups, such as generators must be ready to kick in when needed. Sprinkler systems must be tested regularly to ensure that they will operate automatically should a fire erupt. Storage of oxygen tanks, nitrous oxide gas, and other types of gases must meet specific specifications, or there could be the risk of an explosion. **Heating ventilation air conditioning (HVAC)** systems work to ensure not only temperature control for comfort, but proper ventilation (air exchange) to avoid sick building syndrome. As per the Environmental Protection Agency (EPA), *"The term 'sick building syndrome' (SBS) is used to describe situations in which building occupants experience acute health and comfort effects that appear to be linked to time spent in a building."*

Ongoing maintenance plans must be implemented and equipment must be kept at optimal performance levels to ensure your staff and your patients are kept safe.

facility maintenance
the upkeep of building and equipment.

heating ventilation air conditioning (HVAC)
equipment responsible for control of internal environment.

CORPORATE WELLNESS

The success of the television show *"The Biggest Loser"* has had an unexpected and wonderful impact on offices and companies all across the United States. Offices of all sizes are having their own weight-loss competitions that include weekly meetings to discuss food choices and challenges. Co-workers are getting together to take walks during lunch hours (Figure 5-3 ■), taking the stairs instead of the elevator, and helping each other quit smoking. This is not about companies taking over the obligations for staff personal responsibilities. However, it is in the company's best interests, both financially and morally, to do whatever possible to ensure its workforce stays healthy—or gets healthier.

Morally, it is a good thing to encourage good eating habits without sacrificing good taste, fitting exercise into employees' already overloaded schedules, managing stress, helping employees quit smoking, and making other smart choices for better health. These are proven methods, based on scientific research, for creating a **workforce health promotion (WHP)**.

Financially, your organization will benefit in many ways. The most obvious may be that healthy workers come to work—reducing the number of sick days and increasing productivity. According to the U.S. Bureau of Labor Statistics, the average total compensated cost for sick pay, for all levels of workers, is 23 cents per work hour. Based on a 40-hour workweek,

workforce health promotion (WHP)
education and activity efforts to assist staff members in better health methodologies.

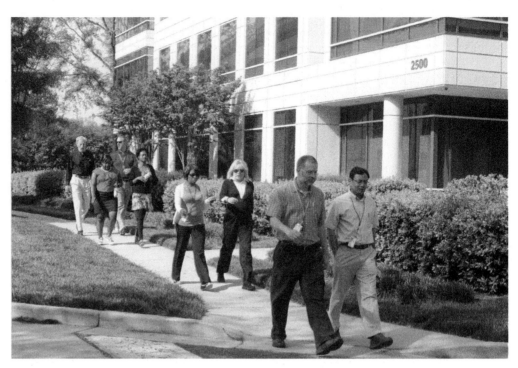

FIGURE 5-3 Co-workers walk together during lunchtime.

Photo credit: CDC/Debora Cartagena.

sick pay costs $478.40 per year for each staff member. When employees stay healthy, there is no cost for sick pay. There is no need to pay temporary workers or pay overtime to others to cover for someone who calls in sick. In addition, when employees are healthier, they suffer fewer chronic illnesses such as hypertension and diabetes or these conditions are more easily controlled to reduce potential manifestations. When these and other systemic conditions are controlled, health insurance premiums for coverage go down, saving additional monies from the corporate budget. All of these elements not only increase productivity, they increase the quality of the work being done.

The Centers for Disease Control and Prevention (CDC) has great, downloadable toolkits that provide step-by-step guidance for promotion of nutritious eating, physical activity, sponsoring preventive health screenings, and making healthy choices. Look at an example in Box 5-5 ■.

BOX 5-5 **Moving into Action: Promoting Heart-Healthy and Stroke-Free Communities**

What Is Moving into Action?
Moving into Action is a series of action items designed to help governors, state legislators, local officials, employers, and health care leaders promote heart-healthy and stroke-free communities. Each item suggests ways to encourage general interest and awareness of these health issues to specific policies that promote healthy behaviors and reduce risks associated with heart disease and stroke. Included are examples gathered from states and communities that are working to reduce these risks and a summary of the science underlying heart disease and stroke prevention.

Suggested actions are based on current national guidelines, scientific evidence, and existing efforts from states throughout the country. For example, some actions are supported by years of research from leading public health, public policy, and medical organizations, while others stem from efforts by communities and organizations to address unhealthy behaviors related to heart disease and stroke.

Moving into Action can help policy makers, employers, and health care leaders assess what actions are most appropriate for their communities and can lend support to the efforts of individuals to prevent, manage, and control their risks for heart disease and stroke.

Source: Centers for Disease Control and Prevention.

COST TO THE ORGANIZATION

Despite all the good reasons to keep workers safe and healthy, there are some organizations that cannot see past the upfront cost for following all the safety precautions prescribed. As an administrator, you should learn how to look beyond the upfront costs to the return on the investment. Even beyond the reward of healthy staff members, there is money—actual money—that will be realized.

Workers' Compensation Insurance

Although each state may have its own requirements, the U.S. Department of Labor's Office of Workers' Compensation Programs (OWCP) does provide guidance as well as specific benefits to employees of the federal government, and their dependents, who are found to be injured during the performance of their job or are diagnosed with an occupational-caused illness. However, virtually all workers' compensation programs provide the following when a work-related injury or illness has occurred:

- Wage replacement—the program will replace a portion of salary lost when an individual cannot work due to the injury or illness
- Payment for medical treatment of the injury or illness
- Vocational rehabilitation in cases when the lasting effects of the injury or illness results in an inability to return to original job classification

In many states, all employers are required to contribute money based on a percentage of total payroll into the state's workers' compensation pool of monies used to provide the aforementioned benefits. The percentage will increase based on the number of workers' compensation claims paid out to that organization's employees. Therefore, when companies do everything possible to provide a safe workplace, they will pay less into the fund—saving money. Some larger organizations will self-insure rather than participate in the state program. Again, the fewer claims paid, the less money the facility will have to pay.

Paid Time Off (PTO) Sick Leave

Earlier, it was pointed out that healthy employees do not call in sick, saving the money otherwise spent for the replacement worker or possible overtime pay for those who must work longer to make up for the missing staff member. This does not include any added danger to patients for fewer than needed staff members on duty or inexperienced fill-in help.

At this time, there are no legal requirements, on the federal level, for an employer to offer paid time off for sick leave. Under the provisions of the Family and Medical Leave Act (FMLA), some employees may be eligible for unpaid leave under certain medical circumstances. While this may appear to cost the company nothing because the employee is not collecting salary, you must remember that the work must still be done. And the individual that fills in must have the appropriate qualifications and skills. Remember, in a health care facility, you can't get just anyone to do any job.

OSHA Violations

In 2012, one company was charged with a total of $702,300 in proposed OSHA fines for 18 alleged violations of workplace safety standards while another faced proposed penalties of over $1 million, including 13 citations of failure to properly maintain equipment, each of which carried a $70,000 penalty. Box 5-6 ■ shows you the section of the law pertaining to OSHA penalties for failure to ensure a safe workplace for your staff. Not only do you have to deal with injured or ill workers, you have to deal with the financial impact, as well.

As the administrator, what could you do, what programs could you implement to ensure your facility does not fail an OSHA inspection? Yes, there are many regulations an organization must follow. Yes, it can seem difficult at times. However, you must look at the big picture. The company may save some money by not complying fully with the recommendations. However, as these examples show, the company will pay a great deal later. Of course, there is also the moral issue that surrounds the failure to comply with a regulation that results in the injury, illness, or death of a staff member.

BOX 5-6   **OSHA Penalties**

(a) Any employer who willfully or repeatedly violates the requirements of section 5 of this Act, any standard, rule, or order promulgated pursuant to section 6 of this Act, or regulations prescribed pursuant to this Act, may be assessed a civil penalty of not more than $70,000 for each violation, but not less than $5,000 for each willful violation.

(b) Any employer who has received a citation for a serious violation of the requirements of section 5 of this Act, of any standard, rule, or order promulgated pursuant to section 6 of this Act, or of any regulations prescribed pursuant to this Act, shall be assessed a civil penalty of up to $7,000 for each such violation.

(c) Any employer who has received a citation for a violation of the requirements of section 5 of this Act, of any standard, rule, or order promulgated pursuant to section 6 of this Act, or of regulations prescribed pursuant to this Act, and such violation is specifically determined not to be of a serious nature, may be assessed a civil penalty of up to $7,000 for each violation.

(d) Any employer who fails to correct a violation for which a citation has been issued under section 9(a) within the period permitted for its correction (which period shall not begin to run until the date of the final order of the Commission in the case of any review proceeding under section 10 initiated by the employer in good faith and not solely for delay or avoidance of penalties), may be assessed a civil penalty of not more than $7,000 for each day during which such failure or violation continues.

(e) Any employer who willfully violates any standard, rule, or order promulgated pursuant to section 6 of this Act, or of any regulations prescribed pursuant to this Act, and that violation caused death to any employee, shall, upon conviction, be punished by a fine of not more than $10,000 or by imprisonment for not more than six months, or by both; except that if the conviction is for a violation committed after a first conviction of such person, punishment shall be by a fine of not more than $20,000 or by imprisonment for not more than one year, or by both.

(f) Any person who gives advance notice of any inspection to be conducted under this Act, without authority from the Secretary or his designees, shall, upon conviction, be punished by a fine of not more than $1,000 or by imprisonment for not more than six months, or by both.

(g) Whoever knowingly makes any false statement, representation, or certification in any application, record, report, plan, or other document filed or required to be maintained pursuant to this Act shall, upon conviction, be punished by a fine of not more than $10,000, or by imprisonment for not more than six months, or by both.

(h)(1) Section 1114 of title 18, United States Code, is hereby amended by striking out "designated by the Secretary of Health and Human Services to conduct investigations, or inspections under the Federal Food, Drug, and Cosmetic Act" and inserting in lieu thereof "or of the Department of Labor assigned to perform investigative, inspection, or law enforcement functions."

(2) Notwithstanding the provisions of sections 1111 and 1114 of title 18, United States Code, whoever, in violation of the provisions of section 1114 of such title, kills a person while engaged in or on account of the performance of investigative, inspection, or law enforcement functions added to such section 1114 by paragraph (1) of this subsection, and who would otherwise be subject to the penalty provisions of such section 1111, shall be punished by imprisonment for any term of years or for life.

(i) Any employer who violates any of the posting requirements, as prescribed under the provisions of this Act, shall be assessed a civil penalty of up to $7,000 for each violation.

(j) The Commission shall have authority to assess all civil penalties provided in this section, giving due consideration to the appropriateness of the penalty with respect to the size of the business of the employer being charged, the gravity of the violation, the good faith of the employer, and the history of previous violations.

(k) For purposes of this section, a serious violation shall be deemed to exist in a place of employment if there is a substantial probability that death or serious physical harm could result from a condition which exists, or from one or more practices, means, methods, operations, or processes which have been adopted or are in use, in such place of employment unless the employer did not, and could not with the exercise of reasonable diligence, know of the presence of the violation.

(l) Civil penalties owed under this Act shall be paid to the Secretary for deposit into the Treasury of the United States and shall accrue to the United States and may be recovered in a civil action in the name of the United States brought in the United States district court for the district where the violation is alleged to have occurred or where the employer has its principal office.

Source: Occupational Safety and Health Administration.

Bad Reputation as an Unsafe Employer

The shortage of nurses and doctors in the United States continues, a fact that translates to a longer, more difficult search for the right candidate. If the facility gains the reputation for being an unsafe place to work, it will make this process even more challenging. Higher salaries and more extensive benefits will be required to encourage the best and brightest. Turnover, the term used to describe the frequency with which employees join and leave a company, will be high. High employee turnover costs even more money because the same position must be advertised, interviewed, provided with an orientation, and then, before the company can gain benefit from this staff member, the new staff member leaves, and the whole process must start all over again. In addition, an unstable staff results in inconsistent and lower quality of care for the patients.

WORKPLACE SAFETY PLAN

There are so many things you, as the administrator, must do to ensure the safety of your staff, and we have only reviewed some of the highlights here. It is important to create an organized and efficient written plan that will provide clear communication about all elements of concern and the details of compliance. Begin with the main sections of the plan:

- *Applicable Elements to Be Addressed*
  In this section, you create an outline of all applicable considerations. Begin by determining those elements mandated or recommended by federal or state law. Add anything tradition- ally covered in your organization along with credible ideas from the staff.
- *Current Status*
  Evaluate not only the presence of an item but all aspects involved. For example, the ele- ment listed in column one is: "gloves must be worn in the patient examination rooms."
  In addition to determining if every examination room has a stockpile of gloves, evaluate where the stockpile of gloves is located. Is it in a location that is easily and quickly acces- sible? Are all sizes available? Are nitrile gloves available for those with latex allergies? Determine and document whose responsibility it is to refill or replace empty boxes.
- *Assessment for Modifications*
  Identify those elements that are found not in compliance with state or federal law, autho- rizing agency, or accrediting organization. Include in this section, any reasonable sugges- tions from staff members. Sometimes company policies and procedures seem logical in the boardroom yet do not work well in day-to-day action. It is wise to get input from those who are, or will be, involved in compliance.
- *Plan*
  Create an action list to ensure that everything identified for modification in the previous section will get done. Identify the responsible department, and as specifically as possible, the individual responsible. Do not forget to specify the deadline for completion along with consequences for missing that deadline. This is very important because without a deadline, the hectic, day-to-day workday will never allow the individual responsible to find time to get anything extra done.
- *Confirmation*
  Once the deadline has arrived, an authorized individual—usually from the administrative team—should perform a final evaluation to ensure all modifications have been completed and meet standards.

In health care, documentation provides verification of the core of what we do—care for patients. In addition, documentation is critical to workplace safety. Remember the preliminaries of the OSHA investigation that you read about in Box 5-1, specifically the second and third bul- lets: *employer recognition* and *existence of feasible means of abatement*, respectively. Employer recognition refers to evidence that the employer recognized the potential risk factor. A rule or regulation suggesting that the organization do something to address a known risk factor is evi- dence that the risk factor was brought to the company's attention—so you knew about it. Is there any evidence that the organization recognized this by creating a policy or procedure to either avoid or at least minimize this risk? Means of abatement refers to evidence that the organization put into place specific elements to prevent or reduce the negative impact.

Let's look at an example:

Applicable Element to Be Addressed: All staff members need to get flu shots. Place and date documented.

Current Status: Only 91 percent of staff members have provided documentation of receiving a flu shot.

Assessment for Modification: Staff members who have not had shots state the reason is lack of accessibility. Due to schedule conflicts and other issues, they cannot get to the clinic to get the shots.

Plan: Assign Mabel Tucker, RN, to provide a mobile flu shot clinic. On two different days of the week, at different shift times, Ms. Tucker will travel from department to department, floor by floor, and provide flu shots for all those who have not yet had one. She will docu- ment each administration. This will be completed no later than April 1.

Confirmation: On April 3, Joseph Vales, office manager, reviewed all documentation submitted by Nurse Tucker. Flu vaccination rate is now 100 percent.

CHAPTER REVIEW

SUMMARY

Working in health care can be very rewarding; however, it can also be dangerous. It is an employer's responsibility to ensure that every staff member has a workplace safe from violence and illness. In addition, it is beneficial to encourage all employees to live healthier lives. It has been proven that employer-sponsored wellness programs reduce incidents, or severity, of obesity, diabetes, and hypertension, as well as other diseases and conditions. Creating a workplace safety plan supports the corporate objective of ensuring a safe and compliant workplace.

REVIEW QUESTIONS

MULTIPLE CHOICE

Choose the most accurate answer.

1. Protecting the health and well-being of staff members is a requirement of
   a. legal regulations.
   b. accrediting organizations.
   c. moral obligations.
   d. all of the above

2. _____ has identified health care as a "high-incidence industry" for workplace violence.
   a. AMA
   b. OSHA
   c. ECP
   d. HVAC

3. John was upset that he was not promoted to office manager because he really needed the extra money. One day he got drunk and went to Dr. Jones' office with a gun to show them how wrong they were to not promote him. He shot two co-workers and wounded three others. John would be categorized as a _____ workplace violence perpetrator.
   a. Type 1
   b. Type 2
   c. Type 3
   d. Type 4

4. Installation of _____ at corners or intersections will prevent staff members from walking into a blind spot.
   a. personal alarms
   b. password-protected locks
   c. shatterproof glass
   d. curved mirrors

5. Using _____ to all authorized personnel will prevent access to strangers.
   a. photo identification badges
   b. quiet rooms

   c. bright lighting
   d. mandatory training for staff

6. Exposure to bloodborne pathogens can be reduced with the implementation of an ECP. ECP stands for _____.
   a. Environmental Control Protocol
   b. Economically Classified Pathogens
   c. Exposure Control Plan
   d. Equipment and Catalyst Program

7. PPE includes all of the following EXCEPT
   a. gloves
   b. masks
   c. vaccinations
   d. gowns

8. A needlestick injury prevention plan should be included in every
   a. facility maintenance program.
   b. exposure control plan.
   c. workplace violence prevention program.
   d. workforce health promotion.

9. HVAC stands for
   a. heaters, ventilators, and catheters
   b. hepatitis, varicella administration controls
   c. housekeeping, vacuuming, abatement, and catalysts
   d. heating ventilation air conditioning

10. To be safe, any broken glass should be picked up with
    a. a gloved hand.
    b. a brush and dustpan.
    c. an ungloved hand.
    d. paper towels.

FILL-IN-THE-BLANK

Fill in the blank with the accurate answer.

11. The first step when creating a Workplace Violence Prevention Program is to perform a _____ of the physical property.

12. Bacteria and viruses contracted by exposure to infected blood are known as _____.

13. The acronym MMR when referring to recommended vaccinations refers to _____, _____, and _____.

14. OSHA requires that only _____approved disinfectants be used to clean all work surfaces.

15. Housekeeping employees should be reminded that _____can also carry pathogens.

16. Improper storage of oxygen tanks could risk _____.

17. When employees are healthier, premiums for health insurance go _____.

18. A man came into the clinic with a knife, looking to steal drugs. He cut one of the nurses who tried to stop him. The man is a _____workplace violence perpetrator.

19. Creating a workforce _____ is beneficial to individual wellness and therefore beneficial to the company as a whole.

TRUE/FALSE

Determine if each of the following statements is true or false.

20. Building maintenance evaluations should cover all property assets interior and exterior.

21. Employers do not really have a duty to care about their employees.

22. There is no reason why a workplace violence event could occur at a small physician's office.

23. Hepatitis B vaccine has successfully reduced the number of health care workers infected.

24. Mary was trying to administer a vaccination to a five-year-old boy who got upset, flung his arms, and hit Mary in the nose. This is a case of workplace violence.

25. Costs to the company increase when employees actively try to be healthier.

26. Electricity, water, and building maintenance are of no concern to health care provides who rent their space and have a landlord to handle maintenance

27. After an accidental needlestick, NIOSH recommends that the area be washed with soap and water.

28. Some furnishings, such as lamps or ashtrays, can be used as impromptu weapons.

29. Providing panic buttons for staff members will only worry them. It is a wasted cost.

30. Work schedules should be designed to have all staff members working alone because they are adults who can take care of themselves.

WHEN YOU ARE THE ADMINISTRATOR . . .

Critical Thinking and Analysis

Case Study #1

Workplace Injuries

Read the following excerpt. **What can you do, as the administrator, to reduce the potential for injury to this important group of staff members? Be specific.**

"Most of the nursing aides, orderlies, and attendants who were injured or became ill were women suffering sprains and strains to the back due to overexertion related to lifting or moving patients."

Source: Occupations with the Most Injuries and Illnesses with Days Away from Work, 2002; William J. Wiatrowski, Bureau of Labor Statistics.

Case Study #2

Workplace Violence

Read the following article. **Imagine that you have just been hired as the administrator for ResCare Ohio. One of your first responsibilities is to get the organization back on track to ensure the safety of all staff members as well as the patients. What are some of the actions you might take?**

U.S. Labor Department's OSHA fines ResCare Ohio for inadequate workplace violence safeguards at residential care facility in Fairfield, Ohio

An investigation was initiated March 26 under OSHA's Site-Specific Targeting Program and a national emphasis program targeting nursing home facilities with a days away, restricted, transfer, or

(Continued)

"DART," rate of 10 or higher per 100 full-time workers. Camelot Lake accumulated a total of 20 workplace violence cases from 2009–2012, resulting in 53 days away from work and 37 days of restricted duty. Employees have been exposed to physical assaults during routine interaction with residents who have a history of violent behavior.

A serious violation of OSHA's "general duty clause" involves failing to provide a workplace free from recognized hazards likely to cause serious injury or death. A serious violation occurs when there is substantial probability that death or serious physical harm could result from a hazard about which the employer knew or should have known.

OSHA established the National Emphasis Program for Nursing and Residential Care Facilities to provide guidance to agency compliance staff on policies and procedures for targeting and conducting inspections focused on the hazards associated with nursing and residential care. In 2010, according to the department's Bureau of Labor Statistics, nursing and residential care facilities experienced one of the highest rates of lost workdays due to injuries and illnesses of all major American industries.

ResCare Ohio employs more than 270 workers, including 50 at the Camelot Lake facility who provide daily care for up to 36 clients. ResCare is a human service company that provides residential, therapeutic, job training and educational support to people with developmental and other disabilities, seniors who need in-home assistance and youth with special needs. Based in Louisville, Ky., ResCare and its nearly 45,000 employees serve some 57,000 people daily in 42 states, Washington, D.C., Canada and Puerto Rico.

Source: Excerpted from: OSHA, U.S. Department of Labor.

Case Study #3

Preventing Needlestick Injuries

Using this case study as an example, prepare a presentation on steps employees can take to prevent needlestick injuries that will be shown to all new staff members at their orientation at your facility.

A hospitalized patient with AIDS became agitated and tried to remove the intravenous (IV) catheters in his arm. Several hospital staff members struggled to restrain the patient. During the struggle, an IV infusion line was pulled, exposing the connector needle that was inserted into the access port of the IV catheter. A nurse at the scene recovered the connector needle at the end of the IV line and was attempting to reinsert it when the patient kicked her arm, pushing the needle into the hand of a second nurse. The nurse who sustained the needlestick injury tested negative for HIV that day, but she tested HIV positive several months later.

Source: Centers for Disease Control and Prevention: NIOSH.

 ## INTERNET CONNECTIONS

National Institute for Occupational Safety and Health (NIOSH)—Workplace Safety and Health Topics

More than 18 million workers are at risk for illness and injuries because of long hours, changing shifts, lifting and repetitive tasks, violence, stress, and exposures to infectious diseases and hazardous chemicals. It is important that every employer—whether a nonprofit or for-profit organization—do everything possible to keep everyone safe. This website contains many ideas for creating a safe place to work or volunteer.

http://www.cdc.gov/niosh/topics/safety.html

Occupational Safety and Health Administration– Hospital eTool

This OSHA-created website provides detailed information about common hazards in health care facilities and follows each with recommended safe work practices to ensure employee safety and health.

http://www.osha.gov/SLTC/etools/hospital/index.html

Centers for Disease Control and Prevention

"Healthier Worksite Initiative"

You can find toolkits on this website that support the creation and implementation of corporate wellness programs. Corporate wellness can be accomplished in the smallest of health care facilities and yet provide huge benefits for everyone within.

http://www.cdc.gov/nccdphp/dnpao/hwi/toolkits/index.htm

HEALTH CARE TECHNOLOGY

LEARNING OBJECTIVES

Upon completion of this chapter, you should be able to:

- Define commonly used terms, abbreviations, and acronyms.
- Understand the use of administrative and clinical technology to enhance health care operations.
- Review the benefits and challenges of health information exchanges.
- Identify the importance for management of mobile device usage.
- Evaluate the ways to use telehealth, cloud computing, and radio frequency identification technology to benefit health care delivery.

WHEN YOU ARE THE ADMINISTRATOR . . .

When you are the administrator, you will be responsible for:

- Research, analysis of data, and determination of recommendations for the addition, expansion, or reduction of specialized services currently provided by the organization.
- Provision of leadership and promotion of effective and efficient integration of services in a worker-friendly environment.
- Analysis of data to identify trends of improvement and/ or areas of concern and maintenance of processes designed to follow up on areas of concern.

INTRODUCTION

Technology is everywhere, and it is here to stay. You are certainly aware of the benefits and challenges of computers and the computerization of virtually everything. Now, the administrative side of health care is taking a big leap forward with the nationwide implementation of **electronic health records (EHRs)**, mobile devices, and health information exchange networks. The clinical side of health care has been advanced with surgical robotics, mechanical prosthetics, and new methodologies for noninvasive procedures.

electronic health record (EHR)
software used to create and maintain patient charts; a computerized record of health care information and associated processes.

ADMINISTRATIVE HEALTH CARE TECHNOLOGY

The business aspect of health care has found many benefits by incorporating various types of technology to support their responsibilities of managing the provision of health care services.

Electronic Health Records (EHR)

Word processing software was the entry point for many into the world of technology. So, it is logical that electronic health records mark one of the biggest entryways for individuals working in health care to use computers.

electronic medical record (EMR)
software used by hospitals to create and maintain patient charts; a computerized record of medical information and associated processes.

You may have heard the term **electronic medical record (EMR)**. The difference between EHR and EMR is the difference between health and medicine, or more specifically health care and medical care—the way the industry uses these terms. Medical care is that which works to diagnose and treat diseases, injuries and other conditions, while health care is medical care plus preventive care. Most often, you will hear and see EMR in hospitals because an acute care facility will rarely become involved in providing preventive care, like vaccinations or annual physicals. Instead, EHR is more likely to be used in a physician's office, when one health care professional provides, and therefore documents, both preventive care and medical care to patients. An example of a screen from an EHR is shown in Figure 6-1 ■.

TECHNICAL ASPECTS   From the technical perspective, EHR and EMR are the same—a category of software programs used to computerize patient records. Both are electronic documentation of patient care. Different companies offer similar software packages with a variety of features that

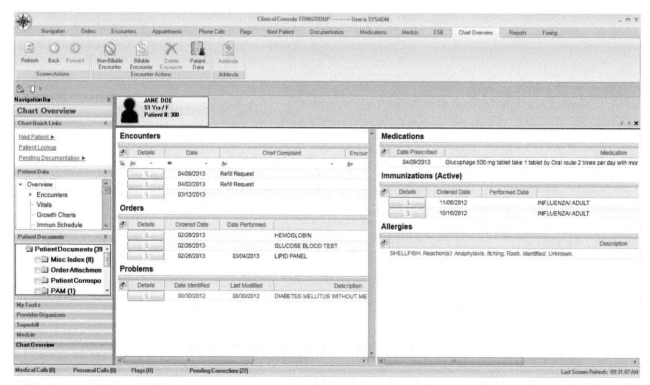

FIGURE 6-1   An example of one screen within an electronic health care record.
Source: Success EHS. Used with permission.

may or may not be of benefit to each specific facility. It is a challenge for any ongoing organization to switch from paper to electronics, especially when dealing with individual staff members' fear of change, adapting personal work habits from pen to keyboard, as well as the overall cost for equipment, software, setup, training, and lost productivity during the adaptation time line.

There is fear amongst many administrators about the adoption of EHR related to **interoperability**—the ability for the software to communicate and exchange data with other software programs. If the EHR cannot share data with the **practice management system (PMS)**—the software used to create, submit, and manage claims to third party payers—then the data must be entered separately, increasing the opportunity for error. One of the benefits about computerizing patient records is the ability to limit the potential for error. Every time data must be typed and entered, there is a new opportunity for a mistake to be made. When different software programs can share data, there is no need to reenter the same data again. This way, the data is entered once—correctly—and it will be correct a thousand times, for the next office visit as well as for the next claim.

Beyond just the internal use, it would be logical and beneficial to ensure that the EHR that is used at the physician's office would be able to communicate and exchange data with the EMR at the hospital where the physician performs surgery and other procedures. Only then would the patient's chart at the hospital and the patient's chart at the office match and enable seamless continuity of care. You, as the administrator, can ensure interoperability by confirming that the EHR software your facility purchases and implements has been certified by the Certification Commission for Health Information Technology (CCHIT), an independent, not-for-profit, volunteer organization set up to establish criteria standards for electronic health information technology. CCHIT stated in March 2013 that it would begin a testing program to establish certification of health information exchanges (HIEs) for their ability to provide *"plug and play"* connectivity with each other and with EHRs. The certification will be provided under a contract with the Interoperability Work Group (IWG) and the eHealth Exchange, the successor to the Nationwide Health Information Network Exchange (NwHIN).

CONFIDENTIALITY AND SECURITY   The Health Insurance Portability and Accountability Act (HIPAA) includes a section known as the *Security Rule* that governs the protection of patient's confidential health information. The rule incorporates three specific standards for security of electronic information:

- *Administrative safeguards* refer to the policies and procedures that must be developed and maintained by an organization's intent to protect electronic health information. These internal policies must include assessment of the security that is in place to protect the information, actions to correct any holes in that security's ability to keep the data secure, and training for all staff members as to how to ensure patient data is kept private from those who have no right to see it.
- *Physical safeguards* direct the facility to ensure that everything is done to protect electronic health information from intrusion, such as computer hackers, gossipy staff members, or dissatisfied patients and their families. Also included is the directive to shield the data from physical threats such as fire, flood, computer failure, electrical surges, and other disturbances to the proper function of the system, ensuring there would be no data loss or corruption. You, as the administrator, should ensure the facility has an organizational policy mandating that all computer files are backed up regularly (at least once every twenty-four hours) and that backup files are stored off-site, perhaps in another state or by use of cloud computing.
- *Technical safeguards* are those designed to control access to data so that only those who have a legal right can see it. This standard includes the mandate for password protection as well as firewalls, antivirus software, and confirming that all data transmissions are encrypted. The Health Information Technology for Economic and Clinical Health (HITECH) Act reinforces the requirement to use available technology to secure electronic health information by use of encryption.

BENEFITS OF EHR   The benefits of EHR far outweigh the obstacles. EHR has demonstrated improvement in the quality of patient care by enabling health care professionals access to not only more information but more *accurate* information, faster. This increases the opportunity for a more precise and quicker diagnosis and treatment plan. Fewer errors are made due to the elimination of misinterpretating poor handwriting. **Computer physician order entry (CPOE)**

interoperability
the ability for software to communicate and exchange data with other software programs.

practice management system (PMS)
the software used to create, submit, and manage claims to third party payers.

computer physician order entry (CPOE)
interactive electronic documentation of physician's orders and prescriptions electronically sent to pharmacies, imaging centers, and laboratories.

systems have been shown to save thousands of patient lives by preventing prescription mistakes made by pharmacists that could not read the prescription accurately. Patients benefit from a reduction in the time necessary for testing, both pathology testing (i.e., blood tests, urinalyses, cultures) and imaging (i.e., x-rays, MRIs, ultrasound), as well as lower costs because this system also reduces the need for repeated tests later on.

EHR enables multiple individuals to view and work in a patient's chart at the same time. Imagine that a patient chart is being viewed in the billing department for creating the claim form, while the nurse is speaking with the patient on the phone answering a question, and while the patient care coordinator is scheduling the patient for an MRI—all at the same time. This could not possibly happen with a paper chart.

EHR increases the probability for patient documentation to be complete because electronic reminders can be inserted to prevent the omission of required information. Having electronic alerts inserted in key locations in the electronic chart can prevent certain mistakes. For example, reminding the physician about a patient's allergy to penicillin or preventing a female patient from being scheduled for a prostate exam. Charts and graphs can be created with patient data, so a physician can more easily see that a patient's blood pressure has been increasing over the last year or that his or her weight has been staying steady. Features such as these, only available in electronic records and not paper records, support better health care, especially for those with chronic illness such as diabetes mellitus or hypertension.

When it comes to patient information, everyone must be vigilant to protect confidentiality and privacy. Password protection and firewalls are only a couple of the tools available to EHR, whereas there are few fortifications that can be taken to completely protect paper records, especially when one is left unattended on a desk.

INCENTIVE PROGRAMS FOR COMPLIANCE   HITECH, a portion of the American Recovery and Reinvestment Act (ARRA), supports the adoption of health information technology and the concept of meaningful use of such technology. Specifically, one section, known as *Subtitle D*, directly addresses methodology for keeping patient data secure and private during electronic transmission.

CMS created the *Medicare and Medicaid EHR Incentive Programs* to help with the financial aspects of computerizing health information management. An eligible professional (EP) can qualify for a financial incentive and receive as much as $44,000 through Medicare or $63,750 through Medicaid for achieving meaning use of EHR. Eligible hospitals can realize incentive payments totaling $2 million. Box 6-1 ■ shows a list of eligible professionals and hospitals who may earn an incentive payment.

The criteria for receiving the incentive payments include the need to show specific evidence that the EP is accessing their EHR system to share information with other providers and to connect

---

BOX 6-1   **Eligible Professionals**

Medicare EPs
- Doctors of medicine or osteopathy
- Doctors of dental surgery or dental medicine
- Doctors of podiatric medicine
- Doctors of optometry
- Chiropractors
- Medicare Advantage (MA) hospitals
- Critical access hospitals
- Subsection (d) hospitals that are paid under the Hospital IPPS

Medicaid EPs
- Physicians
- Nurse practitioners
- Certified nurse-midwives
- Dentists
- Physician Assistants (PAs) in PA-led federally qualified health centers (FQHC) or those in rural health clinics (RHC)
- Children's hospitals (no Medicaid volume required)
- Acute care hospitals (Including CAHs) with at least 10 percent Medicaid patient volume

Source: U.S. Government Health Information Technology Web Site.

more productively with patients. **Meaningful use** of certified EHR technology is measured by objectives that connect to health care outcomes classified into one of five patient-driven domains:

1. Improve Quality, Safety, Efficiency
2. Engage Patients and Families
3. Improve Care Coordination
4. Improve Public and Population Health
5. Ensure Privacy and Security for Personal Health Information

There are many health care providers who have successfully incorporated EHR into their practices and found they were able to truly improve their ability to care for their patients, despite the challenges of this adoption. Box 6-2 ■ has one of many case studies from the Health IT website.

In addition to the *Medicare and Medicaid EHR Incentive Programs* to provide funding to support an EP's transition to digital health information management, the Affordable Care Act (commonly termed *Obamacare*) includes more than $18 million in grants available to community health centers across the country. More than 600 health centers will be able to afford the benefits of EHR and other technology to support improved operational and clinical functions.

CHOOSING AN EHR VENDOR   With hundreds of different vendors offering hundreds of different EHR software programs, deciding which vendor to choose can be very intimidating. HealthIT. gov suggests these nine steps to use as a checklist to support your facility's decision in choosing an EHR vendor:

1. Site visits for EHR solution
2. Develop and distribute request for proposals (RFPs)
3. Review vendor proposals
4. Conduct vendor demonstrations
5. Review specialty specific functionality and general usability
6. Identify hardware and IT support requirements
7. Rank EHRs and compare functionality, usability, and pricing
8. Negotiate contract and licensing agreements
9. Purchase an EHR solution

The website also offers several templates to guide this complex decision, including an RFP template and the Vendor Meaningful Use Compare Tool, shown in Figure 6-2 ■.

meaningful use
a set of standards set by the HITECH Act and used by CMS to determine qualification for financial incentives connected to the adoption of EHR.

BOX 6-2	**Engaging Patients with Diabetes**

Meaningful use has helped to improve diabetes care at both practices [BSHC and Family Medicine Clinic of Danville]. At BSHC, the certified diabetes educator, Angie Conley, RN, BSN, CDE, CPT, uses the EHR system to identify patients who need assistance to better manage their condition. BSHC runs monthly reports of patients who have out-of-range hemoglobin A1c (HbA1c) values and targets them for diabetes education. The diabetes educator works with patients individually and conducts diabetes management classes. The classes are promoted to patients through the patient portal and to the broader community through the local media, the health department, Facebook, and posters and flyers at community locations.

Overall, relatively few patients currently use secure messaging, but the practices are finding it helpful for engaging patients in their diabetes care. Patients can easily communicate with the diabetes educator (at the Family Medicine Clinic of Danville) and providers between visits to let them know how they are doing—for example, to report glucose levels or symptoms, to ask questions, and to get help with self-management.

One patient explained the value of this communication: "It's provided a great deal of peace of mind for me, to know that my doctor knows what's happening with me."

Providers similarly find that using secure messaging between visits helps them to have a more complete understanding of how the patient is managing their diabetes and any issues that need to be addressed.

Both practices provide diabetes education materials to their patients, which are automatically generated based on a diabetes diagnosis entered into the EHR. At BSHC, the educational materials are routinely printed and given to patients at checkout together with the clinical summary, which explains action steps for diabetes care. One ongoing challenge is finding materials that are suitable for patients with limited education and lower literacy.

Source: Health IT.

National Learning Consortium
Advancing America's Health Care

HealthIT.gov

Vendor Meaningful Use Compare Tool

Instructions: Score each vendor on a scale from 1 (poor) to 5 (excellent) on each item. Total up your ratings for each vendor to help make your comparisons. Write the names of the vendors you are comparing in the watermark space provided in vendor columns. Use the blank rows at the end of the worksheet to ask your own questions.

Vendor	Vendor 1	Vendor 2	Vendor 3	etc.		
1 Demographics/Care Management						
1.1 The system has the capability to record demographics including: Preferred language, insurance type, gender, race, ethnicity, and date of birth.						
2 Patient History						
2.1 The system has the capability to import patient health history data from an existing system.						
2.2 The system presents a chronological, filterable, and comprehensive review of patient's EHR, which may be summarized and printed, subject to privacy and confidentiality requirements.						
3 Current Health Data, Encounters, Health Risk Appraisal, and Coordination of Care						
3.1 The system can exchange key clinical information among providers of care and patient authorized entities electronically.						
3.2 The system obtains test results via standard HL7 interface from: laboratory.						
3.2.1 The system obtains test results via standard HL7 interface from: radiology/imaging.						
3.2.2 The system obtains test results via standard HL7 interface from: other equipment such as Vitals, ECG, Holter, Glucometer.						
3.3 The system can record and chart changes in vital signs including: heights, weight, blood pressure, calculate and display BMI, plot and display growth charts for children 2–20 years including BMI.						
3.4 The system provides a flexible, user modifiable, search mechanism for retrieval of information captured during encounter documentation.						
3.5 The system provides a mechanism to capture, review, or amend history of current illness.						
3.6 The system enables the origination, documentation, and tracking of referrals between care providers or healthcare organizations, including clinical and administrative details of the referral.						
3.7 The system can track and provide a summary care record for each transition of care and referral visit.						
4 Encounter – Progress Notes						
4.1 The system records progress notes utilizing a combination of system default, provider-defined templates.						
4.2 The system includes a progress note template that is problem oriented and can, at the user's option be linked to either a diagnosis or problem number.						
5 Problem Lists						
5.1 The system creates and maintains patient-specific problem lists of current and active diagnoses based on ICD9/10 CM or SNOMED CT.						
5.2 For each problem, the systems has the capability to create, review, or amend information regarding a change on the status of a problem to include, but not be limited to, the date the change was first noticed or diagnosed.						
5.3 The system can record smoking status for patient 13 years or older.						
6 Care Plans						
6.1 The system provides administrative tools for organizations to build care plans, guidelines, and protocols for use during patient care planning and care.						
6.2 The system generates and automatically records in the care plan document, patient-specific instructions related to pre- and post-procedural and post-discharge requirements. The instructions must be simple to access.						
7 Prevention						
7.1 The system has the capability to display health prevention prompts on the summary display. The prompts must be dynamic and take into account sex, age, and chronic conditions.						
7.2 The system includes user-modifiable health maintenance templates.						
7.3 The system includes a patient tracking and reminder capability (patient follow-up) updatable by the user at the time an event is set or complied with.						
7.4 The system has the capability to send reminders to patients per patient preference for preventive/follow up care.						
8 Patient Access to Personal Health Information/Patient Education						
8.1 The system can provide patients with an electronic copy of their health information.						
8.2 The system can provide patients with timely electronic access to their health information.						
8.3 The system can provide clinical summaries to patients for each visit						
8.4 The system has the capability to create, review, update, or delete patient education materials. The materials must originate from a credible source and be maintained by the vendor as frequently as necessary.						
8.5 The system has the capability of providing printed patient education materials in culturally appropriate languages on demand or automatically at the end of the encounter. Please provide current list of available languages.						
9 Alerts/Reminders						
9.1 The system includes user customizable alert screens/messages, enabling capture of alert details.						
9.2 The system has the capability of forwarding the alert to a specific provider(s) or other authorized users via secure electronic mail or by other means of secure electronic communications.						

FIGURE 6-2   The Vendor Meaningful Use Compare Tool is focused on the evaluation of functionalities of Meaningful Use guidelines within the EHR using a rating scale from 1 (poor) to 5 (excellent).

Source: Health IT.

#	Item						
10	**Orders**						
10.1	The system includes an electronic Order Entry module that has the capability to be interfaced with a number of key systems depending on the health center's existing and future systems as well as external linkages, through a standard, real-time, HL7 two-way interface.						
10.2	The system displays order summaries on demand to allow the clinician to review/correct all orders prior to transmitting/printing the orders for processing by the receiving entity.						
11	**Results**						
11.1	The system has the capability to route, manage, and present current and historical test results to appropriate clinical personnel for review, with the ability to filter and compare results.						
11.2	Results can be easily viewed in a flow sheet as well as graph format.						
11.3	The system incorporates clinical lab-test results into EHR as structured data						
11.4	The system accepts results via two way standard interface from all standard interface compliant/capable entities or through direct data entry. Specifically – Laboratory, Radiology, and Pharmacy information systems.						
11.5	The system includes an intuitive, user customizable results entry screen linked to orders.						
11.6	The system has the capability to evaluate results and notify the provider.						
11.7	The system allows timely notification of lab results to appropriate staff as well as easy routing and tracking of results.						
11.8	The system flags lab results that are abnormal or that have not been received.						
12	**Medication**						
12.1	The system identifies drug interaction warnings (prescription, over the counter) at the point of medication ordering. Interactions include: drug-drug, drug-allergy, drug-formulary, drug-disease, and drug-pregnancy.						
12.2	The system alerts providers to potential administration errors for both adults and children, such as wrong patient, wrong drug, wrong dose, wrong route, and wrong time in support of medication administration or pharmacy dispense/supply management and workflow.						
12.3	The system supports multiple drug formularies and prescribing guidelines.						
12.4	The system provides the capability to generate and transmit permissible prescriptions electronically (eRx) pharmacy and other appropriate organization for dispensing.						
12.5	The system creates and maintains active medication list.						
12.6	The system is able to keep a history of Rx changes for a specific drug a patient is taking, and this is visible both to the clinician and to an auditor/QA person.						
12.7	The system maintains active medication allergy list.						
12.8	For maintenance drugs for chronic conditions the system can remind the provider about any prescriptions expiring or running out.						
12.9	The system has capability to perform medication reconciliation at relevant encounters and each transition of care.						
13	**Confidentiality and Security**						
13.1	The system provides privacy and security components that follow national standards such as HIPAA and PHI.						
13.2	The system provides privacy and security components that follow Nebraska state-specific laws and regulations.						
13.3	The system hardware recommendations meet national security guidelines.						
13.4	The system protects electronic health information created or maintained by the certified EHR technology through the implementation of appropriate technical capabilities.						
13.5	The system has hardware recommendations for disaster recovery and backup.						
14	**Clinical Decision Support/Quality Improvement**						
14.1	The system provides the capability to implement a minimal of 5 clinical decision support rules relevant to specialty or high clinical priority.						
14.2	The system has ability to generate lists of patients by specific condition to use for quality improvement, reduction of disparities and outreach.						
14.3	The system offers prompts to support the adherence to care plans, guidelines, and protocols at the point of information capture.						
14.4	The system triggers alerts to providers when individual documented data indicates that critical interventions may be required.						
15	**Reporting**						
15.1	Are standard clinical reports built into the system for the user to query aggregate patient population numbers?						
15.2	The system can generate lists of patients by specific conditions to use for quality improvement.						
15.3	The system has the capability to report ambulatory quality measures to CMS or the state.						
15.4	The system supports disease management registries by:						
15.4.1	Allowing patient tracking and follow-up based on user defined diagnoses.						
15.4.2	Providing a longitudinal view of the patient medical history.						
15.4.3	Providing intuitive access to patient treatments and outcomes.						
15.5	What reporting engine is utilized within the software?(ex. Crystal Reports, Excel, proprietary).						
15.5.1	If utilizing Crystal Reports do you provide a listing of all reportable data elements?						
15.6	Does the end user have the ability to create custom reports?						
15.7	Can reports be run on-demand during the course of the day?						
15.8	Can reports be set up to run automatically as well as routed to a specific person with in the office?						
16	**Cost Measuring/Quality Assurance**						
16.1	The system has built-in mechanism/access to other systems to capture cost information.						
16.2	The system supports real-time or retrospective trending, analysis, and reporting of clinical, operational, demographic, or other user-specified data including current and future UDS reports.						
16.3	The system allows customized reports or studies to be performed utilizing individual and group health data from the electronic record.						
16.4	The system will provide support for third-party report writing products.						

FIGURE 6-2 *(Continued)*

17	Chronic Disease Management / Population Health								
17.1	The system can submit immunization data electronically to immunization registries.								
17.2	The system can provide electronic syndromic surveillance data to public health agencies and actual transmission according to applicable law and practice.								
17.3	The system provides support for the management of populations of patients that share diagnoses, problems, demographic characteristics, etc.								
17.4	The system has a clinical rules engine and a means of alerting the practice if a patient is past due.								
17.5	The system generates follow-up letters to physicians, consultants, external sources, and patients based on a variety of parameters such as date, time since last event, etc. for the purpose of collecting health data and functional status for the purpose of updating the patient's record.								
17.6	At minimum, the system is able to generate a variety of reports based on performance measures identified by the Physician Consortium for Performance Improvement (AMA/Consortium), the Centers for Medicare & Medicaid Services (CMS), and the National Committee for Quality Assurance (NCQA) for chronic diseases. Information on these measures can be found at: http://www.amaassn.org/ama/pub/category/4837.html. The system follows measures approved by NQF (national quality form) and prompted by the AQA (ambulatory quality alliance) as well as those identified by the HRSA's Health Disparities Collaborative http://www.healthdisparities.net/.								
18	Consents, Authorizations, and Directives								
18.1	The system has the capability for a patient to sign consent electronically.								
18.2	The system has the capability to create, maintain, and verify patient treatment decisions in the form of consents and authorizations when required.								
18.3	The systems captures, maintains, and provides access to patient advance directives.								
19	Billing								
19.1	The system provides a bidirectional interface with practice management systems.								
19.2	The system can check insurance eligibility electronically from public and private payers. List clearinghouses with which this functionality exists.								
19.3	The system can submit claims electronically to public and private payers.								
20	Document Management								
20.1	The system includes an integrated scanning solution to manage old charts and incoming paper documents.								
20.2	Scanned documents are readily available within the patients chart.								
20.3	Scanned documents can be attached to intra office communication and tracked.								
20.4	The system has the ability to bulk scan and easily sort old patient charts for easy reference later.								
20.5	Images and wave files can also be saved and stored in the document management system.								
20.6	Insurance cards and drivers license can be scanned and stored in patient demographics.								
20.7	Scanned documents can be attached to visit notes.								
20.8	In a multiple location environment can each office scan in the same manner?								
	Total Score								

FIGURE 6-2　(Continued)

Health Information Exchange (HIE)

Earlier in this chapter, you learned about interoperability—the concept regarding software programs, such as EHR, and their ability to communicate and share data with other facilities' EHR and PMS programs. The federal government created the **Health Information Exchange (HIE)** to furnish both health care professionals and patients with protected access to the patient's electronic health information and the ability to share the information securely.

With HIE, patients no longer have to request copies of their records at one physician's office and hand carry or mail those records to another physician or the hospital. What happens when the patient cannot physically do this and the receiving health care professional must attempt to properly care for the patient without all of the applicable information? A lack of completeness of information, such as the absence of accurate patient history, recent test results, current medications and over-the-counter drugs being taken, can unnecessarily hamper a physician's ability to be efficient and effective for the patient. The industry has already seen proof that timely sharing of a patient's vital information at the time that care is provided will:

- Diminish the opportunity for medication errors, especially reducing drug interactions
- Contribute to more accurate diagnoses that result in more effective treatments
- Reduce the need for duplicate testing, lowering health care costs
- Help to avoid readmissions—patients being admitted into the hospital for the same reason for which the patient had been recently discharged (Figure 6-3 ■)

At this time, there are three types of HIEs for health care providers to use. All three of these exchanges have been tested and are currently available for use.

health information exchange (HIE)
a technical network enabling different providers to access patient information.

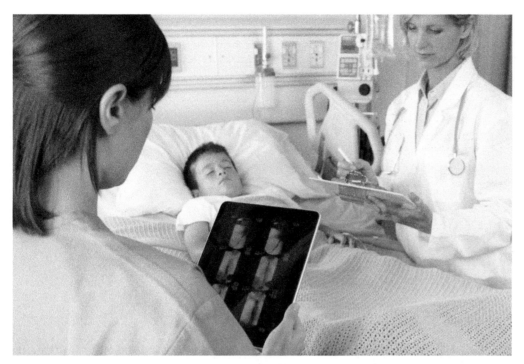

FIGURE 6-3 Timely sharing of patient information contributes to more effective treatments, therefore reducing readmissions.

Photo credit: Monkey Business Images/Shutterstock.

Directed Exchange: Used to share information between providers. These are especially beneficial for continuity of care between providers. For example, between a pharmacy and a physician's office regarding prescriptions, refills, or contraindications; or between a physician's office and a laboratory to ensure well-defined testing orders and rapid results. This type of exchange is also useful for reporting immunization data to the public health department or reporting quality measures to CMS in compliance with the Physicians Quality Reporting System.

Query-based Exchange: Used to share information for support care. This system enables a professional to search for specific data about a patient, most frequently used during unplanned medical encounters. For example, a trauma surgeon in an emergency department can use this to get answers to key elements regarding the patient's health, such as drug allergies or current diagnoses.

Consumer-Mediated Exchange: Used by patients to control dissemination of their health information. Patients can send their health information to other providers; track their own health data, such as weight, blood pressure, or cholesterol levels; identify and correct erroneous health information; fill in any missing information related to health, such as family history; and update billing information, such as a new health insurance policy.

The ability to share information instantaneously, using this technology, is an example of how computers have improved the delivery of care to patients. Streamlining, in a fashion, the processes of health care, such as patient histories, test results, allergies, current medications, and so on. The entire health care system functions on a foundation of information. The more accurate and complete the information provided, the more accurate and complete the diagnosis can be. In turn, the physician can make better decisions about treatment options, and this can all lead to more favorable outcomes.

Mobile Technology

Smartphones and tablets have put virtually the whole world of technology into the palm of our hands. Computers have been in the administrative offices of health care facilities for quite some time. Then, nurses' stations were connected. Now, the physician can be standing at the patient's bedside and access an incredible quantity of important information. Most mobile devices have

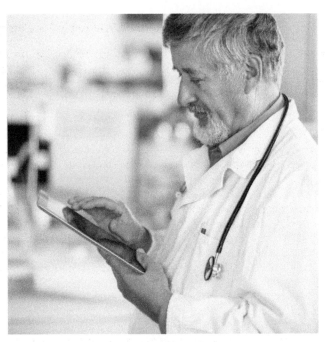

FIGURE 6-4   Mobile technology has put evidence-based medicine and other key research materials literally into the palm of the physician's hand.

Photo credit: lightpoet/Shutterstock.

the ability to connect with evidence-based medicine research, Physician's Desk Reference (PDR), and other key resource materials with just a touch of the finger (Figure 6-4 ■).

The benefits are numerous. Uncertain about a possible drug interaction, the physician just touches an **app**, and the information is literally at hand. Whether the data available is patient-specific or evidence-based medicine, more and more health care providers are saving time, saving money, and saving lives by engaging smartphone and tablet apps into their processes for providing care to patients.

As of January 2013, there were over 14,000 medical apps approved by the U.S. Food and Drug Administration (FDA) and more than 17,000 health and fitness apps on the market. In May 2012, the FDA approved *iBGStar Diabetes Manager*, an iPhone-enabled blood glucose meter so patients with diabetes can not only test their blood sugar, they can send the data to their physician electronically. According to the FDA, "*Development of mobile medical applications is opening new and innovative ways for technology to improve health and health care. …Health care professionals are using these applications to improve and facilitate patient care. These applications include a wide range of functions from allowing individuals to monitor their calorie intake for healthy weight maintenance, to allowing doctors to view a patient's X-rays on their mobile communications device.*" Box 6-3 ■ shows which mobile medical apps the FDA intends to regulate.

Cloud computing is already being used by a number of health care organizations. There are debates about the privacy and security issues that health care providers must be concerned about, however, the ability to reduce information technology operational costs is a strong motivator to adoption. Virtually all mobile apps are backed by a "cloud." You may be familiar with Google's Suite, including gmail, online document management, and more. This is an example of cloud computing.

Health care facilities of all sizes may benefit from the cloud-based technologies, such as cloud storage, backup, and data resiliency. The ability for document sharing can be very beneficial when multiple providers are caring for one patient. This, in turn, allows for consolidation of patient data, reducing clutter and enhancing communication between providers, resulting in better medical decision making. Storage in the cloud is abundant.

Can a patient's privacy be protected in the cloud? Some believe the data is safer in the cloud then it is on a hospital server. Many cloud providers have systems that comply with HIPAA's Security Rule as well as the Federal Information Security Management Act (FISMA). FISMA has over 400 audited controls for data security.

app

short for application, a mini software program used mostly on mobile devices.

| BOX 6-3 | **Mobile Medical Apps for Which FDA Will Apply Regulatory Oversight** |

Mobile apps may take a number of forms, but it is important to note that the FDA will apply its regulatory oversight to only the subset of mobile medical apps as expressed in this guidance.

Similarly, mobile medical apps that transform a mobile platform into a regulated medical device may do so by using attachments, display screens, sensors, or other such methods.

The following examples represent apps that the FDA considers to be mobile medical apps and therefore, will be subject to its regulatory oversight:

- Mobile apps that are an extension of one or more medical device(s) by connecting to such device(s) for purposes of controlling the device(s) or displaying, storing, analyzing, or transmitting patient-specific medical device data. Examples of displays of patient-specific medical device data include remote display of data from bedside monitors, display of previously stored EEG waveforms, and display of medical images directly from a Picture Archiving and Communication System (PACS) server, or similar display functions that meet the definition of an MDDS. Examples of mobile apps that control medical devices include apps that provide the ability to control inflation and deflation of a blood pressure cuff through a mobile platform and mobile apps that control the delivery of insulin on an insulin pump by transmitting control signals to the pump from the mobile platform.
- Mobile apps that transform the mobile platform into a medical device by using attachments, display screens, or sensors or by including functionalities similar to those of currently regulated medical devices. Examples include a mobile app that uses a mobile platform for medical device functions, such as attachment of a transducer to a mobile platform to function as a stethoscope, attachment of a blood glucose strip reader to a mobile platform to function as a glucose meter, or attachment of electrocardiograph (ECG) electrodes to a mobile platform to measure, store, and display ECG signals; or, a mobile app that uses the built-in accelerometer on a mobile platform to collect motion information for monitoring sleep apnea.
- Mobile apps that allow the user to input patient-specific information and—using formulae or processing algorithms—output a patient-specific result, diagnosis, or treatment recommendation to be used in clinical practice or to assist in making clinical decisions. Examples include mobile apps that provide a questionnaire for collecting patient-specific lab results and compute the prognosis of a particular condition or disease, perform calculations that result in an index or score, calculate dosage for a specific medication or radiation treatment, or provide recommendations that aid a clinician in making a diagnosis or selecting a specific treatment for a patient.

Source: Federal Drug Administration.

Another benefit of cloud computing can be its flexibility, especially evident in the inexpensive, speedy upgrades and improvements, provided with little-to-no downtime. Installation of new software programs, new features, and an IT staff with enough time to focus on responsibilities with far more value to the organization all make cloud computing a viable asset to any health care facility.

Bar Codes and RFID Systems

Consumers have been familiar with bar codes for years, as they track every item in the supermarket and other retail stores. Of course, health care facilities have been using them to track inventory of equipment, supplies, and pharmaceuticals. The technology has been expanded to the patient side. Nurses can use handheld scanners or an app on an iPhone or other mobile device using the built in camera to read the bar code on a patient's wrist band and then a medication bottle or IV bag to ensure the right patient is getting the right drug.

Radio frequency identification (RFID) technology can not only be used to track equipment but also the movements of doctors, nurses, patients, and others in real time. Alzheimer patients can be found instantly and continuously. Some of these systems can be designed to electronically link patient data using Wi-Fi (wireless technology) providing important patient information immediately at bedside or in the exam room. In addition, RFID tags attached to staff ID badges can ensure that only authorized personnel are permitted to enter secured locations. Restricting access to specific areas can be important for locations such as the neonate nursery, pediatrics, the infectious disease ward, or the emergency department. Furthermore, as RFID tags

radio frequency identification (RFID)

a wireless technology used to track specific items, such as medications, patient charts, and patient identification.

can track locations, if there is ever a question of missing drugs, for example, the facility's system would be able to identify exactly which staff member was in that cabinet.

There are many real life examples of how this technology can help to save lives. One such case involved actor Dennis Quaid's newborn twins. Admitted to the hospital with a staph infection, the nurse grabbed the wrong strength of medication bottle and administered 10,000 units of Heparin (a blood thinner) instead of the 10 units that were prescribed by the attending physician. Blame was abundant and included reproaching the pharmaceutical manufacturer of the medication for making the 0.01 bottle and the 1.0 bottle appear too similar: one light blue, the other medium blue. Nurses in a rush—humans in a rush—look quickly, and this is not always very accurate. Imagine if the hospital had been using either bar code scanners or RFID to track the drugs and patients. The computer's alert signal could have easily prevented this mistake. Fortunately, the Quaid twins were not harmed permanently from this medication error; however, there are thousands of patients who were not as lucky.

CLINICAL HEALTH CARE TECHNOLOGY

On the clinical side, technology has enabled physicians and other health care professionals to more accurately diagnose patients, with less invasive methodologies, treat patients with more specific techniques and improved outcomes. The Office for the Advancement of Telehealth (OAT), a part of the Health Resources and Services Administration (HRSA) of the federal government, was created for the specific purpose of promoting the use of telehealth for the improvement of patient and physician education, health information services, as well as the delivery of health care services.

Telehealth

telehealth
any remote telecommunication between health care providers and patients or other providers for the purposes of managing the patient's health care.

Telehealth is the term used to identify the use of telecommunications for managing patient health. This may be a teleconference between physician and patient, a physician offsite remotely connecting with the patient's EHR, a radiologist in Australia providing interpretation and report on an MRI taken in Parma, Ohio, or a blood pressure cuff automatically reading a patient's blood pressure at his or her home and transmitting the data directly to the physician's EHR system.

Remote monitoring devices can extend important monitoring and continuous patient care, especially with populations such as aging seniors who insist on living in their own home rather than with a relative or an organized facility such as an assisted living facility. A patient's vital signs (i.e., respiration, oxygenation, blood pressure, and heart rate) can be measured and transmitted to the physician's office as frequently as necessary, depending upon the patient's health. Earlier in this chapter, you learned about the FDA approved *iBGStar Diabetes Manager*, an iPhone-enabled blood glucose meter so patients with diabetes can not only test their blood sugar, they can send the data to their physician electronically. In these situations, the nurse or physician can review the data and contact the patient if necessary. If the patient's data is within normal limits (WNL), then the patient is being monitored without the cost and inconvenience of an office visit. Now, despite the physician and nursing shortage, that appointment time can be given to another patient who actually needs the face-to-face time.

Remote Presence (RP) Robots

remote presence (RP)
the use of telecommunication devices, such as robots, enabling a physician to meet with and evaluate a patient without being physically at the location.

In November 2012, the FDA announced its first approval of an autonomous-navigation **remote presence (RP)** robot to be used in health care delivery at acute care hospitals. The robot was approved for use in cardiovascular, neurological, prenatal, psychological, and critical care procedures, preoperatively, during surgery, and postoperatively.

The robot, like any other telemedical device, combines navigational technologies with mobility and wireless communications to enable a physician to care for a patient by way of real-time audio and video. A video monitor at the top of the robot provides a human face—of the physician—for a gentler interaction with patients, as well as family members, nurses, and other health care providers and caregivers. Attachments to the unit enable the nurse to provide vital signs data in addition to other test results.

RP robots expand a physician's ability to care for patients without having to be physically present. One hospital in Florida, with three locations, uses RP robots in two of them. With these units, one trauma surgeon can oversee patients at all three facilities at one time. When his presence is required at one specific location, he can then travel to that one location, all the while

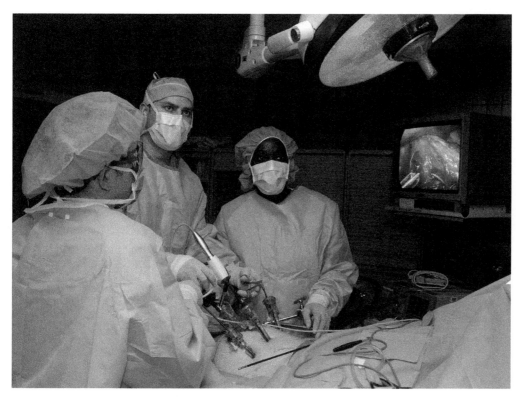

FIGURE 6-5 Laparosopic stomach surgery.
Photo credit: DoD/Staff Sgt. Samuel Bendet.

during this travel, keeping in constant communications with the patient, the nurses, and other support personnel. Costs are reduced, and the patient actually receives better care.

Robotic and Laparoscopic Surgery

Generally, robots and other technological based surgical methodologies such as laparoscopy, are known as **minimal access surgery (MAS)**, also known as minimally invasive surgery (MIS) (Figure 6-5 ■). The *da Vinci Robotic System* has proven to reduce hospital costs for procedures as much as 30 percent because MAS is less invasive, meaning a smaller incision than traditional methods. A smaller incision means less pain for the patient, faster healing, and a smaller scar. All of these factors have contributed into shorter hospital stays, and often, no hospital stay at all. Quite a number of procedures previously approved for inpatient operating room status have been approved for outpatient surgical status further reducing costs and upheaval to the patient and his or her family.

minimal access surgery (MAS) the ability to visualize and treat internal aspects of the patient without the need for a large incision.

The benefits of these procedures are largely on the patient side. These systems are quite expensive, some as much as $1 million for each device. Surgeons require additional training on the system and this takes time, during which that surgeon is not caring for other patients, reducing productivity. The equipment takes up more space in the operating room, making it difficult for assistants and other support personnel to do their jobs.

All elements considered, these highly technical surgical techniques have become more widespread and have found acceptance as the standard of care very quickly with health care professionals and third-party payers alike.

Mechanical Prosthetics

A prosthetic is a device that is designed to take the place, visually as well as functionally, of a human anatomical site, for example an artificial arm or leg. Twenty-first century technology has again come up with tremendous advancements from the wooden legs of decades ago.

There are several types of technologically enhanced prosthetics:

- *Body-powered prosthetics* are strapped to the patient using cables and harnesses. They are designed to enable the patient to mechanically maneuver the artificial limb using their own, existing muscle, shoulder, and arm movements.

- *Externally powered artificial limbs* use battery-packs and an electronic system to control movement of the limb.
- *Myoelectric prosthetics* also use a battery and electronic motors to function; however, myoelectric artificial limbs use suction technology to attach to the stump. Enclosed electronic sensors are programed to detect microscopic muscle, nerve, and EMG activity. The sensors then translate that muscle activity and use it to control the artificial limb's movements. The end result is that the artificial limb moves more like a natural limb, as directed by the mental stimulus of the patient.
- *Mind-controlled prosthetics* are being created by the Defense Advanced Research Projects Agency (DARPA) within the U.S. Pentagon. One example is the DEKA arm. During surgery, the axilla (armpit) nerves are rerouted into the thoracic cavity, changing the location of the "move" command from the patient's brain to the sensors placed into the chest. The sensors then transmit the command to the bionic arm. The patient thinks of the action he or she wants the limb to take. The nerves in the chest are stimulated and transmit the message to the robotic arm or leg, and the action is done. This process is known as targeted muscle reinnervation (TMR). As of December 2012, 35 individuals in the world are using TMR limbs.
- *Modular Prosthetic Limb* is the next level of innovation being worked on currently by the Pentagon using reliable central-nervous-system interfaces (RCI). In these patients, microchips are implanted into the patient's brain so the directions to the artificial limb will mimic real flesh-and-blood arms and legs.

Advances over the years have also been made in the actual materials used to create prosthetics. Moving away from the original wood, carbon fiber has been discovered to provide more comfort with a more lifelike feel externally. Thermoplastics are now used for a more comfortable fit at the socket—the connection point between the prosthesis and the stump. Using titanium has also lengthened both durability and usability. Figure 6-6 ■ shows a U.S. Army soldier using one of these updated prosthetic legs.

The addition of Bluetooth technology is being used to enable a double-amputee's two prosthetic legs to communicate with each other to coordinate the patient's stride, pressure of walk, and speed. Microprocessor knees, through the use of onboard computer technology, enable greater stability when walking and stopping, as well as when walking on inclines, as the

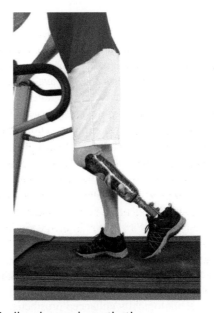

FIGURE 6-6 Technologically advanced prosthetics.
Photo credit: Belushi/Shutterstock.

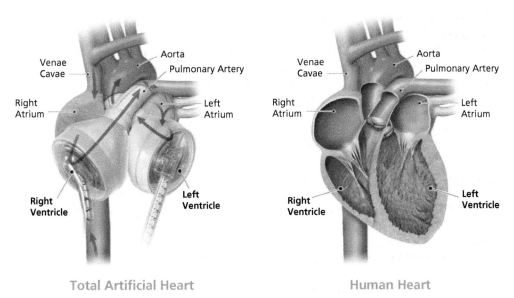

FIGURE 6-7   Comparison of a total artificial heart and a natural heart.
Source: From Wikipedia.

computer evaluates the pressure of the patient's steps and then transfers this data to the prosthetic limb and knee.

Technologically powered artificial limbs are not the only prosthetics being used to help patients. A total artificial heart (TAH) can be used to extend the life of a patient in end-stage heart failure as he or she waits for an available organ for transplant. The TAH attaches to the atria (the upper chambers of the heart), replacing ineffective ventricles (the lower chambers of the heart) to enable complete function of a heart that otherwise could no longer effectively process and pump blood through the cardiovascular system. Figure 6-7 ■ compares a TAH with the natural organ.

Wearable Technology

Technology merged with the textile industry to develop fabrics known as "smart textiles" for the creation of apparel that supports good health in a very new way. Currently, there is a T-shirt that contains ribs in the sleeves which are actually electrodes programmed to measure heart rate, respiration, and skin temperature. Other garments can be made to provide data that would normally be provided by electrocardiography (EKG), electroencephalography (EEG), or electromyography (EMG).

Companies are currently working on wearable sensors that will collect specific information, including the patient's respiration rate and number of hours slept. This information is then transmitted electronically to designated smartphones—the patient's phone, a caregiver's phone, or the physician's phone. Built-in Bluetooth technology records the specific data, such as blood glucose level or blood pressure readings, from the patient's body and sends it to the patient's home base station. The base station is programmed to forward the data to the physician using a secured wireless connection. Many of these devices have an alert system that can be triggered by a predefined threshold so the physician or nurse can react immediately in a case of data that is found to be outside of preset limits. Another company, recently approved by the FDA, has developed a remote monitoring system used to observe patients diagnosed with a cardiac arrhythmia as they go about their daily activities. Mobile phone technology is used in this system, also, to transmit the data to the physician for evaluation.

CHAPTER REVIEW

SUMMARY

Technology is integrally involved in the care of many patients. Electronic health records provide important information about patients to their health care providers, wherever they may be: in a hospital nurses' station, in a physician's office, or at a patient's bedside. Software programs, such as CPOE and PMS, eliminate the potential confusion over poor handwriting and have already saved thousands of patients' lives. Health information exchanges (HIEs) have been created to permit health care professionals to share information about a patient, thereby improving diagnostic and treatment plans that result in better patient outcomes. All this information can be available in the palm of a physician's hand—using a smartphone, an iPad, or other tablet.

Technological advancements help physicians have a remote presence enabling them to care for patients when they are not physically in the same place, and new technological advancements affect the way surgery is performed so patients suffer fewer incisions, little to no hospital stays, less pain, and faster healing. Amputees are finding the new, technologically enhanced prosthetics can replace a missing limb with incredible function and stability. An artificial heart uses technology to keep a patient alive long enough to get a transplant. And a physician can gather data about a patient from the T-shirt being worn to support more accurate diagnostics.

REVIEW QUESTIONS

MULTIPLE CHOICE

Choose the most accurate answer.

1. Interoperability refers to the ability of software to
    a. create a claim form.
    b. diagnose a patient.
    c. perform surgery on a patient.
    d. exchange data with other software programs.

2. HIPAA includes all of the following standards in the Security Rule EXCEPT
    a. administrative safeguards.
    b. security safeguards.
    c. physical safeguards.
    d. technical safeguards.

3. With regard to the Medicare and Medicaid EHR Incentive Program, EP stands for
    a. eligible professional.
    b. effective program.
    c. electronic programs.
    d. elite physicians.

4. Which type of health information exchange would an emergency department physician use to determine if the unconscious patient has any allergies to medication?
    a. Consumer-mediated exchange
    b. Directed exchange
    c. Query-based exchange
    d. None of these

5. Which type of health information exchange would Natalie use if she wants to electronically send her patient information from Dr. Smith's office to Dr. Jansen's office?
    a. Consumer-mediated exchange
    b. Directed exchange
    c. Query-based exchange
    d. None of these

6. Which of the following is an example of telehealth?
    a. A patient phoning a doctor's office for an appointment
    b. A radiologist in California reading an x-ray taken of a patient in Florida
    c. A hospital with free Wi-Fi for patients and visitors
    d. A digital thermometer

7. One downside of implementing a surgical robotic system is
    a. less pain for the patient.
    b. shorter hospital stay for the patient.
    c. the high cost of the equipment.
    d. faster healing time.

8. The use of titanium has lengthened both usability and _____ of prosthetic limbs.
    a. mobility
    b. durability
    c. comfort
    d. lifelike feel

9. Microprocessor knees, using _____ computer technology enables greater stability walking with a prosthetic leg.
   a. Wi-Fi
   b. EHR
   c. onboard
   d. EMR

10. Which type of health information exchange would Dr. Peele use to send a prescription to the pharmacy for a patient?
    a. Consumer-mediated exchange
    b. Directed exchange
    c. Query-based exchange
    d. None of the above

FILL-IN-THE-BLANK

Fill in the blank with the accurate answer.

11. _____ direct the facility to ensure that everything is done to protect electronic health information from intrusion.

12. A software program used to create, submit, and manage claims to third-party payers is called a _____.

13. A set of standards determined by the HITECH Act and used by CMS to determine qualification for financial incentives connected to the adoption of EHR is known as _____.

14. A physician would use a health information exchange, known as a _____, to order specific imaging tests for a patient.

15. An Alzheimer's patient who wandered away from his or her room could be found very quickly using _____.

16. _____, also referred to as MAS, uses smaller incisions, which means less pain and faster healing for the patient.

17. CPOE stands for _____.

18. Technology and the textile industry have developed fabrics known as _____.

19. Nurses can use handheld scanners or an app to read the _____ on a patient's identification band.

20. Use of a _____ robot can enable a physician to treat a patient miles away.

TRUE/FALSE

Determine if each of the following statements is true or false.

21. Electronic health records and electronic medical records catalog the exact same information about a patient.

22. Administrative safeguards refer to elements that control access to data.

23. RFID is wireless technology used to track specific items within a facility.

24. The health care industry has already seen proof that timely sharing of a patient's vital information at the time that care is provided will diminish medication errors.

25. Many physicians can now use their smartphones to access evidenced-based medicine data.

26. Bar codes cannot help ensure the right patient gets the right medication.

27. A prosthetic is a device that supports a weakened or broken limb, such as a cast or brace.

28. The FDA is planning to apply regulatory oversight to mobile medical apps.

29. RFID technology can be used to track doctors, nurses, and patients in real time.

30. The ability to share information instantaneously has not improved the delivery of health care to patients at all.

WHEN YOU ARE THE ADMINISTRATOR . . .

Critical Thinking and Analysis

Case Study #1

Benefits of Electronic Health Records in a Rural Critical Access Hospital

Sierra Vista Hospital is a 25-bed critical access hospital located in the rural city of Truth or Consequences, New Mexico. Sierra Vista Hospital serves approximately 13,000 area residents and provides primary care, outpatient behavioral health care, and community education programs. They need to begin implementation of electronic health records (EHRs).

When the subject of implementation of an EHR system was first broached, the hospital's physicians and staff were skeptical. Many were not comfortable integrating computers into clinical practice and did not recognize how EHR implementation could help improve efficiencies and health care quality.

Imagine that you are the administrator of Sierra Vista Hospital. How will you help the hospital's physicians and staff overcome their skepticism and get on board with the adoption of EHR? What specific benefits can you share with them? What specific objections might they express? How will you overcome their objections and convince them to agree?

Read the complete case study: http://www.healthit.gov/providers-professionals/sierra-vista-hospital

Case Study #2

The Challenges of Interoperability

It is necessary to safely and securely exchange protected health information (PHI) among providers and organizations because this is critical to delivering coordinated, accountable, and patient-centered care, promoting better health and better care at lower costs. The reality is, however, that patient records are often housed in disconnected and dissimilar electronic systems in varied settings across a community: offices of primary care and specialist physicians, clinics, hospitals, long-term care facilities, and home health agencies.

Imagine that you are the administrator of the county health care cooperative. The patient population is small with an average age of forty-five. This means that many patients are older and are being treated by more than one physician group in the area, meaning that your local health care providers have overlapping patient lists (i.e., the cardiology group, women's health center, orthopedic group, physical therapy group, and the hospital all are treating many of the same patients).

What will you do to overcome these challenges of interoperability? What specific actions can you take so a majority of the health care providers in your community can gain the benefits of sharing patient information?

Read the complete case study of the Beacon Community-EHR Vendor Affinity Group on the HealthIT website: http://www.healthit.gov/providers-professionals/vendors-and-communities-working-together-catalyst-interoperability-and-excha

Case Study #3

Florida Physician Uses EHR for Practice Improvement Effort

Dr. Linda Groene is a solo practitioner in Fort Lauderdale, Florida. She practices internal medicine and geriatrics and serves a patient population of about 340. In addition, her practice oversees and manages a certified patient-centered medical home. This designation emphasizes the importance that Dr. Groene's practice has placed on facilitating partnerships and communication between practice and patients/caregivers.

Imagine that you are the administrator of Dr. Groene's practice. How could you use EHR to generate details and statistics on quality measures? What specifically would you recommend to improve communication between your practice and the patients and caregivers of your patients? Think also of adult children of elderly patients who may be out of the area but have important information to share and have a need to get health information about their parents.

Read the complete case study on the HealthIT website: http://www.healthit.gov/providers-professionals/florida-physician-uses-ehr-practice-improvement-effort

---

 # INTERNET CONNECTIONS

Health Information Exchange

This website explains what health information exchanges are, why they are important, and includes several examples of their benefits.
http://www.healthit.gov/providers-professionals/health-information-exchange

Myoelectric Prostheses

This webpage includes an extensive explanation of myoelectric prosthetics along with additional resources for further exploration.
http://www.myoelectricprosthetics.com/

Remote Presence Robots

This is the website for the company that manufacturers the iRobot, one of the first FDA-cleared remote presence device. Read about all of the variations of remote presence devices available to hospitals and physicians.
http://www.intouchhealth.com/products-and-services/products/

CHAPTER 7

INSTITUTIONAL FOOD SERVICES

LEARNING OBJECTIVES

Upon completion of this chapter, you should be able to:

- Define commonly used terms, abbreviations, and acronyms.
- Describe how food operations are handled in the health care industry.
- Discuss the importance of food safety.
- Identify ways to prevent foodborne illness.
- Review policies and procedures related to food hazards.
- Promote healthy eating.
- Consider the impact of incorporating medical nutrition therapy into patient care services.
- Recognize the opportunity for food service to become a revenue-producing department.

KEY TERMS

foodborne hazard
foodborne illness
food preparation area
food safety
microorganism
outsourcing
pathogen
self-operation

WHEN YOU ARE THE ADMINISTRATOR . . .

As the administrator, in order to ensure healthy and safe food and nutrition to patients, employees, and visitors, you must take into account your responsibility to:

- Assess and identify specific services, facilities, equipment, and personnel needed to address the current and future health care needs of the community and the funding required to provide such services.
- Supervise the activities of all departments.
- Perform risk assessments prior to enactment of any improvement plans and/or expansion plans.
- Analyze data to identify trends of improvement or areas of concern and maintenance of processes designed to follow up on areas of concern.

INTRODUCTION

When patients stay at your facility overnight, you will need to feed them. Therefore, if you choose to go to work at an acute care hospital, short-term care or long-term care facility, skilled nursing facility, assisted living facility, or any other inpatient health care facility, you will have to deal with food services. As the administrator, you will need to be aware of what is going on in the kitchen. Hospital food has come a long way from the green gelatin of long ago.

Those individuals who are sick, those who have weakened immune systems, and those who are recovering from an illness together represent one of the most susceptible segments of the population to **foodborne illness**. These individuals are likely to suffer more severe consequences from that illness than the rest of the general population. This is, essentially, your entire patient population. Your facility has an obligation to ensure that patients are well-nourished—a critical factor in healing and recovery. Whether food and nutritional services function as one of your departments or are outsourced, you, as the administrator, need to know enough about this area to effectively oversee these activities and keep your patients safe.

IN-HOUSE OR OUTSOURCE

Food service operations in the health care industry are handled in one of two ways: in-house, also known as **self-operation**, or outsourced, which means contracting with another company to provide all necessary services:

- *Self-operation*: A health care facility, such as a hospital or nursing home, has all food service activities related to the procurement, preparation, and delivery of food items managed and performed by employees of the facility.
- *Outsourcing*: The health care facility contracts with a company that specializes in supplying all food service activities, including managing as well as all required activities related to the provision of edibles for patients, employees, and visitors. In many cases, the outside company will occupy physical space on the premises (Figure 7-1 ■). In these situations, you, as the administrator, will need to oversee the actions of these organizations because, ultimately, the facility will retain a certain liability for any harm that results from these services.

foodborne illness
any illness or disease caused by ingesting contaminated food or drink.

self-operation
procurement, preparation, and delivery of food items managed and performed by employees of the facility.

outsourcing
contracting with another company to provide food services for the facility.

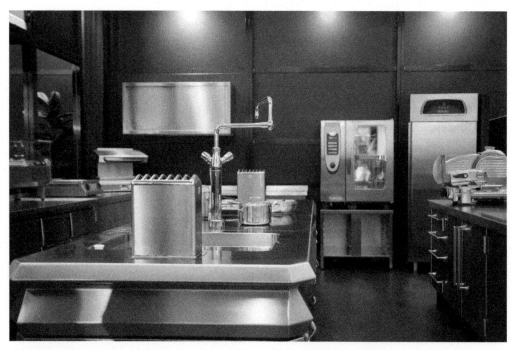

FIGURE 7-1 An industrial kitchen equipped to feed patients, visitors, and employees.
Photo credit: ariadne de raadt/Shutterstock.

FOOD SAFETY

The concept of **food safety** concerns the responsibility and obligation to ensure that all edible substances cannot cause harm. When patients are admitted into your facility, they put their health into your hands. Just as the facility will provide what is needed on the clinical side, you must be just as meticulous providing nourishment.

Legal Requirements

The Food and Drug Administration (FDA), in conjunction with the Centers for Disease Control and Prevention (CDC), publish the "Food Code." The FDA describes this document as "*a model code and reference document for state, city, county and tribal agencies that regulate restaurants, retail food stores, vending operations and foodservice operations in institutions such as schools, hospitals, nursing homes and child care centers.*" State and local governments are permitted to adopt this guidance in whole or in part. It is your facility's responsibility to identify the regulations that govern and ensure all policies and procedures are in compliance. The industry expectation is that you will take reasonable care to document and implement all necessary precautions to avoid violating any of these rules.

All those involved with preparing, serving, and storing food have a legal obligation to ensure that food will not cause illness or harm. The "person in charge" of food service is the individual recognized by law to be responsible for food safety compliance (Box 7-1 ■). Many states require one certified food safety manager to be on the premises at all times while the department is open

---

BOX 7-1	**Responsibilities of the Person in Charge**

The PERSON IN CHARGE shall ensure that:

(A) FOOD ESTABLISHMENT operations are not conducted in a private home or in a room used as living or sleeping quarters as specified under § 6-202.111;

(B) PERSONS unnecessary to the FOOD ESTABLISHMENT operation are not allowed in the FOOD preparation, FOOD storage, or WAREWASHING areas, except that brief visits and tours may be authorized by the PERSON IN CHARGE if steps are taken to ensure that exposed FOOD; clean EQUIPMENT, UTENSILS, and LINENS; and unwrapped SINGLE-SERVICE and SINGLE-USE ARTICLES are protected from contamination;

(C) EMPLOYEES and other PERSONS such as delivery and maintenance PERSONS and pesticide applicators entering the FOOD preparation, FOOD storage, and WAREWASHING areas comply with this Code;

(D) EMPLOYEES are effectively cleaning their hands, by routinely monitoring the EMPLOYEES' handwashing;

(E) EMPLOYEES are visibly observing FOODS as they are received to determine that they are from APPROVED sources, delivered at the required temperatures, protected from contamination, unADULTERED, and accurately presented, by routinely monitoring the EMPLOYEES' observations and periodically evaluating FOODS upon their receipt; Pf

(F) EMPLOYEES are properly cooking POTENTIALLY HAZARDOUS FOOD (TIME/TEMPERATURE CONTROL FOR SAFETY FOOD), being particularly careful in cooking those FOODS known to cause severe foodborne illness and death, such as EGGS and COMMINUTED MEATS, through daily oversight of the EMPLOYEES' routine monitoring of the cooking temperatures using appropriate temperature measuring devices properly scaled and calibrated as specified under § 4-203.11 and ¶ 4-502.11(B);

(G) EMPLOYEES are using proper methods to rapidly cool POTENTIALLY HAZARDOUS FOODS (TIME/TEMPERATURE CONTROL FOR SAFETY FOODS) that are not held hot or are not for consumption within 4 hours, through daily oversight of the EMPLOYEES' routine monitoring of FOOD temperatures during cooling;

(H) CONSUMERS who order raw; or partially cooked READY-TO-EAT FOODS of animal origin are informed as specified under § 3-603.11 that the FOOD is not cooked sufficiently to ensure its safety;

(I) EMPLOYEES are properly SANITIZING cleaned multiuse EQUIPMENT and UTENSILS before they are reused, through routine monitoring of solution temperature and exposure time for hot water SANITIZING, and chemical concentration, pH, temperature, and exposure time for chemical SANITIZING;

(J) CONSUMERS are notified that clean TABLEWARE is to be used when they return to self-service areas such as salad bars and buffets as specified under § 3-304.16;

(K) Except when APPROVAL is obtained from the REGULATORY AUTHORITY as specified in ¶ 3-301.11(D), EMPLOYEES are preventing cross-contamination of READY-TO-EAT FOOD with bare hands by properly using suitable UTENSILS such as deli tissue, spatulas, tongs, single-use gloves, or dispensing EQUIPMENT;

(L) EMPLOYEES are properly trained in FOOD safety, including food allergy awareness, as it relates to their assigned duties; and

(M) FOOD EMPLOYEES and CONDITIONAL EMPLOYEES are informed of their responsibility to report in accordance with LAW, to the PERSON IN CHARGE, information about their health and activities as they relate to diseases that are transmissible through FOOD, as specified under ¶ 2-201.11(A).

Source: Food and Drug Administration, U.S. Public Health Service, 2009 Food Code.

and serving food. This manager is responsible for ensuring that key regulations are followed, including:

- All employees must wash their hands properly and maintain good personal hygiene.
- Foods must be received from approved sources.
- Foods must be kept at required temperatures.
- Foods must be protected from contamination.
- Potentially hazardous foods must be cooked and cooled properly.
- Multi-use equipment and utensils must be cleaned and sanitized before and after each use.
- All measures to prevent cross-contamination of ready-to-eat foods must be implemented.
- All employees must receive proper training in food safety as relevant to their job descriptions.

One of the most frequently used plans is known as Hazard Analysis and Critical Control Point (HACCP).

Hazard Analysis and Critical Control Point (HACCP)

HACCP is an organizational plan designed to focus on food safety, specifically by the creation and implementation of internal processes that analyze the environment and personnel involved with food procurement, preparation, and delivery; identify all hazards; and ensure that biological, physical, and chemical hazards for the entire nutritional process—from raw or original ingredients to the service or delivery of the finished food items—are under control.

HAZARD ANALYSIS   As the administrator, you must create and implement policies and procedures for the ongoing analysis of the entire food services operation. Designate a staff member to perform the analysis at a predetermined frequency (i.e., monthly, bimonthly, quarterly). Use a checklist at every evaluation to ensure that a thorough inspection of all stages of the process is completed. Ensure that analysis is done for each type of foodborne hazard: biological, including potential issues of contamination; physical including the delivery to each patient's room; and chemical.

CRITICAL CONTROL POINTS   The evaluation process should identify the safety and preventive measures in place, such as covering food to prevent physical hazards from dropping in, and using warming trays to prevent bacteria from developing on cooling food. It should confirm that those controls are used correctly and consistently. Direct staff to identify additional food safety control points for future implementation. The idea here is to determine what steps can be incorporated into the daily processes that will effectively prevent a hazard from affecting the food or, at the very least, minimize the negative impact that may result. Some of these steps include:

- Purchasing raw food from a verified vendor
- Storing the raw and ready-to-eat components at the proper temperature in appropriate storage containers
- Preventing contamination of ready-to-eat foods from raw foods
- Cooking foods to the required temperature for safe consumption
- Maintaining necessary temperatures between cooking and serving

IMPLEMENTATION AND MONITORING   Once control points are identified, corrective measures must be taken to achieve a complete food service process that is safe from all potential hazards. Documentation should be maintained to identify what corrective actions are needed, and who is responsible for ensuring they are taken. New standards should be added to the analysis checklist so supervisors can monitor that all systems are in place and being implemented correctly to keep all food stuffs safe and hazard free.

VERIFICATION AND DOCUMENTATION   All processes and systems should be routinely verified as "in place and functional" as required to ensure the safety of all food coming through this department whether delivered to a patient or served to employees and visitors in the cafeteria.

Potential Hazards Involving Food

Foodborne hazards are categorized into three types:

- Biological
- Physical
- Chemical

Just as with virtually any health care concern, prevention is the preference. Preventing contamination is the basis for "reasonable care," the legal definition from the Food Code. You must ensure that employees have a clear understanding of issues that may cause a food hazard so they are more likely to comply with your policies and procedures regarding this issue.

BIOLOGICAL FOODBORNE HAZARDS **Pathogens** cause illnesses acquired through food and include bacteria and viruses, as seen in other areas of health care. In addition, parasites such as tapeworms, roundworms, and protozoa can be transmitted through edibles. Fungi, such as molds and yeasts, can negatively impact a patient's health, especially one particular poison that is produced by some molds known as *mycotoxins*. Some plants, fish, and mushrooms may also carry some naturally occurring poisons. You can see that these potential dangers cover a wide variety of diets or nutritional regimes. This is important for everyone to understand—a healthy diet is not exempt from foodborne hazard.

Bacteria can contaminate food from contact with raw food, particularly those of animal origin. These foods include eggs, shellfish, poultry (chicken, turkey), meat (beef, pork, lamb, etc.) as well as vegetables. Pathogenic **microorganisms** can come from untreated or improperly treated water sources, such as wells, lakes, and rivers. Make certain that the facility has confirmed the water source for the entire building and, specifically, food service areas. Soil can house bacteria and cause foodborne illness when food has not been properly washed, especially with those foods that are ingested raw, such as carrots, lettuce, and other vegetables.

Waste materials that are not disposed of properly can enable bacteria and pests to invade and contaminate the food. Food and other debris, including rotting and decaying food, commonly referred to as food that is "going bad," attract pathogenic bacteria that can travel and settle down on uncovered food or **food preparation areas** (Figure 7-2 ■). In other parts of the facility, proper disposal of medical waste is clearly defined. In the food service department, the waste disposal process must be addressed with equal concern.

There are viruses that are known to be foodborne. For example, hepatitis A, rotaviruses, Norwalk virus, Norwalk-like viruses, and small round structured viruses (SRSVs) can be contracted via edibles, then spread person to person. Foodborne parasites depend upon another organism, referred to as the host organism, to survive and multiply. Three of these are of specific concern to food service operations:

- *Roundworms*: Trichina spiralis is found in hogs, including in pork, where it can cause trichinosis, and in fish, particularly cod and herring, where Anisakis can develop. According to the CDC, anisakiasis is a parasitic disease caused by anisakid nematodes (worms).
- *Flatworms*: found in beef, pork tapeworms, and fish tapeworms
- *Protozoa*: found in water infected by single-cell micro-organisms such as *Giardia lamblia* and *Cryptosporidium parvum*

Naturally occurring food hazards include poisonous mushrooms; the mycotoxins created by some molds, such as those that form on rye bread, some cereals, and nuts, particularly peanuts; and some reef fish, including grouper, mackerel, and snapper, that are carriers of ciguatera toxins. Some of the foods most commonly associated with foodborne illness, according to the CDC, are shown in Box 7-2 ■.

foodborne hazard
any biological, physical, or chemical substance that may get into food and cause harm to individuals who consume that food.

pathogen
bacterium or virus that can cause illness or disease.

microorganism
a tiny life form including some parasites, viruses, bacteria, molds, and yeasts.

food preparation area
any surface touched by food.

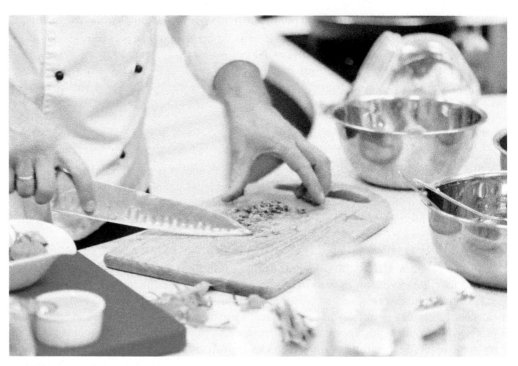

FIGURE 7-2   Food preparation areas must be cleaned before and after each use.

Photo credit: Maksim Shebeko/Fotolia.

> **BOX 7-2**   **Foods Most Commonly Associated with Foodborne Illness**
>
> - Raw foods of animal origin are the most likely to be contaminated; that is, raw meat and poultry, raw eggs, unpasteurized milk, and raw shellfish.
> - Because filter-feeding shellfish strain microbes from the sea over many months, they are particularly likely to be contaminated if there are any pathogens in the seawater.
> - Foods that mingle the products of many individual animals, such as bulk raw milk, pooled raw eggs, or ground beef, are particularly hazardous because a pathogen present in any one of the animals may contaminate the whole batch.
>   - A single hamburger may contain meat from hundreds of animals.
>   - A single restaurant omelet may contain eggs from hundreds of chickens.
>   - A glass of raw milk may contain milk from hundreds of cows.
>   - A broiler chicken carcass can be exposed to the drippings and juices of many thousands of other birds that went through the same cold water tank after slaughter.
> - Fruits and vegetables consumed raw are a particular concern. Washing can decrease but not eliminate contamination, so consumers can do little to protect themselves.
>   - Recently, a number of outbreaks have been traced to fresh fruits and vegetables that were processed under less than sanitary conditions. These outbreaks show that the quality of the water used for washing and chilling the produce after it is harvested is critical. Using water that is not clean can contaminate many boxes of produce.
>   - Fresh manure used to fertilize vegetables can also contaminate them. Alfalfa sprouts and other raw sprouts pose a particular challenge, as the conditions under which they are sprouted are ideal for growing microbes as well as sprouts, and because they are eaten without further cooking. That means that a few bacteria present on the seeds can grow to high numbers of pathogens on the sprouts.
>   - Unpasteurized fruit juice can also be contaminated if there are pathogens in or on the fruit that is used to make it.
>
> *Source: Centers for Diseases Control and Prevention.*

PHYSICAL FOODBORNE HAZARDS   Many physical foodborne hazards can be found in any environmental hazard list. These things are dangerous on the floor or in a patient room; therefore it does not stretch the imagination to understand that these elements do not belong in or near food or food preparation areas. Dust and dirt from the air, rubbish, or equipment that has not been cleaned creates a danger when that dirt gets into food. Broken glass, broken dishware, string, paper, staples, fragments of bone or shell, fingernails, hair, buttons, tops of pens, bandages, nuts, bolts, screws—you get the idea.

Who would not agree that all of these and similar items must be kept away from food? How could these things actually get into food when professionals are working in this area? Things happen in the oddest ways, such as maintenance being done on a piece of equipment next to a food preparation area. A tiny washer drops. The maintenance worker looks for it, cannot find it, and figures it is on the floor somewhere. "What's the big deal?" he reasons. "Washers only cost a penny." And he goes back to fixing the machine. Later that day, a food service employee plops some dough on the board to knead it (Figure 7-3 ■). He has no way of knowing that the stickiness of the dough has "found" the washer and enveloped it. Without anyone knowing, that washer is now embedded in a fresh loaf of bread.

Let's look at another example. The removal of the old light bulb will certainly release dust and dirt that has accumulated over time on the bulb and the light cover. This dirt and dust falls, invisibly, down into an open soup pot on the stove below. If the bulb breaks, the shards may find their way into the smallest locale, as well.

You can see from these two brief examples that all behaviors must be regulated and that all staff members who may interact with the food service area be trained, as necessary. As the administrator, you must ensure that policies and procedures are in place to direct every action and behavior that happens around food and food preparation areas.

CHEMICAL FOODBORNE HAZARDS   Logically, wherever there is food, there is a potential for insects and rodents to come to eat. A clean food service department will need to employ pesticides and other chemicals to keep these unwanted critters at bay. There are very specific guidelines that must be followed to ensure chemical foodborne hazards are prevented by directing the use of chemicals in a manner to protect the area and not contaminate any foods.

Similarly, the regulations (and common sense) require staff members to keep food areas clean. However, many cleaning products contain chemicals not compatible with good health. In this case, searching for and purchasing effective cleaning materials that are approved for use

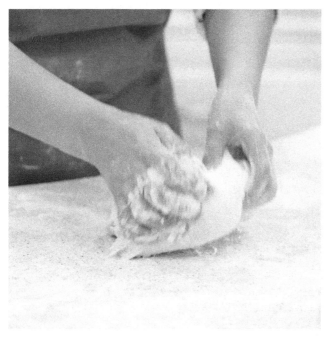

FIGURE 7-3   The stickiness of dough can attract unwanted ingredients.

Photo credit: Maksim Shebeko/Fotolia.

around food would resolve this concern easily. If these are not available, then a clear and direct rule must be in place to ensure that harmful chemicals are kept from contaminating any food.

Another chemical foodborne danger comes from leaving certain foods in open metal containers for a length of time. In these cases, dissolved metals can transfer from the inside of the metal container and leech into the food within, causing a hazard to those who ingest any of the contents. Not only must you create and enforce a policy about transferring the leftover contents of the metal container into a safe storage container but you must also ensure that safe storage containers are available.

PROMOTING HEALTHY EATING

It is logical for people to look to health care facilities for examples of healthy eating. Therefore, the CDC has consulted hospital administrators and public health officials to create initiatives that can be promoted to staff members in addition to patients and visitors at any health care facility (Box 7-3 ■).

All health care facilities need to recognize their role in guiding employees and patients to staying well-nourished and healthy at the same time. The fight against disease, especially chronic disease such as obesity, hypertension, and diabetes, is fueled by the link between food and nutrition. This is nothing new. However, health care organizations, of all sizes, need to set a good example of how food can be healthy, nutritious, and tasty—(Figure 7-4 ■).

BOX 7-3   **Hospital Healthy Eating Initiatives**

- Health sector and public health have an opportunity to address the nation's chronic disease burden and health care costs by promoting healthy hospital food environments.
- Healthy food is to be defined not only by nutrition standards but also by an economically and environmentally sustainable food system.
- Current food environment measurement tools should be further adapted for hospitals.
- Food policies should cover all venues, including cafeterias, vending machines, snack carts, and gift shops.

Source: National Center for Chronic Disease Prevention and Health Promotion, Division of Nutrition, Physical Activity, and Obesity. "Healthy Hospital Choices."

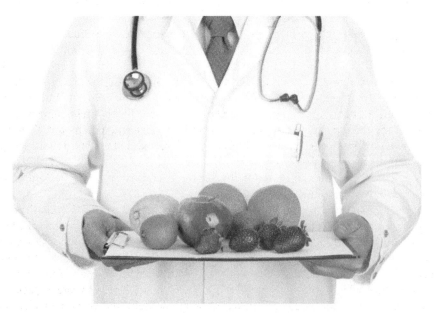

FIGURE 7-4   Health care professionals should reinforce healthy attitudes about eating in every environment.

Photo credit: panco971/Shutterstock.

| BOX 7-4 | **Nutrition Therapy** |

Treatment based on nutrition. It includes checking a person's nutrition status, and giving the right foods or nutrients to treat conditions such as those caused by diabetes, heart disease, and cancer. It may involve simple changes in a person's diet, or intravenous or tube feeding. Nutrition therapy may help patients recover more quickly and spend less time in the hospital. Also called medical nutrition therapy.

Source: National Cancer Institute.

MEDICAL NUTRITION THERAPY (MNT)

The National Guidelines Clearinghouse offers medical nutrition therapy (MNT) guidelines aimed at managing symptoms of heart failure (edema, shortness of breath, fatigue), and maintaining optimal nutrition status. The purposes of these guidelines include those that have measureable clinical outcomes.

The National Cancer Institute has emphasized the importance of implementing nutrition therapy (Box 7-4 ■) to support patient care during cancer treatments. The "healthy eating guidelines" for these patients are different from those for healthy individuals. Cancer patients need nutritional support to maintain their body weight and strength, to support healthy body tissue, and of course, to fight infection. Several studies have found that some cancer therapies actually become more efficacious when the patient remains well nourished.

Medicare Part B (physician and outpatient services), covers medical nutrition therapy services for its beneficiaries who have been diagnosed with diabetes mellitus, kidney disease, those on dialysis, or anyone else the physician believes has a medical necessity for these services.

What impact should this have on you, as the administrator, with regard to the food services provided in your facility? The organization, as a whole, must understand the provision of food is an integral part of the provision of health care.

MANAGING THE MENUS

The days of green gelatin have passed, now replaced with more fresh vegetables and fruits, a greater variety of salads, with more fish, poultry, and meat choices. Menu planning in restaurants is often consumer driven. This is also true for health care food services to an even greater degree.

The largest group of consumers for a health care food service venue is a captive audience. These customers are not eating your food because of good marketing or the reputation of the chef. They are here for other reasons—health care clinical needs—and the food provided is happenstance. As discussed earlier in this chapter, for the patients of the facility, this necessity is part and parcel of the care you provide to that patient. In addition, those patients with health care insurance are not paying for these meals. Reimbursement for food comes from the third party payer at a very specific, predetermined amount. Compounding the challenges of providing meals with good taste are the dietary restrictions for patients with various illnesses, such as low or no salt, low fat, and sugar-free as well as any food allergies noted on the patient's chart. Of course, consideration must also be paid to religious or cultural food requirements.

Decades ago, these factors equated to low quality and low taste meals with the reputation of providing little more than minimum sustenance. Food technologies have innovated salt substitutes, so meals prepared for this dietary restriction are no longer devoid of flavor. Healthier preparation methods can satisfy a low-fat diet with more flavor than ever, and natural sweeteners, such as Stevia, support sugar-free diets while avoiding lackluster meals. Some organizations have implemented what is known as the "room service" model for health care, especially useful in acute care facilities. Meals can be cooked to order and delivered when the patient is ready, rather than the traditional model of preparing mass quantities of batched fixed meals at one time, ready to deliver at a prescheduled time. Under the traditional model, a patient who might be out at x-ray, or some other test, will return to his or her room to find a meal that has been sitting on a tray losing temperature and desirability. Room service menus are typically available all day long, empowering the patient to order what they want in accordance with hunger levels, personal eating times, as well as scheduled medical procedures. These systems result in greater patient satisfaction, improved patient nutrition, and less waste. Food that is tasteless is not consumed, thereby delivering zero nutrition and food that is thrown away.

Menus established for a health care facility, whether short-term or long-term, must keep an eye on food costs and actual meal costs. Retail restaurateurs keep image in mind (expensive, moderately priced, or cheap food restaurants) while determining the menu price for each dish. You do not have to address this concern as the administrator of a health care facility. You do, however, need to ensure that the meals being prepared for your patients provide nutrition, taste, and presentation within the limitations established by third-party payer reimbursement. Components in this calculation include:

- Food components: actual cost (per serving) for meat, fish, vegetables, and so forth.
- Food additives: amortized costs (per serving) of additional recipe ingredients such as spices, oils, butter, flavor extracts (e.g., vanilla extract, almond extract), salt, pepper, and so on.
- Labor: amortized costs (per serving) for all staff members involved with foodservice from managers to cooks, and those who deliver the meals to patient rooms, and so on.
- Equipment: amortized costs (per serving) for all equipment related to food services.

You should evaluate the department's ability to generate revenue and properly control expenses to provide a true analysis of the food service operation, as a stand-alone success within your facility. A relatively simple formula can be used to determine the cost of food as a percentage of sales.

$$Food\ cost\ percentage = \frac{Total\ cost\ of\ food}{Total\ sales}$$

By performing an analysis of the revenue mix, you can calculate this for retail sales (i.e., to staff members and visitors) because determining total sales for patients will be more complex. Ideally, commercial food service operations aim for no more than 30 percent of food costs. Whether or not profit is a goal of this department, it still should be managed efficiently.

Technology has not forgotten this area of the health care business. Many hospitals use software applications that are designed to oversee the entire food service process. Not only costs, but quality and nutritional values, can be integrated with a room service model for providing food to patients. Software programs are available that integrate physician orders related to diet into the patient ordering system, thereby averting a problem of serving a patient meals inconsistent with good health while still enabling a room service type of process where the patient can order from a greater variety of meal choices. Food service carts are available with a heating component on one side and refrigeration on the other, so food can be kept at a safe temperature up to the minute of delivery. No more melted ice cream or room-temperature chicken.

Nursing homes and other residential health care facilities that bring patients into a dining room atmosphere may employ a limited-menu restaurant model. This model is likely to increase nutrition and reduce waste because patients/residents actually eat what they order. And meal service becomes an enjoyable activity. There is also a psychological benefit when patients/residents can make their own decisions. They feel less helpless, more empowered, even when the decision is only about what to have for lunch. This is especially true for older patients who are discovering a loss of many choices in their lives once taken for granted.

FOOD SERVICE: EXPENSE OR REVENUE

As discussed throughout this chapter, food service activities are necessary in inpatient health care facilities. Some administrators look at this as another overhead cost, similar to electricity and telephone. While some revenue is realized from third-party payers reimbursing for patient meals, as well as employees and visitors who pay for what they take from the cafeteria, this is generally not initially intended as a profit-making department. The traditional model for health care food service is becoming old-fashioned in the twenty-first century. Restaurant and room

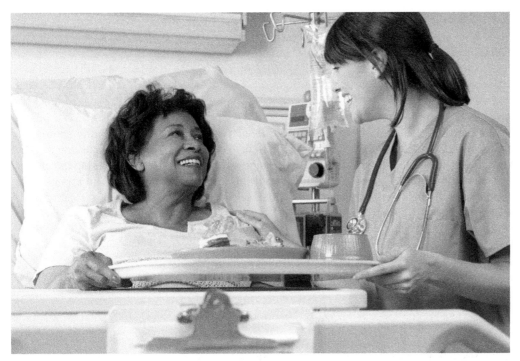

FIGURE 7-5 The necessity of feeding patients can become an asset to the facility.

Photo credit: Monkey Business Images/Shutterstock.

service models are increasing the value of health care food service to the organization's bottom line. A necessity has evolved into an asset (Figure 7-5 ■).

Public and private health care organizations have become focused on patient (customer) satisfaction, and food has a strong influence on the perceptions of those for whom care was provided. Culinary conscientiousness and variety can combine good nutrition and dietary responsibility to become a marketing feature for hospitals, nursing homes, and other health care residential facilities as they battle for a fair share of a growing population's business. Eldercare residential facilities (i.e., skilled nursing facilities, assisted living facilities, short-term and long-term care, etc.) have a golden opportunity now and for the next several decades as baby boomers, the largest segment of the population by age, move into the time of their lives when the need for these organizations increases.

Using food as a marketing device can also be seen in acute care hospitals. Many advertise that an elegant dinner from a custom menu for mom and dad is provided after the baby is delivered in their maternity ward. Many cancer-care centers promote holistic methodologies that include standard of care medical nutritional therapies.

Expanding the room service model used for patient meals can provide a healthy resource for staff and visitors, providing an increased opportunity for revenue. Some hospitals have recently introduced late night menus. Staff members work around the clock, and being able to purchase healthy, hot meals from the facility's food service department means they can eat better and be back at work on time. Many facilities no longer limit visiting hours to early evening. These visitors, and the patients as well, can order from the room service menu and purchase good quality food regardless of the time. Food is delivered to patients, while visitors and staff must go pay and pick up.

Fast food and other retail-type restaurants have set up inside of hospitals. McDonald's and Starbucks are two of the many tenants providing food and beverage service to staff, visitors, and hospital administration. These vendors provide food that is "not hospital food," while they contribute to the revenue stream. Needless to say, there are many against this infusion of what they perceive as nourishment without nutrition. They believe that the presence of such questionable food items within the walls of a health care facility is contradictory to the tenets of good health, thereby appearing that the organization has sold its soul for the money received; however, these restaurants increase patient, visitor, and staff satisfaction.

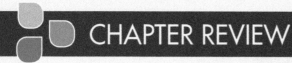

CHAPTER REVIEW

SUMMARY

Inpatient and resident health care facilities are obligated to provide food for their patients. As the administrator, you must be aware of what is going on in the kitchen and ensure that food safety procedures are followed and everything that can be done to prevent foodborne illness and hazards is being done. Consideration must be given to providing patients with food that provides good nutrition, good taste, and is safe, whether the service is provided by in-house staff members or by a contracted outside vendor. Health care facilities of all types should educate patients, visitors, and staff by promoting healthy eating and investigate the value of incorporating medical nutrition therapy into the services provided. In addition to increasing the quality of the food, updating to restaurant style or room service style menus and processes can expand the appeal of the entire facility. Increased patient satisfaction often equates to increased revenues. Food service can offer more than simple, required food to the patients; it can actually become a profitable concern within the facility.

REVIEW QUESTIONS

MULTIPLE CHOICE

Choose the most accurate answer.

1. Which of the following individuals may suffer more severe consequences from a foodborne illness than the rest of the general population?
    a. Individuals who are sick
    b. Individuals who have weakened immune systems
    c. Individuals who are recovering from an illness
    d. All of these

2. Health care food service activities include all of the following EXCEPT
    a. procurement.
    b. preparation.
    c. packaging.
    d. delivery.

3. Which of the following actions might result in a food hazard?
    a. Purchasing raw food from a verified vendor
    b. Storing raw food and ready-to-eat foods together
    c. Cooking foods to the required temperature
    d. Maintaining necessary temperatures between cooking and serving

4. Viruses, such as _____ are known to be foodborne.
    a. hepatitis A
    b. mycotoxins
    c. protozoa
    d. *Trichina spiralis*

5. Medical Nutrition Therapy has been shown to support patients diagnosed with
    a. heart failure.
    b. cancer.

    c. Neither a or b
    d. Both a and b

6. Meal costs are calculated using the actual costs for
    a. salt, pepper, and other spices.
    b. meat, fish, chicken.
    c. labor.
    d. equipment.

7. It can be a challenge to provide meals with good taste that comply with physician-ordered
    a. budget.
    b. time schedule.
    c. dietary restrictions.
    d. reimbursement.

8. The mold on rye bread and cereals is one type of _____ foodborne hazard.
    a. biological
    b. physical
    c. chemical
    d. parasitic

9. HACCP stands for
    a. Health and Clinical Consumer Provisions.
    b. Health care Avoidance to Clinical Contamination Procedures.
    c. Hazard and Contamination Control Plan.
    d. Hazard Analysis and Critical Control Point.

10. The FDA describes the Food Code as a
    a. legally binding document.
    b. reference document.
    c. legal obligation.
    d. key legislation.

FILL-IN-THE-BLANK

Fill in the blank with the accurate answer.

11. Food and nutritional services may function as self-operational or _____.

12. The _____ of food service is the individual recognized by law to be responsible for food safety compliance.

13. One of the most frequently used plans is known as Hazard _____.

14. The FDA, in conjunction with _____ publishes the "Food Code."

15. _____ such as tapeworms and roundworms can be transmitted through edibles.

16. The fight against disease, especially chronic disease, is fueled by the link between food and _____.

17. Restaurant and room service models can evolve food service from just a necessity into an _____.

18. A hospital that permits a patient to order what he wants to eat, when he wants to eat it from a menu is using the _____ model for food service.

19. The largest group of consumers for a health care food service venue is a _____ audience.

20. Naturally occurring food hazards include _____ mushrooms.

TRUE/FALSE

Determine if each of the following statements is true or false.

21. Your facility has an obligation to ensure your patients/residents are well-nourished.

22. When a health care facility outsources foodservices, it no longer has any liability for these activities.

23. The industry expects that you will take "reasonable care" to document and implement all necessary precautions to avoid violating rules of the Food Code.

24. A rubber band found in the soup is an example of a biological foodborne hazard.

25. Food left inside an open metal container may be contaminated with a chemical foodborne hazard.

26. Medicare Part A (hospital/major medical) covers medical nutrition therapy services for beneficiaries diagnosed with diabetes mellitus.

27. Reimbursement to hospitals and nursing homes for food is always completely paid for by the patient. No third-party payers cover food.

28. Computer software programs can integrate a patient's food order with physician orders to ensure all dietary restrictions are followed for the good health of the patient.

29. Expanding the room service model used for patient meals can provide a healthy resource for staff and visitors.

30. Everyone in the industry and throughout the country agree that fast food restaurants should be permitted to open inside of a hospital.

WHEN YOU ARE THE ADMINISTRATOR . . .

Critical Thinking and Analysis

Case Study #1

Nutrition Therapy in Cancer Care

The National Cancer Institute at the National Institutes of Health states, "*Early nutrition screening and assessment help find problems that may affect how well the patient's body can deal with the effects of cancer treatment. Patients who are underweight or malnourished may not be able to get through treatment as well as a well-nourished patient. Finding and treating nutrition problems early can help the patient gain weight or prevent weight loss, decrease problems with the treatment, and help recovery.*"

Source: http://www.cancer.gov/cancertopics/pdq/supportivecare/nutrition/Patient/page2

How would you use this advisory to create a policy in your facility? How could this knowledge support better care for cancer patients in active therapy at your facility? What might you direct your foodservice manager to do?

(Continued)

Case Study #2

Food Safety

The U.S. Department of Agriculture published these four items for preparing food safely.

- Always wash hands with warm water and soap for twenty seconds before and after handling food.
- Don't cross-contaminate. Keep raw meat, poultry, fish, and their juices away from other food. After cutting raw meats, wash cutting board, utensils, and countertops with hot, soapy water.
- Cutting boards, utensils, and countertops can be sanitized by using a solution of 2 tablespoons of unscented, liquid chlorine bleach in 1 gallon of water.
- Marinate meat and poultry in a covered dish in the refrigerator.

Source: http://www.fsis.usda.gov/Fact_Sheets/
Basics_for_Handling_Food_Safely/

Create a PowerPoint presentation that you can use to teach your food service staff members how to prepare food safely. Include a plan for regular assessments to ensure compliance.

Case Study #3

Fast Food in Hospitals

The Institute of Food Technologies identified twelve new trends and innovative ideas emerging in acute care facilities (hospitals). One of these is permitting fast food restaurants to operate in the building or an adjacent outparcel.

Identify the benefits and concerns about permitting a fast food franchise to set up an outlet in your facility. How would you address the controversies connected with the "poor nutrition" image of this sector of the food service industry?

 INTERNET CONNECTIONS

Nutrition and Food Services; U.S. Department of Veterans Affairs

The Veterans Administration believes in the connection between good health and nutrition.
http://www.nutrition.va.gov/

Association of Nutrition and Foodservice Professionals

The Association of Nutrition and Foodservice Professionals (ANFP) is a national not-for-profit association of professionals dedicated to providing optimum nutritional care through foodservice management.

ANFP members work in hospitals, long-term care, as well as other noncommercial food service locations such as schools and correctional facilities.
http://www.anfponline.org/

Association for Healthcare Foodservice (AHF)

The Association for Healthcare Foodservice (AHF) is a national trade organization for self-operated food service professionals who work within health care-oriented facilities.
http://www.healthcarefoodservice.org/

COMPLIANCE PLANS

INTRODUCTION

Department of Health and Human Services (DHHS)
the principal agency for protecting the health of all Americans.

Federal Register
the daily publication for rules, proposed rules, and notices of the federal government.

Office of the Inspector General (OIG)
an investigative branch of the US federal government.

compliance
observance of laws and policies; behaviors and actions directly following rules and regulations.

consequence
result or outcome of behavior.

qui tam lawsuit
a feature of HIPAA that entitles an individual citizen to file a lawsuit on behalf of the government; used in cases of whistleblowers uncovering fraud.

Whether you are working in a small physician's office or in a large hospital, it will be part of your responsibility as the administrator to make certain that both your clinical and administrative staff understand the importance of complying with rules, regulations, policies, and laws. Whether it is a statutory law passed by the federal or state legislature, an administrative law from the **Department of Health and Human Services (DHHS)**, or an initiative from The Joint Commission (TJC), all regulations must be interpreted, translated into easily understood language, and incorporated into internal policies that will guide each member of your staff in complying.

June Gibbs Brown, the inspector general, was quoted in the February 11, 1998, issue of the **Federal Register** as saying, "*Ultimately, it is the* **OIG**'s *hope that a voluntarily created compliance program will enable hospitals to meet their goals, improve the quality of patient care, and substantially reduce fraud, waste and abuse, as well as the cost of health care to Federal, State, and private health insurers*" [FR Doc. 98-4399 Filed 2-20-98; 8:45 a.m.]. In volume 65, No. 194 (October 5, 2000) of the Federal Register, it is noted that physicians and small group practices are encouraged, but not mandated, to develop compliance programs. However, the Patient Protection and Affordable Care Act of 2010 requires physicians who treat Medicare and Medicaid beneficiaries to create and implement a compliance program.

◗ WHAT DOES A COMPLIANCE PLAN DO?

You would expect that all those in your facility have sufficient education to know the applicable laws and what they require. However, in the hectic environment of a typical day in health care, it is not always easy to determine what action is legal to take. Therefore, it will be necessary to enact a continuous awareness campaign to remind them what to do. A **compliance** plan lays out the details of precisely how the organization as a whole will go about educating the staff, explaining what they need to do under various circumstances, and the **consequences** of failing to follow the policies of the organization and the laws of the governing authorities.

Specifically, your compliance plan should:

- Enable all staff members to comprehend the elements involved. Keep in mind that your staff is comprised of highly educated individuals as well as those with less formal education. In addition to regular training sessions, include some type of assessment to ensure comprehension. This is a good thing to document.
- Determine explicit guidelines for behavior under all foreseeable circumstances, and provide for contingency planning. Use examples that provide clear illustrations of situations that may occur along with precisely how the organization expects the employee to handle things. Not every circumstance can be predicted, so include directions for what staff members should do when they are uncertain.
- Create a secure process for individuals to report alleged violations without fear of repercussions. Virtually everyone in your facility can see and hear things that you cannot. They are the front-line individuals who really know what is going on. Patients, patients' family and friends, and your employees know the truth, and you want them to be able to trust enough to be honest and open. You need to encourage them to come to you so you will have the opportunity to fix the problem before it gets to a point so serious that someone might file a **qui tam lawsuit**. (See the note on page 142.) A toll-free phone number for anonymous reports and a web-based complaint form are two of the most popular methods. Of course, you must make certain that all complaints are investigated and proper action is taken as a result. Ignoring obvious infractions will breed contempt and complacence—neither of which are ingredients for quality of care.
- Describe consequences for failure to comply and implement them when noncompliance has been found. You must make certain that your policies and procedures are taken seriously and that all staff members are aware of the penalties if they do not. An absence of consequences from wrong doing makes your policies meaningless.
- Implement methodologies for adjusting behaviors and/or processes before external agencies get involved. As soon as a breach has been discovered, you must take action. Investigate, apply corrective action to the staff member or members involved, and if

necessary, adjust internal policies and procedures to make it easier for everyone to comply. Sometimes a policy makes sense on paper yet encounters logistical problems when put into the workday. For example, you might create a policy that all documentation must be presented to the director's office no later than end of shift. This may be difficult for those working at another location, so those getting off at midnight are consistently noncompliant. Therefore, it would make sense to change the policy to make it easier to comply. Possibly, enabling them to e-mail the reports, or giving them a twenty-four-hour window to deliver them.

- Establish regularly performed **internal audits.** These investigations should be designed to identify quality as well as human error or specific wrongdoing. Unless you are in a large organization that has the financial strength to hire a team dedicated to conduct internal audits, analyze the results, make recommendations for corrections, and implement approved corrections, you will need to designate a member of the current staff. Deadlines must be established and met; otherwise, day-to-day tasks will push them aside, and your facility will never be able to benefit from this important information about the internal workings of your organization (Figure 8-1 ■). In many cases, you will find opportunities for praise as well as improvement.

internal audit
an assessment to determine compliance performed by, or initiated by, the organization or facility itself, to look for improprieties, errors, and other wrongdoing.

A well-implemented compliance plan will often provide outcomes that will benefit everyone and are not solely limited to satisfying legal requirements. This document will create a blueprint for your organization as it establishes a mindset, from the top down, of how to treat patients and each other. The foundation of establishing an environment of honorable actions is often a true understanding of what is required and is built into a culture of what is expected. When an attitude of excellence is, indeed, proliferated throughout the organization, everyone benefits: patient care is improved; staff members treat each other with respect, thus reducing employee turnover; and financial loss and liability are decreased.

Make note that this culture of honorability and respect must be actuated by everyone in the organization, from the board of governors to the president/CEO to the managers and supervisors through the clinical staff (physicians included) all the way to environmental services and security staff. Otherwise, your employees will see this entire process as a charade and you will lose cooperation.

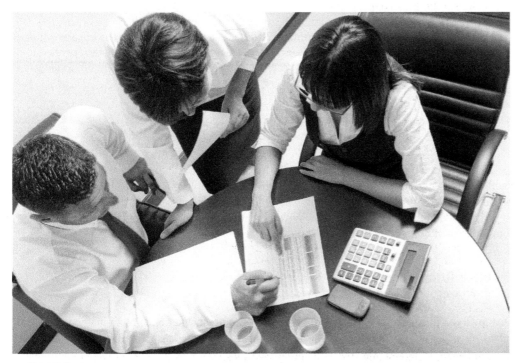

FIGURE 8-1 Internal audits are worth all the work.
Photo credit: Ersler Dmitry/Shutterstock.

BOX 8-1	**Whistleblowers not only stop fraudulent activities, they share in the monies recouped by the government.**

Justice Department Announces Largest Health Care Fraud Settlement in Its History

Pfizer to Pay $2.3 Billion for Fraudulent Marketing

WASHINGTON—American pharmaceutical giant Pfizer Inc. and its subsidiary Pharmacia & Upjohn Company Inc. (hereinafter together "Pfizer") have agreed to pay $2.3 billion, the largest health care fraud settlement in the history of the Department of Justice, to resolve criminal and civil liability arising from the illegal promotion of certain pharmaceutical products, the Justice Department announced today.

Pharmacia & Upjohn Company has agreed to plead guilty to a felony violation of the Food, Drug and Cosmetic Act for misbranding Bextra with the intent to defraud or mislead. Bextra is an anti-inflammatory drug that Pfizer pulled from the market in 2005. Under the provisions of the Food, Drug and Cosmetic Act, a company must specify the intended uses of a product in its new drug application to FDA. Once approved, the drug may not be marketed or promoted for so-called "off-label" uses—i.e., any use not specified in an application and approved by FDA. Pfizer promoted the sale of Bextra for several uses and dosages that the FDA specifically declined to approve due to safety concerns. The company will pay a criminal fine of $1.195 billion, the largest criminal fine ever imposed in the United States for any matter. Pharmacia & Upjohn will also forfeit $105 million, for a total criminal resolution of $1.3 billion.

In addition, Pfizer has agreed to pay $1 billion to resolve allegations under the civil False Claims Act that the company illegally promoted four drugs—Bextra; Geodon, an anti-psychotic drug; Zyvox, an antibiotic; and Lyrica, an anti-epileptic drug—and caused false claims to be submitted to government health care programs for uses that were not medically accepted indications and therefore not covered by those programs. The civil settlement also resolves allegations that Pfizer paid kickbacks to health care providers to induce them to prescribe these, as well as other, drugs. The federal share of the civil settlement is $668,514,830 and the state Medicaid share of the civil settlement is $331,485,170. This is the largest civil fraud settlement in history against a pharmaceutical company.

As part of the settlement, Pfizer also has agreed to enter into an expansive corporate integrity agreement with the Office of Inspector General of the Department of Health and Human Services. That agreement provides for procedures and reviews to be put in place to avoid and promptly detect conduct similar to that which gave rise to this matter.

Whistleblower lawsuits filed under the qui tam provisions of the False Claims Act that are pending in the District of Massachusetts, the Eastern District of Pennsylvania and the Eastern District of Kentucky triggered this investigation. As a part of today's resolution, six whistleblowers will receive payments totaling more than $102 million from the federal share of the civil recovery.

"This historic settlement will return nearly $1 billion to Medicare, Medicaid, and other government insurance programs, securing their future for the Americans who depend on these programs," said Kathleen Sebelius, Secretary of Department of Health and Human Services. "The Department of Health and Human Services will continue to seek opportunities to work with its government partners to prosecute fraud wherever we can find it. But we will also look for new ways to prevent fraud before it happens. Health care is too important to let a single dollar go to waste."

Source: Department of Health and Human Services (DHHS).

Note: A qui tam lawsuit is covered by the Whistleblower's Statute, a part of HIPAA. This statute permits current and former employees to file a complaint in court against the accused institution on behalf of the government. The whistleblower can be rewarded with as much as 30 percent of all monies recouped by the government. Some whistleblowers have been rewarded with millions of dollars (see Box 8-1 ■).

ELEMENTS OF AN EFFECTIVE COMPLIANCE PLAN

Creating a compliance plan is a large project and will require the participation of many within your organization. The good news is, once it is done, it only has to be updated once every year thereafter.

This section will provide you with an outline of the components of an effective compliance plan, upon which you and your team can build. This document is expected to provide your staff with the guidance to complete their tasks and job responsibilities legally and ethically at all times.

In addition, advice should be included to guide your staff as to what to do when encountering a legal or ethical gray area—a situation where the right thing to do is not clear-cut.

The Federal Sentencing Guidelines (FSG) include seven steps to ensure **due diligence** is properly carried out. These steps must be followed by all facilities to meet the minimum requirements necessary to avoid criminal conduct and the resulting liability by staff and all others under the control of the organization.

1. Establish compliance standards and procedures.
2. Assign overall responsibility to specific high-level individual(s).
3. Use due care to avoid delegation of authority to individuals with an inclination to get involved in illegal actions.
4. Effectively communicate standards and procedures to all staff.
5. Utilize monitoring and auditing systems to detect noncompliant conduct.
6. Enforce adequate disciplinary sanctions when appropriate.
7. Respond to episodes of noncompliance by modifying the program, if necessary.

due diligence
complete and thorough background checks; proof that everything possible was done, every reasonable precaution was made to prevent a wrong from occurring.

Identify Applicable Laws and Regulations

You can use the FSG steps as the framework for creating a compliance plan that covers all the bases. However, before you can begin, you must meticulously identify all of the laws (federal and state), regulations, standards, and policies by which your facility must abide. Some laws will affect all facilities, regardless of their size, such as HIPAA (Health Insurance Portability and Accountability Act) and the federal False Claims Act. Other laws may not impact physician's offices or clinics, such as the Emergency Medical Treatment and Active Labor Act (EMTALA), a law that directs specific care responsibilities to Medicare-participating hospitals only. You may consider engaging an attorney who specializes in health care law to create this list or review a list that might already exist. Ignorance of the law is never a viable defense, and this is an excellent motivator to do some serious research in this area.

SPECIAL CIRCUMSTANCES/CRISIS MANAGEMENT   In addition to laws and regulations, you and your team should consider any special circumstances that would challenge your staff. When a celebrity arrives in the emergency department or is admitted, even the most staid adult can behave outside professional norms. When another type of crisis, such as a hurricane, impacts your facility, your guidance will help your employees know how to divide their loyalties between job obligations and family concerns. An established policy, such as inviting immediate family to have **safe harbor** at your facility when they have nowhere else to go, would alleviate distractions and enable your staff to focus only on their patients. Advance planning is the key to managing a crisis effectively (see Figure 8-2 ■).

safe harbor
a location protected from storm or other crisis.

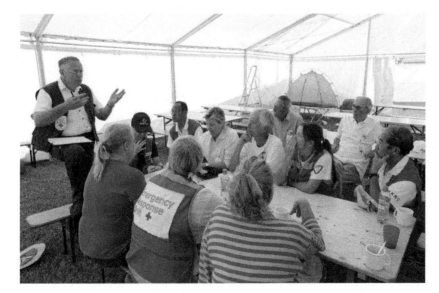

FIGURE 8-2 Emergencies require coordinated efforts.
Photo credit: © Caro/Alamy.

Establish Policies and Procedures

Once you have completed a list of the laws, statutes, and guidelines applicable to your facility, you have the foundation for establishing your organizational policies and procedures that will provide your staff with solid direction for compliance. Your staff will perceive it as a sign of respect if you to explain the foundational issues for your policies rather than just telling them what to do or what not to do. Employees may gripe about a specific policy whose purpose is unexplained, constantly discussing how stupid it is, listing the reasons why it should not be followed, and generating dissatisfaction amongst others. However, once the thought process or the basis for the policy is explained, dissatisfaction is often replaced by understanding and ultimate compliance. Individuals are more likely to follow a policy when they understand its foundation.

As you determine these policies, you will also need to determine appropriate consequences for violating the policy. These consequences should be documented specifically for various levels of failure to comply. Not all offenses are worthy of firing the individual, yet some may be. At the same time, a verbal warning is not a strong enough punishment for other infractions. All of these variations should be worked out ahead of time to avoid any appearance of personal prejudice toward a specific employee.

Create Reporting Systems

Everyone on the staff should be on board with your corporate culture of honesty and respect. When this is the belief system upon which your organization is built, you will be able to have the confidence that employees will feel a moral obligation to make a report when someone breaks the rules. However, you will need to make it easy for them to do this.

Creating a reporting system will permit any member who witnesses a violation to let you know so you can investigate and do something to lessen the impact of that breach. Of course, you want to ensure that all members know they can file a report with their manager or supervisor. However, some may be afraid to do this. In addition, you must take into consideration that it may be the manager who is behaving inappropriately. As mentioned earlier in this chapter, you might set up a phone line so a report can be called in anonymously. A special e-mail box might also be established so the violation can be reported electronically, or a link to a form that can be completed and filed online might be posted on your facility's intranet website.

It is a good idea to emphasize assurances that no one has the power to get someone else in trouble or fired (Figure 8-3 ■). Accentuate the fact that all individuals reporting a potential infraction will not be subjected to any repercussions or backlash. It is simply a matter of a person

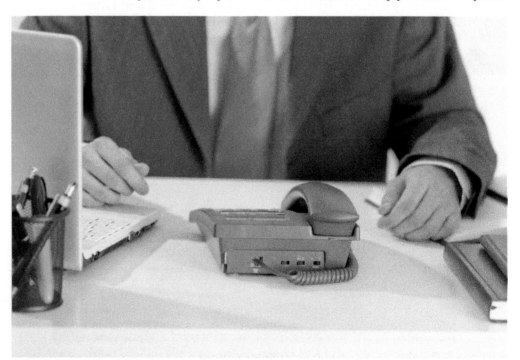

FIGURE 8-3 Realize that even good people will hesitate to report a co-worker.

Photo credit: Alliance/Shutterstock.

sharing an issue of concern that someone else may need to explore. You want to make every effort to help everyone feel comfortable about sharing their observations without feeling like a tattletale. Reassure them that a report to the hotline is for the greater good.

Investigate All Suspected Occurrences of Noncompliance

Every report coming into the phone line, e-mail box, website form, and to a manager must be investigated. There are certain to be false accusations along with some cases of actual noncompliance that cannot be proven. However, you must investigate them all without any prejudgment for the program to have any meaning.

Remember, it is one thing to have the concept of investigations and quite another to actually conduct them. You must determine, ahead of time, precisely who on your staff or which outside company will handle these probes and ensure it gets done in a timely and proper fashion.

Implementing Monitoring Procedures

While it is important to have your people watching out to protect each other and the facility, you will need some objective monitoring devices to support the effort. For example, most electronic health records (EHR) programs create a log of who opens and views a patient's record. If this individual is not a health care professional assigned to the patient, this could be a violation of HIPAA's Privacy and/or Security Rule. Regularly checking the report will notify you of any violation. Paper charts can be implanted with radio-frequency identification (RFID) chips that are able to electronically track the folder throughout the facility—similar to a GPS tracker.

Conducting regularly scheduled audits will reveal any violations relating to billing and claims. Discovering this type of violation may save the organization millions of dollars in potential penalties and fees from a charge that your facility is submitting fraudulent claims (see Box 8-2 ▇).

BOX 8-2	HHS Settles HIPAA Case with BCBST for $1.5 million

Blue Cross Blue Shield of Tennessee (BCBST) has agreed to pay the U.S. Department of Health and Human Services (HHS) $1,500,000 to settle potential violations of the Health Insurance Portability and Accountability Act of 1996 (HIPAA) Privacy and Security Rules, Leon Rodriguez, Director of the HHS Office for Civil Rights (OCR), announced today. BCBST has also agreed to a corrective action plan to address gaps in its HIPAA compliance program. The enforcement action is the first resulting from a breach report required by the Health Information Technology for Economic and Clinical Health (HITECH) Act Breach Notification Rule.

The investigation followed a notice submitted by BCBST to HHS reporting that fifty-seven unencrypted computer hard drives were stolen from a leased facility in Tennessee. The drives contained the protected health information (PHI) of over 1 million individuals, including member names, social security numbers, diagnosis codes, dates of birth, and health plan identification numbers. OCR's investigation indicated BCBST failed to implement appropriate administrative safeguards to adequately protect information remaining at the leased facility by not performing the required security evaluation in response to operational changes. In addition, the investigation showed a failure to implement appropriate physical safeguards by not having adequate facility access controls; both of these safeguards are required by the HIPAA Security Rule.

"This settlement sends an important message that OCR expects health plans and health care providers to have in place a carefully designed, delivered, and monitored HIPAA compliance program," said OCR Director Leon Rodriguez. "The HITECH Breach Notification Rule is an important enforcement tool and OCR will continue to vigorously protect patients' right to private and secure health information."

In addition to the $1,500,000 settlement, the agreement requires BCBST to review, revise, and maintain its Privacy and Security policies and procedures, to conduct regular and robust trainings for all BCBST employees covering employee responsibilities under HIPAA, and to perform monitor reviews to ensure BCBST compliance with the corrective action plan.

HHS Office for Civil Rights enforces the HIPAA Privacy and Security Rules. The HIPAA Privacy Rule gives individuals rights over their protected health information and sets rules and limits on who can look at and receive that health information. The HIPAA Security Rule protects health information in electronic form by requiring entities covered by HIPAA to use physical, technical, and administrative safeguards to ensure that electronic protected health information remains private and secure.

The HITECH Breach Notification Rule requires **covered entities** to report an impermissible use or disclosure of protected health information, or a "breach," of 500 individuals or more to HHS and the media. Smaller breaches affecting fewer than 500 individuals must be reported to the secretary on an annual basis.

Source: Department of Health and Human Services (DHHS).

covered entities
individuals and organizations obligated to abide by the Privacy Rule of HIPAA.

BOX 8-3	**UCLA Health System Settles Potential Violations of the HIPAA Privacy and Security Rules**

Following an investigation by the Department of Health and Human Services (HHS) Office for Civil Rights (OCR), the University of California at Los Angeles Health System (UCLAHS) has agreed to settle potential violations of the HIPAA Privacy and Security Rules for $865,500 and has committed to a corrective action plan aimed at remedying gaps in its compliance with the rules.

The resolution agreement resolves two separate complaints filed with OCR on behalf of two celebrity patients who received care at UCLAHS. The complaints alleged that UCLAHS employees repeatedly and without permissible reason looked at the electronic protected health information of these patients.

OCR's investigation into the complaints revealed that from 2005–2008, unauthorized employees repeatedly looked at the electronic protected health information of numerous other UCLAHS patients. Through policies and procedures, entities covered under HIPAA must reasonably restrict access to patient information to only those employees with a valid reason to view the information and must sanction any employee who is found to have violated these policies.

"Covered entities are responsible for the actions of their employees. This is why it is vital that trainings and meaningful policies and procedures, including audit trails, become part of the every day operations of any health care provider," said OCR Director Georgina Verdugo. "Employees must clearly understand that casual review for personal interest of patients' protected health information is unacceptable and against the law."

The corrective action plan requires UCLAHS to implement Privacy and Security policies and procedures approved by OCR, to conduct regular and robust trainings for all UCLAHS employees who use protected health information, to sanction offending employees, and to designate an independent monitor who will assess UCLAHS compliance with the plan over three years.

"Covered entities need to realize that HIPAA privacy protections are real and OCR vigorously enforces those protections. Entities will be held accountable for employees who access protected health information to satisfy their own personal curiosity," said Director Verdugo.

Source: Department of Health and Human Services (DHHS).

Educate the Staff

The next step is to educate everyone about the policies so the facility will be able to avoid the costly repercussions of noncompliance (Box 8-3 ■). This must be more than simply publishing and distributing an *Employee Policies and Procedures* manual. You need to ensure that they are well versed in the importance and impact of compliance. This may be one of your greatest challenges, as most staff members feel these educational sessions interfere with the real reason they are employed at your facility—to care for patients.

Perhaps, rather than make these sessions a separate event, they could be integrated into each and every job description and the responsibilities that go with each job. Department heads should be made responsible for including these topics in their department meetings on a predetermined schedule (e.g., once a month, once a quarter). Rather than focus on the big picture of compliance, narrow the scope to that which affects each subgroup of your organization. Connect the dots, if you will, for them to be able to understand their individual role in compliance and how to ensure these concerns are diligently followed.

Corrective Actions

As you can see from the articles shown in Box 8-1 and Box 8-2, consequences for noncompliance will be implemented. You can do this internally and minimize the possibility of the issue literally becoming a federal offense. As sad as it is, some people follow the rules to avoid punishment rather than view them as guidelines to correct behavior. As mentioned earlier, the consequences of noncompliance must be determined and published in advance, and then applied as circumstances require.

1. *Initiate an investigation.* An investigation may sound more serious than it is. However, someone must check reports, logs, and any related documentation; interview employees and visitors in the area who may have witnessed a questionable action; and evaluate the evidence to determine what caused the breach.

2. *Determine if the cause of the breach is the employee or the policy.* As the plan is developed, you and your team need to acknowledge that some theories sound great on paper but are difficult to put into effect on the job. Therefore, it is important to seek out feedback from staff members directly involved in following the rules. You don't want policies to get in the way of quality care. Everything needs to work together, whenever possible, with a natural flow. As necessary, you will need to adjust the details of the policy until it works within the organization as well as protects the organization as a whole.

3. *Implement predetermined consequences for confirmed occasions of noncompliance.* As you and your team establish each policy and procedure, you need to determine what internal consequences will be initiated should a staff member fail to comply. Some common punishments are:

   * *Verbal warning*: Speak privately with the individual found to have breached the policy as a warning against repeating the bad behavior, to reinforce the appropriate actions, and to provide reinforcement of the consequences of failing to correct their conduct.
   * *Written warning*: Document a second breach in the employee's record and provide a copy to the employee. Establish a following step. For example, two written warnings may result in mandatory additional training, suspension (with or without pay), or termination.
   * *Additional training/education*: Certain circumstances may be best served by having the staff member attend remedial education on the policies and procedures of the facility.
   * *Suspension with pay*: A breach that has serious consequences, such as harm to a patient, may require you to suspend the employee from working while the investigation is being conducted. Until guilt can be confirmed, it would be improper to suspend the individual without pay. However, the situation may make it unwise to have this person continue on the job until innocence or guilt can be documented.
   * *Suspension without pay*: If a serious breach is made by an employee with a good track record who has proven their value to the facility, suspension without pay may be a fair option. The need for corrective action is reinforced while retaining the staff member for future benefit to the organization.
   * *Termination*: There are some actions that cannot be forgiven or improved with retraining. Some examples might be coming to work while intoxicated, stealing medication or equipment, or abandonment of patient(s) without a **mitigating circumstance** or reason.

mitigating circumstance
an event that partially excuses a wrong or lessens the result.

PROJECT MANAGEMENT: THE PATH TO COMPLETION

Creating a compliance plan is a large undertaking, as you have learned throughout this chapter. Even if you only need to update an existing plan, the work required is extensive and intense. Employing project management skills can support your success.

1. Begin with an overview of the entire project: The section of this chapter titled *Elements of an Effective Compliance Plan* can be used as an outline. Take each section and preliminarily determine what needs to be done—a path to completion, step by step. For example, the first component is "Identify the applicable laws and regulations." The path to completion would start by checking the federal and state websites, the Centers for Medicare and Medicare Services (CMS) website, as well as your major third-party payers for laws that impact your type of health care facility (i.e., hospital, nursing home, physician's office, etc.). Also, check with national trade organizations and their state chapters, such as the American Medical Association or American Hospital Association. Often, they post articles covering new legislation and how it will impact its members. If this is a new plan, you will need to research all applicable laws, regulations, and guidelines. When you are updating an existing plan, you only need to identify those laws that are new since the last update. Be alert to longstanding regulations with recent updates.

2. Delegate the work to be done: Each member of the team should have a specific list of tasks assigned. Whenever possible, try to match the individual's skill set to their assignment responsibilities. Matching skills to tasks will improve the outcomes and make it less tedious. Avoid staff with any **propensity** for negative behavior.

propensity
a tendency to demonstrate particular behavior.

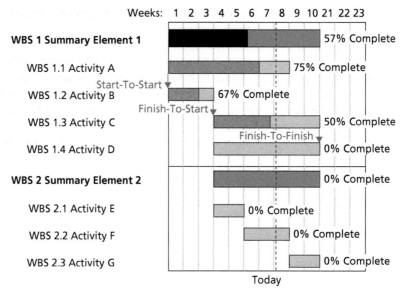

FIGURE 8-4 Using a Gantt project management chart can help keep the project on track. *Source:* From Wikipedia.

3. Establish quality standards: Each step and section of the plan should have tangible measures to ensure the quality of the information within. Resources must be confirmed as credible, reliable sources of applicable data. As the team works together, everyone should understand the need to trust each other to do a quality job, however verification is required.

4. Create the timeline: Deadlines must be set, not only for the completion of the project but for each and every step, each and every section. Impress upon everyone the importance of meeting the deadlines to ensure the well-balanced flow of the project from beginning to end. If the components of the project are delayed, then a serious bottleneck in workflow may occur. When work is done in a rush, there is an increased opportunity for error. Use an organizational or project management chart such as a Program Evaluation and Review Technique (PERT) or a Gantt Chart (Figure 8-4 ■) to help you manage this type of large project.

5. Keep team communications open: When working on a huge project, it is critical that all the members of the team feel free to share any concerns, frustrations, or blocks with you, the team leader. If there is the chance that problems may arise, you need to know about them sooner rather than later. It is a good idea to schedule regular meetings—weekly or biweekly—to help keep everyone on track. Sometimes an individual needs to be coaxed in the right direction or reassured that he or she is on the right path.

6. Build in contingencies: There is always the chance that one component or another will not go according to the plan. A team member unexpectedly gets promoted and can no longer work on the project. Another may become overwhelmed with his or her part. You must arrange for the unexpected. Keep a list of potential alternates to step in to finish that assignment. This same list may be helpful if the timeline gets into crunch mode. You can bring in additional staff members to get the job done on time.

7. Work smarter, not harder: Remember, you are not the first health care facility to create a compliance plan. In addition to this textbook, you may find support in the Federal Register, the OIG website, or from CMS. These resources can give your project a jump-start and get you going in the right direction.

◗ THE BOTTOM LINE

fraud
using dishonest or inaccurate information with the intention of wrongly gaining money or other benefit.

A compliance plan is a precise blueprint for the prevention of **fraud** and abuse, the reduction of occurrences of medical misadventures, and the overall better health of the organization. It is the map of preventive medicine. Annual updates are like a personal annual physical, and training and educational programs are like vaccinations against the disease of malfeasance and criminal behaviors. There will be fewer concerns potentially audited by the government and third-party payers, reduced liability, and better care for your patients.

The bonus is that, in some situations, a properly created and implemented compliance plan may reduce the assessment of fines and penalties should an audit uncover some criminal behaviors. This plan can be evidence of the honest intent of the organization to function within the laws and regulations involved. The United States Sentencing Commission, in their published *Federal Sentencing Guidelines* may give organizational defendants "good corporate behavior credits" resulting in a reduction of fines and penalties by as much as 70 percent when a compliance plan has been created and implemented using their seven steps to ensure due diligence (discussed earlier in this chapter).

CHAPTER REVIEW

SUMMARY

Creating and implementing a compliance plan is a major undertaking that will take many hours over the course of several weeks. It does not have to be completed all at once, so this task can be worked into a job description for an administrator or assistant administrators. Even when a compliance plan already exists, it must be updated. New laws are enacted, crises occur, and you must confirm that policies and procedures are in place so that every member of your staff can do the right thing. A reporting system should permit individuals to bring violations to your attention without fear of repercussion, and then the administration must confirm that a full investigation is done. As the administrator, you must be certain that every member of your staff is aware of the policies, knows the importance of compliance, and is cognizant that, in those situations when procedures are not followed, consequences will be assessed.

Prevention is a valuable thing. Proper and complete preparation of your staff members is important and can actually support your facility's functioning more effectively and efficiently.

REVIEW QUESTIONS

MULTIPLE CHOICE

Choose the most accurate answer.

1. A compliance plan should
   a. educate staff about paid time off.
   b. establish regularly performed employee reviews.
   c. create a secure way for reporting an observed violation.
   d. provide staff with acceptable excuses for noncompliance.

2. A qui tam lawsuit can be filed by a
   a. competitor.
   b. current employee.
   c. former employee.
   d. either b or c.

3. One of the FSG seven steps to ensure due diligence is to
   a. enforce adequate disciplinary sanctions when appropriate.
   b. establish methods for faking compliance reports.
   c. effectively prevent staff from seeing the plan's contents.
   d. respond only to episodes of serious noncompliance.

4. HIPAA is a law that is applicable to
   a. only Medicare-participating hospitals.
   b. only Medicare-participating physicians.
   c. all health care providers.
   d. all hospitals with more than 100 beds.

5. All of the following are acceptable reporting systems for noncompliance except
   a. telephone hotline.
   b. dedicated e-mail.
   c. online form.
   d. All of the above are acceptable.

6. Coming to work while intoxicated and thereby endangering the lives of patients might be cause for
   a. verbal warning.
   b. written warning.
   c. additional training.
   d. termination.

7. Once a report has been received that a possible infraction has occurred, the first step an administrator should take is
   a. initiate an investigation.
   b. terminate the suspected employee.
   c. phone the police.
   d. contact the department of Health and Human Services.

8. According to the FSG, when a compliance plan structured on their seven steps of due diligence is being used, the facility may receive a discount of _____ off penalties and fines.
   a. 20 percent
   b. 45 percent
   c. 70 percent
   d. 90 percent

9. Implementing a compliance plan can establish your facility as
   a. uncaring about patient care.
   b. honest and respectful.
   c. greedy.
   d. afraid of the authorities.

10. Compliance plans must address how to properly behave according to
    a. federal and state laws.
    b. administrative laws.
    c. initiatives.
    d. all of the above.

FILL-IN-THE-BLANK

Fill in the blank with the accurate answer.

11. The _____ Act requires a physician who treats Medicare and Medicaid beneficiaries to create and implement a compliance program.

12. It is important to create a _____ process for individuals to report alleged violations without fear of repercussions.

13. As the administrator, you should establish regularly scheduled _____ audits to ensure compliance.

14. The Federal Sentencing Guidelines include seven steps to ensure _____ is done properly.

15. Consequences should be documented, specifically for various levels of _____.

16. Create a _____ that will enable any member who witnesses a violation to inform administration.

17. Education of the staff requires more than just publishing a(n) _____.

18. Certain circumstances of noncompliance may best be served by having the staff member attend _____ on policies and procedures.

19. A complete compliance plan includes specific _____ for failure to comply.

20. All laws and regulations must be interpreted and incorporated into internal _____ procedures.

TRUE/FALSE

Determine if each of the following statements is true or false.

21. Compliance plans are only useful to large organizations, such as hospitals.

22. A compliance plan lays out the details of precisely how each individual staff member should go about completing their individual tasks and responsibilities.

23. Internal policies and procedures should be adjusted to make it easier for everyone to comply.

24. A qui tam lawsuit is covered by the Whistleblower's Statute, a part of HIPAA.

25. Advance planning is the key to managing a crisis effectively.

26. Consequences should be vague so you can punish each individually differently.

27. Once a violation has been discovered, you will need to determine if the breach is the employee or the policy.

28. A compliance plan is a general overview for the ethical conduct of staff members.

29. A properly created and implemented compliance plan may reduce the assessment of fines and penalties.

30. Of all the reports coming into the company's hotline, only those that seem credible and worthwhile should be investigated.

WHEN YOU ARE THE ADMINISTRATOR . . .

Critical Thinking and Analysis

Case Study #1

Hospice Employee Fraud

Review and analyze the facts in the *OIG* press release shown in Box 8-4 ■. **Discuss what you would do had you been the administrator of this hospice and these five nurses worked for you. If you discovered this fraud prior to the government audit, how would you handle this situation internally? Be specific about what actions you would take. What might you do to prevent future staff members from perpetrating this same type of fraud at your facility?**

BOX 8-4	Multi-Million Dollar Hospice Health Care Fraud Scheme Alleged

PHILADELPHIA - An indictment was unsealed today charging five nurses in a health care fraud conspiracy arising from their employment at Home Care Hospice, Inc. ("HCH"), a hospice care provider in Philadelphia, between 2005 and 2008, that resulted in a multi-million dollar fraud on Medicare. Patricia McGill, 64, of Philadelphia, was a registered nurse and served as the Director of Professional Services for HCH. She allegedly authorized and supervised the admission of inappropriate and ineligible patients for hospice services, resulting in approximately $9.32 million in fraudulent claims. She is charged, along with Natalya Shvets, 42, of Southhampton, PA, Giorgi Oqroshidze, 36, of Philadelphia, Yevgeniya Goltman, 42, of Newtown, PA, and Alexsandr Koptyakov, 39, of Bensalem, PA, with one count of conspiracy to commit health care fraud and numerous counts of health care fraud. All five defendants were arrested this morning.

HCH was co-owned by Matthew Kolodesh, who is charged separately in an indictment unsealed October 12, 2011, and "A.P." the Hospice Director for HCH. HCH was a for-profit business at 1810 Grant Avenue, and later 2801 Grant Avenue, in Philadelphia, that provided hospice services for patients at nursing homes, hospitals, and private residences. According to the indictment, announced by United States Attorney Zane David Memeger, McGill authorized nursing staff and supervisors, including her co-defendants, to fabricate and falsify documents in support of hospice care for patients who were not eligible for hospice care, or for a higher, more costly level of care than was actually provided to the patients. Between January 2005 and December 2008, approximately $9,328,000 in fraudulent claims for inappropriate patients were submitted to Medicare as authorized by AP and McGill. Defendants Shvets, Oqroshidze, Goltman, and Koptyakov created fraudulent nursing notes for approximately 150 patients indicating hospice services were provided for patients, when, in reality, they were not.

In February 2007, HCH was notified that it was subject to a claims review audit. According to the indictment, in anticipation of this audit McGill assisted A.P. in reviewing patient charts, sanctioning false documentation by the nursing staff, and authorizing the alteration of charts. In September 2007, HCH was notified that it had exceeded its cap for Medicare reimbursement and would have to repay $2,625,047 to the government program. At that point, A.P. and McGill directed staff to review patient files and discharge hospice patients. This resulted in a mass discharge of patients. In one month, 79 hospice patients were discharged in October 2007 and a total of 128 discharged by January 2008, some of whom had been ineligible for hospice or inappropriately maintained on hospice service in excess of six months. Some of the patients discharged were shifted to another hospice business owned by Kolodesh. In the Spring of 2008, approximately 20% of the discharged patients were placed back on hospice service at HCH with McGill's knowledge. McGill is charged in 14 counts; Shvets is charged in eight counts; Oqroshidze is charged in seven counts; Goltman is charged in four counts, and Koptykov is charged in eight counts.

If convicted of all charges, McGill faces a potential advisory sentencing guideline range of 108 to 135 months in prison, a fine of up to $150,000, and a $1400 special assessment; Shvets, Goltman, and Koptykov each face a potential advisory sentencing guideline range of 27 to 33 months in prison, a fine of up to $60,000, and an $800 special assessment; Oqroshidze faces a potential advisory sentencing guideline range of 21 to 27 months in prison, a fine of up to $50,000 and a $700 special assessment.

The case was investigated by the Federal Bureau of Investigation and the Department of Health and Human Services Office of Inspector General. It is being prosecuted by Assistant United States Attorney Suzanne B. Ercole and Trial Attorney Margaret Vierbuchen of the Organized Crime and Gang Section in the Justice Department's Criminal Division.

Source: United States Department of Justice.

(Continued)

Case Study #2

Home Health Fraud

An investigation by the Medicare Fraud Strike Force resulted in the discovery and ultimate sentencing of a registered nurse who defrauded her home health agency and the federal government. Read Box 8-5 ▪ **If you were the administrator of this home health agency what could you have done to prevent this individual, or any staff member, from committing fraud of this nature? What policies or procedures could you implement? What actions could you enforce, within your organization that could have uncovered this illegal behavior sooner?**

| BOX 8-5 | Registered Nurse Pleads Guilty in Connection with Detroit Medicare |

Fraud Scheme

A registered nurse who fabricated nursing visit forms in connection with a $24 million home health care fraud conspiracy in Detroit pleaded guilty today for her role in the scheme, announced Acting Assistant Attorney General Mythili Raman of the Justice Department's Criminal Division, U.S. Attorney for the Eastern District of Michigan Barbara L. McQuade, Special Agent in Charge Robert D. Foley III of the FBI's Detroit Field Office and Special Agent in Charge Lamont Pugh III of the U.S. Department of Health and Human Services Office of Inspector General (HHS-OIG), Chicago Regional Office.

Beverly Cooper, 59, of Detroit, pleaded guilty before U.S. District Judge Victoria A. Roberts in the Eastern District of Michigan to one count of conspiracy to commit health care fraud.

Cooper admitted that she and others conspired to defraud Medicare through home health care companies operating in the Detroit area, including Reliance Home Care LLC, First Choice Home Health Care Services Inc. and Accessible Home Care Inc. According to court documents, Cooper fabricated nursing visit notes and other documents to give Medicare the impression that she had provided home health care services, when, in fact, home health care was not needed and/or was not being provided. Cooper also admitted that while at these companies, she signed nursing visit notes for home visits made by other unlicensed individuals to give Medicare the false impression that she had provided home health care. Court documents reveal that Cooper understood that the documents she created would be used by these companies to submit claims to Medicare for home health services that were not medically necessary and/or not provided.

Court documents show that when home health companies were inspected by state regulatory agencies, Cooper and her co-conspirators participated in staged home health visits, posing as employees of these companies and treating fake patients, all to give inspectors the false impression that these companies' operations were legitimate and that home health services were in fact being provided.

Court documents allege that between 2006 and May 2012, Cooper's conduct caused Reliance, First Choice and Accessible to submit claims to Medicare for services that were not medically necessary and/or not provided, causing Medicare to pay these companies approximately $5,403,703.

At sentencing, scheduled for July 23, 2013, Cooper faces a maximum penalty of 10 years in prison and a $250,000 fine.

This case is being prosecuted by Trial Attorney William G. Kanellis and Assistant Chief Gejaa Gobena of the Criminal Division's Fraud Section. It was investigated by the FBI and HHS-OIG, and was brought as part of the Medicare Fraud Strike Force, supervised by the Criminal Division's Fraud Section and the U.S. Attorney's Office for the Eastern District of Michigan.

Since its inception in March 2007, the Medicare Fraud Strike Force, now operating in nine cities across the country, has charged more than 1,480 defendants who have collectively billed the Medicare program for more than $4.8 billion. In addition, HHS's Centers for Medicare and Medicaid Services, working in conjunction with HHS-OIG, is taking steps to increase accountability and decrease the presence of fraudulent providers.

Source: United States Department of Justice.

Case Study #3

Administrator of Clinic Commits Fraud

Read Box 8-6 ■. **What could you do if you suspected your supervisor of committing fraud? Is there something you can do other than quitting? Explain** **what you would do if you worked for Carol and Michael Ryser and you discovered this fraud before the federal government had that opportunity.**

BOX 8-6	**Medical Clinic Director, CEO Plead Guilty to Health Care Fraud, False Tax Return**

KANSAS CITY, Mo.—Tammy Dickinson, United States Attorney for the Western District of Missouri, announced that the married owner/director and chief executive officer of a Kansas City, Mo., medical clinic pleaded guilty in federal court today to health care fraud and filing a false tax return.

Carol Ann Ryser, 76, and Michael Earl Ryser, 68, both of Mission Hills, Kan., pleaded guilty before U.S. District Judge Greg Kays to the charges contained in a June 26, 2012 federal indictment.

Carol Ryser owned Health Centers of America-Kansas City, LLC (HCA), a medical clinic in Kansas City, Mo., that was closed yesterday as part of today's plea agreement. HCA purported to specialize in the diagnosis and treatment of chronic diseases such as Lyme disease, chronic fatigue syndrome, fibromyalgia, and other auto immune diseases.

Carol Ryser, who was a medical doctor and the clinic's medical director, surrendered her medical license today as a condition of her plea agreement. Carol Ryser may never again seek licensing to practice medicine in the United States and she may never be involved as an owner or employee (or in any other capacity) with any medical clinic, hospital or other health care provider. Michael Ryser was the CEO, chief administrator and vice-president.

Health Care Fraud

By pleading guilty today, the Rysers admitted that they engaged in fraudulent billing by "upcoding" and falsifying claims submitted to insurers (including Blue Cross Blue Shield, Cigna, United Healthcare and others, as well as government programs such as Medicare and Tricare) in an effort to be paid more than the amount to which HCA was entitled.

The Ryser's scheme included: (a) billing for physician office visits when Carol Ryser was out of town; (b) billing for physician office visits when Carole Ryser had little or no involvement with the patient; (c) billing for physician office visits when the patient contact was by telephone call; (d) billing for physician-supervised services when no physician was on duty at the clinic; and (e) improperly billing for consultation services.

The federal indictment describes six variations of billing fraud and includes tables of claims demonstrating each type of billing fraud. For those claims specifically included in the indictment, the total amount billed on those claims was $359,168. The total amount that was actually paid on those claims by health care benefit programs was $51,789.

False Tax Return

The Rysers also admitted that they willfully filed a false tax return for the year 2006. They understated their gross receipts and substantially overstated their expenses for 2006.

The indictment included three tax counts alleging that the Rysers operated their business as a sole proprietorship and gross receipts were deposited into two bank accounts that Michael Ryser maintained and controlled. However, they reported only the gross receipts deposited into one bank account and just part of the gross receipts deposited into the second bank account.

The Rysers understated their $10,060,012 in combined gross receipts for 2006-2008 by a total of $2,501,802—nearly 25 percent of the gross receipts for these three years. They overstated their expenses for 2006 by $9,462,145. The total tax loss for 2006-2008 was $615,749.

Under the terms of today's plea agreements, Michael Ryser will be sentenced within a range of 24 to 30 months in federal prison without parole. Carol Ryser will receive a sentence of three years of probation, including six months of home detention. The Rysers must pay $51,789 in restitution to the health care benefit programs that were defrauded. Sentencing hearings will be scheduled after the completion of presentence investigations by the United States Probation Office.

This case is being prosecuted by Assistant U.S. Attorneys Thomas M. Larson and Lucinda Woolery. It was investigated by the Health and Human Services Office of Inspector General, the Department of Labor Employee Benefits Security Administration, the FBI, IRS-Criminal Investigation, the Defense Criminal Investigative Service and the Food and Drug Administration.

Source: United States Department of Justice.

INTERNET CONNECTIONS

Federal Register

This is the daily journal of all actions, proposed rules, final rules, presidential documents, discussions, and the like, of the U.S. federal government.

https://www.federalregister.gov/

Office of the Inspector General (IOG)

The OIG provides guidance to the health care industry to support the prevention of fraud and abuse of relevant laws. In addition, the agency has the authority to investigate, prosecute, and punish those found guilty of illegal actions. The OIG supports compliance with several documents focused on specific sectors of health care, such as nursing homes, hospitals, and third-party payers.

https://oig.hhs.gov/compliance/compliance-guidance/index.asp

Centers for Medicare and Medicaid Services (CMS)

The CMS website provides complete guidance for compliance, including their Medicare Learning Network (MLN).

http://www.cms.gov/Outreach-and-Education/Medicare-Learning-Network-MLN/MLNGenInfo/index.html

Federal Sentencing Guidelines – Overview of Organizational Guidelines

The United States Sentencing Commission (USSC) issued this overview of organizational guidelines to support efforts to created effective compliance programs.

http://www.ussc.gov/Guidelines/Organizational_Guidelines/ORGOVERVIEW.pdf

CHAPTER 9

STRATEGIC PLANNING

LEARNING OBJECTIVES

Upon completion of this chapter, you should be able to:

- Define commonly used terms, abbreviations, and acronyms.
- Recount the benefits of creating and implementing a strategic plan.
- Identify the components of a strategic plan.
- Recognize the value of staff buy-in.
- Understand how to evaluate and modify the plan, as needed.

WHEN YOU ARE THE ADMINISTRATOR . . .

As the administrator, you will need to be able to:

- Structure and execute a cohesive strategic plan designed to ensure the effective and efficient delivery of services.
- Analyze data to identify trends of improvement or areas of concern and maintain processes designed to follow up on areas of concern.

KEY TERMS

buy-in
executive summary
long-term goals
mission statement
objective
psychographics
short-term goal
strategic goal
strategic plan
SWOT analysis

INTRODUCTION

A health care facility is a living thing. Whether a one-physician office, a fifty-bed assisted living facility, or a 500-bed medical center, a **strategic plan** establishes the identity of the facility, defines its purpose, and illuminates its **objectives**. This is the map that shows "*You Are Here*" as well as "*This Is Where You Are Headed*" and "*How to Get There*" for one department or the entire organization. Needless to say, this is a comprehensive document and for it to provide benefits and value to your facility, it requires the critical investigation of every aspect of how this facility defines the term *success*.

This strategic plan can be a large one—for an entire organization or facility. In these cases, you will go through all the sections of this very important document in an effort to realize that, essentially, you are building the framework of the future, starting with a foundation that will answer these questions:

- *Who* is this organization to its patients, staff, and the community?
- *What* is our true purpose for existing?
- *Where* do we want to go: continue this purpose; expand our purpose; change our purpose?
- *When* do we want to achieve these purposes?
- *How* do we accomplish this?

The process of strategic planning can also be used on a smaller scale, for example when launching a project or single program. In these cases, a three-step approach can condense this process while still producing important results, using the CAP format:

- *Circumstance*: Analyze the context, situation, or event.
- *Aim*: Define the objectives this program or project seeks to accomplish.
- *Path*: Diagram the steps needed to accomplish the aim or objective.

BENEFITS OF HAVING A STRATEGIC PLAN

Creating a strategic plan is a great deal of work. This document will enable you to take every action and activity required each and every day in your facility, organize them with a logical and rational eye, and evaluate them to ensure that each works as an effective building block in the structure of your organization; that each functions optimally; and that each is the best option for moving the facility closer to accomplishing its mission (Figure 9-1 ■).

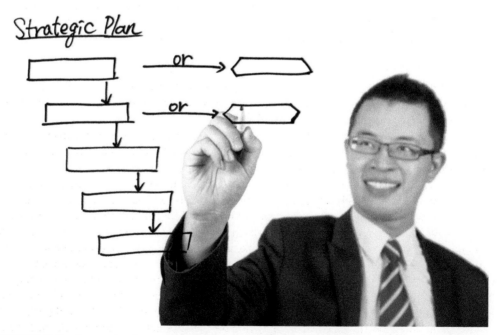

FIGURE 9-1   Strategic plans create a map of which path is best for your organization, and include alternatives, or contingencies.

Photo credit: Tom Wang/Shutterstock.

When you are beginning a program, a project, or getting ready to open a new facility, it makes sense to create a plan of action. An effective plan will list all the necessary steps you need to take to ensure your project is a success. Doing this is logical and efficient and will make sure that you don't forget anything. Over the course of the life of that program, project, or facility, it makes sense to look at that list and update it to ensure all the steps are still logical and necessary; add any new steps that are now required, such as compliance with a newly passed law; and confirm that everyone and everything are working at an optimal level.

Strategic plans, also known as five-year or ten-year plans, are commonplace in large corporations. Smaller organizations and facilities are smart when they adopt these organizational templates to use in support of their success—present and future.

GETTING STARTED

There are certain facts and other pieces of information that you should gather before technically starting the project. Understanding and completing these tasks first will make the process go more smoothly. Strategic plans are complex tools that are intended to provide a guide for the future of the organization. It would be foolish to attempt to plan the future of your facility in a day or two. In short, the more thought and work you put into the plan, the more useful and impressive it will be.

Helpful Lists

Before you start working on the plan, it is advisable to make a list of each of the following groups in your geographic area:

1. Competitors and the services they provide. You need to identify the other choices available to patients in your area when they need these services. Itemize all of the services each competitor offers to your patient population.
2. Groups or clusters that might be interested in or need your services, now or in the future, such as a nearby large retirement community or college campus. Include nearby health care facilities that are not direct competition. For example, if you are creating this plan for a skilled nursing facility (SNF), an acute care hospital in the area should be included on this list. Or a local running club would be a community group interested in or possibly needing the services of a podiatry group or orthopedic practice.
3. Suppliers or vendors with whom you have or may establish a relationship. No facility stands on its own, especially in health care. Pharmaceutical representatives, durable medical equipment companies, and so on, can provide insight and support in their own ways.
4. Other community elements that directly relate to your facility's services.

Research Methodology

Whenever possible, you need to use primary research methods. Therefore, you should first identify your sources, so, as you go through each section of the document, you will already know where to turn to get the information you need.

Primary research methods are those that involve direct interaction with the market you seek to describe. Business markets, like other social groups, typically have spheres of influence that help shape perceptions and direct the future in their industry. These persons may be vendors to the industry, consultants to the industry, members of industry media, patients, and so on. Conversations with these influential people will provide valuable market research information, capable of providing answers to questions about your typical patient population. When in contact with these individuals, always take care to document your conversation and correspondence in order to substantiate claims you may wish to make in the strategic plan as a result. Confidentiality is very important in these situations. Do not assume that persons will want to be quoted or referenced by name; you should always ask their preference and offer the veil of confidentiality. If he or she does not desire to be identified by name, it is recommended that you should note that the information was taken from "a reputable consultant to the industry" or " a well-positioned vendor to the industry." If questioned, you will have the substantiation to your claim. Patient surveys are an excellent primary research method frequently used by hospitals. The quality of the information you receive will improve if you make the provision of personal information (i.e., name, patient number) optional.

Secondary research methods are those from which you gather details from someone else's primary research. The Agency for Healthcare Research and Quality (AHRQ), CMS, CDC, and the National Center for Health Statistics (NCHS) are just a few of the available organizations from which you can collect secondary research. In addition, you can discover a wealth of information from local newspapers, trade/industry newspapers/magazines/journals such as the *New England Journal of Medicine*, the *Journal of the American Medical Association* (JAMA), *Hospitals & Health Networks* (H&HN) from the American Hospital Association, and *Hospital Compare/Nursing Home Compare* from CMS. You are also certain to gather excellent quality information from your state government or organizations within your state. For example, in the state of Florida, the Agency for Health Care Administration as well as the Florida Hospital Association can provide quality, credible data.

Make certain the research is complete before you proceed with creating the plan itself. Keep these efforts coordinated and organized; always reminding yourself what the point is of your research. What questions are you trying to answer and what information will provide real value to your planning process? Coordinate your informational gathering activities. For example, try to make phone calls to primary research sources like vendors while you are doing secondary research on vendors in the industry. Paralleling your research efforts will assist you in asking the best possible questions to your primary sources, and it will give you immediately usable and fresh leads for your secondary information sources.

Facts and Relevant Data Only

Collect only necessary and relevant information. This is not a marketing document, so you will need to set aside slogans and publicity that do not truly represent fact. Include only the facts. Limit the amount of information based on opinion or assumption. Problems occur in plans in which the writers are focusing in on what they perceive as the main issues in the plan, and, as a result, the rest of the plan sections are not adequately supported. A thorough analysis of all the elements included in the plan is necessary to have a strategic plan of value.

COMPONENTS OF A STRATEGIC PLAN

There are many popular variations used for strategic planning methodologies, such as:

PEST = Political, Economic, Social, and Technological

STEER = Socio-cultural, Technological, Economic, Ecological, Regulatory

EPISTEL = Environment, Political, Informatic, Social, Technological, Economic, Legal

The parts of the strategic plan, shown in the following sections, track one of the most frequently used formats and each contains questions that can help you and your team investigate the perception of the organization, inside and out, to find the truth. Once this is determined, corrections, if necessary, can be made to get everyone back on track.

The Executive Summary

executive summary
the first section of a strategic plan that contains summaries of all other sections within that same plan.

This first section is the **executive summary**. It contains an overview of each of the other sections of the strategic plan. The executive summary should be concise and to the point, yet still include sufficient detail to allow the reader to quickly comprehend the key factors within. Although this is the first section of the final document, for some people it is easiest when written last, so the other sections are completed and easier to summarize.

In addition to those strategic goals identified in the plan, it is a good idea to include a time line to highlight what is planned to be accomplished and by what dates. This will provide a strong visual. In this section, it is important to include an explanation of the following elements:

mission statement
an all-encompassing long-term goal or objective.

- *Mission statement.* **Mission statements** are concise one or two-sentence explanations of what this organization does and why (Figure 9-2 ■). If a mission statement already exists, review it carefully to make certain it still applies. It is not uncommon for a facility to begin with one focus and have that change over time.

Vision Statement, Mission Statement, and Core Values

The mission and vision statements are critical to the strategic planning process since they provide clear, guiding principles that further define who the health center is as an organization and why the center exists. Mission and vision statements create the foundation for action planning and a basis for accountability with the community. The mission is the *what*, while a vision is the *why*.

Vision Statement—Why do we pursue the mission everyday? We pursue it to see the vision someday becomes reality. The vision of an organization is the *dream*, the type of statement that answers the questions "where are we going" and "what can we achieve?" It is a concise word picture of what the organization strives to be, and should always be the roadmap that drives, inspires, and motivates those affiliated with the organization. This is the *real purpose* for going to work everyday . . . how the world will be different because of the organization?

Mission Statement—Mission is a statement that specifies an organization's purpose or "reason for being." The mission should capture the essence of who the center is, what the center does, and for whom. The mission should guide each day's activities and decisions. It is the primary standard against which the organization's plans and programs should be evaluated. The mission statements use simple and concise terminology, speak loudly and clearly, and generate enthusiasm for the organization. The mission is the core, it is the purpose of the organization.

It is the board's responsibility to adopt a written mission statement, which articulates the organization's goals, means, and primary constituents served. The statement should serve as a guide to the organization planning, board and staff decision making, and setting priorities among competing demands for scarce resources.

Core Values—Values are the principles and ideals that bind the organization together including the customers, employees, vendors, and all stakeholders. They are developed to frame an ethical context for the organization, and to many they are the "ethical standards" of the organization—the foundation for decision making within the organization.

All leadership must operate from the same ethical frame of reference so that decisions of one will mirror the decisions of others.

Values are critically important to organizations because those who have the same value systems, or core values, tend to succeed within the organization, while those who do not share that set of values generally do not succeed. As employees are faced with daily decision-making, the core values will serve as the guidelines. When managers' and employees' values do not match those of the organization—stated or implied—the results could be turnover, decreased productivity, dissatisfaction.

Example of CHC Vision Statement, Mission Statement, and Core Values

Vision Statement:
Community Health Center will eliminate all health disparities in our community.

Mission Statement:
Community Health Center will provide quality, primary health care services, accessible to all persons in our community including the medically underinsured and uninsured.

Core Values:
Community Health Center's Core Values are:

- Accessibility
- Availability
- Accountability
- Collaboration
- Equality
- Integrity
- Meaningful Value
- Professionalism/Leadership/Personal and Professional Growth
- Quality
- Respect
- Teamwork

FIGURE 9-2 Vision statement, mission statement, and core values.

Source: Primary Care: The Health Center Program, U.S. Health Resources and Services Administration.

- *Unique features of the facility*. Identify those specific services, procedures, or other features that are offered by no other facility in the area, or not done in the same way. For example, all hospitals may perform laparoscopic surgeries, but your chief thoracic surgeon may have more experience than any other in the area.

- *Stakeholders of the facility*. Stakeholders are all those individuals, and on occasion organizations, that have an interest in the success of your facility—patients, staff, and the community as a whole. If this is a private facility, there may also be owners and investors. None of these groups can be overlooked. They have specific expectations about this facility's purpose and some may have very specific interest in any strategic plan that takes the organization in a different direction. These are the individuals who, at least in part, will need to buy in to whatever plans are created and implemented.

- *Market overview*. This is a statistical, demographic, **psychographic**, and economic profile of the community that is served by this facility. This information is most often gathered easily from state governmental agencies. Check area projections to identify major changes—growth or reduction—expected to occur in the area. You must know the basis for your patient population—who they are, what they do, their age and occupations, their education, and other aspects of their lives. This will all come together to create a picture of who uses your facility and what services they are most likely to require.

- *Expected accomplishments*. As this plan takes form, certain specific goals and accomplishments will reveal themselves. These may be grand, such as becoming the number one facility for hip replacements in the Midwest, or they may be more personalized, such as to provide terminally ill patients and their families with the support they need, while mitigating fear and physical pain.

psychographics
four descriptors: geographical location; job title or position; education level; and mind set used to identify specific groups of consumers.

Current Situation

The current situation is a complete description of the company and its products or services. There is an old saying, "You need to know where you are before you can decide where to go." This section describes where the facility now stands. Begin with a history of the company, explaining who founded it and why. There is much to be learned from the inception—the planning and goals at that time. If you are creating this for a hospital, you might try to locate the original certificate of need filed with the state.

Follow the history of the organization with a thorough explanation of the facility's current standing in the industry. This description of the here and now should support the answers to the question: "*Who* is this organization … to its patients, staff, and the community?" Interviews with patients, vendors, owners/investors, and community leaders, as appropriate, may provide great insights into this. What is the facility's reputation in the community? How is the facility rated by authorizing agencies: CMS, Joint Commission, and so forth?

Itemize the services that you provide and to whom. Currently, does your practice focus on Medicare patients, infants and children, only those referred by a specific agency, or some other? While doing this, you might naturally think of ideas for additional services or additional groups. Write them down for later because these new ideas will not go in this section.

SWOT analysis
an evaluation of the strengths, weaknesses, opportunities, and threats relative to the facility's business activities.

SWOT ANALYSIS   Part of the current situation will be the results of what is known in management as a **SWOT analysis.** SWOT stands for Strengths, Weaknesses, Opportunities, and Threats and illuminates the four elements of an analysis important to the current standing of the facility. In order to have any value, this investigation must be conducted with great depth and honesty. Do not stop with just the obvious, or the strategy created will be equally superficial. You want to reveal specifics and perceptions about all four aspects. For example, a specific weakness may be having no x-ray machine on the premises, while an overall perception of the facility's weaknesses may be that the staff members are not friendly.

Strengths. Among your facility's strengths, there will be one or two that are key to the facility's success or failure. The business has one or more unique features that can and should be stressed in the plan and, perhaps, built upon. These key elements, reappearing in appropriate places, will provide a backbone for the organization, a core around which the other essential ideas of your strategic plan will evolve. Be certain to include the top strengths identified by internal shareholders (staff members), and compare these to the top strengths as identified by external shareholders (patients and vendors).

Weaknesses. As you analyze weaknesses, be certain to consider all points of view: the patients may see or experience weaknesses that the staff members do not see as such. In addition, the staff may be conscious of weaknesses of which the administration is unaware. In this document, all must be uncovered and laid on the table for discussion and possible action. Do not prejudge anything. It may be easy to dismiss a weakness perceived by patients as the result of their lack of knowledge of medical procedures. While this may be true, it still should be addressed, perhaps with a brochure to provide facts that will educate the patients so they can understand. Perceptions are reality to those who have them. If they are wrong, this document can help you uncover them and correct them—an important accomplishment.

Opportunities. In every community, there are opportunities previously unidentified or ignored that can be served. Keep in mind that an opportunity might be for new growth or expansion, a potential partner for a project or initiative, or an opportunity to solve a problem currently at issue. Do not dismiss any from this section. It is important to document any and all opportunities that your facility might address. You can evaluate and prioritize them all later.

Threats. One benefit from this process is the identification of threats to your facility's success that might otherwise go by unnoticed until it is too late. It has happened so often to large companies who took a huge hit from which the company could not recover because they did not pay attention to the threat on the horizon. Rather than ignoring a threat, a strategic plan can help to turn a threat into an opportunity. At the very least, the strategic plan can support actions that may lessen the negative impact.

Strategic Goals

Strategic goals are the statements of how the organization will accomplish the objectives and eventually, the mission. The mission statement presents the ultimate objective. In this step, you will need to enumerate the individual objectives that will enable the accomplishment of that mission—the staircase containing all of the steps along the path, made up of **short-term goals** and **long-term goals**.

Action items should be specific, so those individuals assigned to complete them will be clear as to what needs to be done. When a project or the mission is complex, it may be beneficial to organize the list of objectives into hierarchies. You might use a tiered model that creates a linear path to completion (Figure 9-3 ■): do this first, then this, then this. This works best when each subsequent goal depends upon the successful completion of the one prior. For example, in

strategic goal
a statement of how the organization expects to achieve an objective.

short-term goal
action and accomplishment intended to be realized within one to three years.

long-term goal
action scheduled for completion in five to ten years from the plan's implementation.

Linear Time Line of Tasks					

Project: Hire a Phlebotomist   Deadline: March 30

Dept: Immunology   Manager: H.C. Pearson

Task	Week 1	Week 2	Week 3	Week 4	Week 5
Determine state requirements and write job description					
Place classified ad					
Review all resumes received					
Interview top ten candidates					
Hire and have employee go through orientation					

FIGURE 9-3 Linear time line.

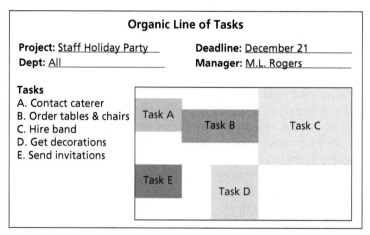

FIGURE 9-4   Organic time line.

a step toward a mission of establishing a full-service health center for patients, a phlebotomist needs to be hired, so blood specimens can be taken right at the physician's office as soon as the physician orders tests to be done. First, research must be done to determine the state and federal requirements for a phlebotomist, an ad must be placed, résumés reviewed, interviews held, and a hiring decision made. All of these mini-goals must be done in this order. You cannot hire anyone until you know the legal requirements, and you cannot interview a candidate until you advertise.

Other projects may be more organic, involving small, medium, and large tasks—all of which need to be completed, however, not necessarily in a specific order (Figure 9-4 ■). For example, you are planning a holiday party for the staff members. A caterer must be hired, chairs and tables must be rented, and decorations must be ordered. As long as all of these tasks are completed by the date of the party, it doesn't matter in which order they are done.

IMPLEMENTING THE PLAN

Once the plan is complete and the team feels that it represents the facility's objectives and clearly defines what must be done to accomplish them, it is ready to implement. This should be done in two steps: obtaining consensus and delegating action-oriented assignments.

Obtaining Consensus

The best method for ensuring compliance with the strategic plan is to first obtain consensus from the staff members. This is commonly known as getting the **buy-in**. Technically, the organization has no obligation to explain itself to its staff members. When the organization gives an order for something to be done, the staff members are obligated to act accordingly and get it done. However, this type of tyrannical management style does not promote excellence. In reality, staff members forced to do things they don't understand or with which they disagree, will often result in unhappy employees doing as little as possible. When working to get employee buy-in, you will need to present the plan to the staff members and explain the thinking behind the actions. Take the time to convince them, just as you may have had to convince the board of governors. You are not seeking their permission; you are seeking their understanding that hopefully will lead to their agreement.

Psychologically, when you explain your reasoning and provide the big picture, you are treating them with respect. When they can understand how their task or responsibility fits into that big picture, they gain a sense of importance and a sense of belonging. For example, method A—the administrator comes into a department's weekly meeting and hands over a large stack of papers (patient surveys) and tells them that all patients treated by this department must complete a survey no later than the end of the month. Can you imagine the resentment these staff members may feel? Typically, they will feel overloaded, and some may feel abused—another task added onto an already too-full workday. Or perhaps they will worry

buy-in
obtaining consensus from participants before putting a plan into action.

Organic Line of Tasks

Project: <u>Staff Holiday Party</u>   **Deadline:** <u>December 21</u>
Dept: <u>All</u>   **Manager:** <u>M.L. Rogers</u>

Tasks
A. Contact caterer
B. Order tables & chairs
C. Hire band
D. Get decorations
E. Send invitations

Task A   Task B   Task C
Task E   Task D

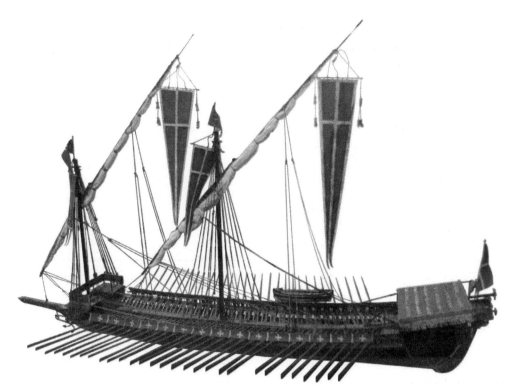

FIGURE 9-5 The oarsmen of a galley ship had to row in the same direction or the ship would not arrive at its destination efficiently.

Photo credit: Maria Thyes.

that the administration will use the patient surveys against them at their next performance review or possibly use them to fire a few people or even close the department. Now, consider method B—the administrator comes into a department's weekly meeting and hands over a large stack of papers (patient surveys). You (the administrator) explain to the group why the organization has decided to survey the patients of this department. You go over the questions on the survey with them and give them insight into why that question is being asked and what data you are hoping to gain from the answers. You tell them what you will do with the information they are gathering via these surveys. Then, you ask them to *help* by getting their patients to complete the surveys by the end of the month. Can you feel the difference? So can your staff members.

Some say all this comes down to semantics. Use different words, but the action is the same. Actually, it comes down to respect. When you share your vision with your employees, they can help you get there more effectively and efficiently. Do you remember those old boats with many oars (Figure 9-5 ■)? Think about how smoothly the boat glides through the water with all of the oars pulling in the same direction at the same time. Now, imagine half of the oarsmen are rowing in the opposite direction. The boat may get nowhere. The boat may move in circles. One thing is for certain—the boat will have more difficulty getting to its destination. When you treat your staff with respect and help them be a part of the team, you will gain the benefit of their knowledge, skill, and energy. This is working smarter, not harder.

Delegating Action-Oriented Assignments

Once you have built consensus, distribute the assignments. You will need to manage this project and keep everyone on task and on time. Make certain every task has a deadline for completion. Larger activities should have intermediate deadlines for individual steps to be completed. This will help ensure that the project does not fall behind.

Keep communications open with your team by scheduling regular meetings, weekly or biweekly, so you can answer any questions that may arise from the implementation. Direct each person to complete a status update sheet, so you have documentation tracking his or her activities.

Action or Activity	Action or Activity Deadline for Completion	Status: 1= Untouched; 2 = Started; 3 = Halfway Completed; 4 = Almost Completed; 5 = Completed	Status Description	Date of This Status Report
Allergy Clinic: Patient surveys/ patients signed up for weekly shots	December 25	3	65% completed	October 1
Allergy Clinic: Staff surveys/ Full time	November 15	5	100% completed	October 1

FIGURE 9-6 Strategic plan project status sheet.

You might use something like the status sheet shown in Figure 9-6 ∎. This will also give you the opportunity to identify problems with logistics, implementation, or an individual staff member who might be unable to complete his or her assigned task.

For example, let's take our previously mentioned patient surveys. It comes up in a meeting that many patients are on vacation due to a holiday between now and the end of the month. What should be done? Should the staff mail the surveys to the patients and hope they will mail them back in time? Should they not worry about these patients and focus on only those patients who come in? Should you move the survey period to the next month when there are no holidays and you can get data from more patients? These are issues that may only come to light during implementation, and you, as the administrator, need to provide the answers. Without regular meetings, you might never have known.

MEASUREMENT AND EVALUATION OF PERFORMANCE

Putting the plan into action is not the end of the project. Throughout the implementation of the plan, you should take notes on how the process is going. Were there any interruptions or difficulties in processing any of the activities, start to finish? Are any systems in place that could be adjusted so they run more smoothly? Within the course of the project, did anything come to light that needs to be modified, altered, or adjusted to make things better? The strategic plan must be a flexible document. It all must be a continuous stream of improvement, as processes are integrated into everyday work.

Strategic plans are typically designed around those short-term goals—one to three years—or the long-term goals—five to ten years. Whichever range of planning is chosen for your facility's plan, updates should be scheduled and the organization should be firm about keeping to this schedule. This will provide the organization the opportunity to learn, and benefit, from the observations of the implementation thus far.

CHAPTER REVIEW

SUMMARY

A strategic plan is a comprehensive document, and for it to provide benefits and value to your facility, it requires the critical investigation of every aspect of how this facility defines the term *success*. This document will enable you to organize and evaluate every activity to ensure that each works as an effective building block in the structure of your organization. Strategic plans are complex tools that are intended to provide a guide for the future of the organization. A thorough analysis of all the elements included in the plan is necessary to have a strategic plan of value.

Strategic goals are the statements of how the organization will accomplish the objectives and, eventually, the mission. The mission statement presents the ultimate objective. Once the plan is complete and the team feels that it represents the facility's objectives and clearly defines what must be done to accomplish them, it is ready to implement. This should be done in two steps: obtaining consensus and delegating action-oriented assignments.

Annual updates should be scheduled for the plan so as to provide the organization the opportunity to learn from the observations of the implementation so far, and benefit from the results of putting theory into action.

REVIEW QUESTIONS

MULTIPLE CHOICE

Choose the most accurate answer.

1. When administration seeks "buy-in" from staff members, it means they are looking for
   a. an investment in the company.
   b. consensus from the staff.
   c. staff to chip in cash to pay for a new project.
   d. enrollment in a payroll deduction plan.

2. A market overview includes
   a. pharmaceutical representatives.
   b. unique features of the facility.
   c. psychographic profiles.
   d. a mission statement.

3. SWOT stands for
   a. strategy, withdrawal, onset, termination.
   b. structure, weakness, offensive, technological.
   c. social, weakness, objective, tactical.
   d. strengths, weaknesses, opportunities, threats.

4. Strategic goals are a statement of _____ the organization expects to achieve an objective.
   a. how
   b. when
   c. why
   d. who in

5. Which of the following describes primary research?
   a. Surveying the patients
   b. Downloading statistics from NCHS
   c. Reading an article in JAMA
   d. All of the above

6. Which of the following describes secondary research?
   a. Surveying the patients
   b. Downloading statistics from NCHS
   c. Reading an article in JAMA
   d. b and c only

7. An all-encompassing long-term goal is known as the _____ statement.
   a. buy-in
   b. action
   c. mission
   d. demographic

8. The executive summary includes all of the following EXCEPT
   a. SWOT analysis.
   b. market overview.
   c. unique features of the facility.
   d. stakeholders of the facility.

9. A CAP plan includes which of the following three sections?
   a. Clinical coverage, accomplishments, projections
   b. Circumstantial, action, plan
   c. Control, achievements, plans
   d. Circumstance, aim, path

10. When a task must be completed before the next task begins, this can be illustrated in
   a. an organic line of tasks.
   b. a linear time line of tasks.
   c. both a and b.
   d. neither a nor b.

FILL-IN-THE-BLANK

Fill in the blank with the accurate answer.

11. Obtaining the consensus of staff is known as getting the _____.

12. Some _____ to the organization can be turned into an opportunity.

13. A goal planned to be accomplished within one to three years is considered a _____ goal.

14. An organic line of tasks can be accomplished in _____ before the deadline.

15. _____ can be kept open with weekly or biweekly meetings.

16. A Strategic Plan _____ Sheet can document the accomplished steps and those lagging behind within a project.

17. Actions scheduled for completion in five to ten years from the plan's implementation are considered _____.

18. Identification of education, social status, income, and political affiliation of a specific sector of the population are data elements categorized as part of the _____ profile.

19. A cohesive _____ can help ensure effective and efficient delivery of services.

20. A strategic plan creates a foundation with answers to the questions: Who? What? _____ When? and How?

TRUE/FALSE

Determine if each of the following statements is true or false.

21. For a strategic plan to provide benefits, it requires the critical investigation of every aspect of how this facility defines the term *success*.

22. An objective is a statement of how a goal will be accomplished.

23. Creating a strategic plan should not take more than a day or two.

24. Getting statistics directly from an AHRQ study is known as primary research.

25. Paralleling your research efforts will assist you in asking the best possible questions.

26. A brief analysis of all the elements included in the plan is sufficient to have a strategic plan of value.

27. The executive summary is the last section of the plan, but should be written first.

28. Unique features of the facility are those services, procedures, or other features that are done by no other facility in the area.

29. A market overview will include a demographic profile of the community that is served by the facility.

30. The Current Situation section of the plan should answer the question, "How do we accomplish these goals?"

WHEN YOU ARE THE ADMINISTRATOR . . .

Critical Thinking and Analysis

Case Study #1

Clinical Public Health Group Mission

The Veterans' Administration, Clinical Public Health Group has a strategic plan that includes this mission:

"We improve the health of Veterans through the development of sound policies and programs related to several major public health concerns. This includes HIV infection, hepatitis C infection, seasonal influenza, smoking and tobacco use cessation, health-care associated infections, and other emerging public health issues.

Our primary focus is the health of Veterans. In order to achieve this goal, we work with Veterans and their families, organizations that represent and support Veteran health care needs, and the variety of providers who deliver clinical, preventive, and support services to Veterans.

Our mission is accomplished through a variety of efforts, including: education and outreach, policy development, clinical demonstration projects, quality improvement initiatives, population based surveillance, performance measurement, clinical practice guidelines, and research."

Source: Clinical Public Health Group, United States Department of Veterans Affairs.

How would you use this mission statement to create an outline for a strategic plan? Come up with at least three action steps that you could include in a strategic plan to accomplish at least one of these visions.

Case Study #2

Strategic Plan for Health Care for Increased Population of Young Women in the Military

Based on statistics cited in the Women's Health Sourcebook, the VA documents, "*The number of young women in VHA [Veterans Health Administration] has been growing rapidly in recent years. This rapid demographic shift highlights the need to assure ample capacity for clinical services necessary for women in their reproductive years and to assure that healthcare providers' knowledge and skills are up to date in this clinical domain.*"

Source: Sourcebook: Women Veterans in the Veterans Health Administration, U.S. Department of Veterans Affairs.

Write a mission statement that will provide a foundation for a strategic plan designed to address the specific health issues for which young women may require services. Specifically emphasize those services different than those needed by men of the same age. Be certain to include attention to what health care professionals need to provide those required services.

Case Study #3

Tobacco Use Cessation Treatment Guidance

The Veterans Health Administration has issued a plan for health care professionals to implement supporting patient reduction of tobacco use. The program is called "The 5 A's" (ask, advise, assess, assist, arrange) (Figure 9-7 ■). Perform a SWOT analysis for the development of a successful Tobacco Use Cessation initiative.

Source: U.S. Department of Veterans Affairs Office of Public Health and Environmental Hazards.

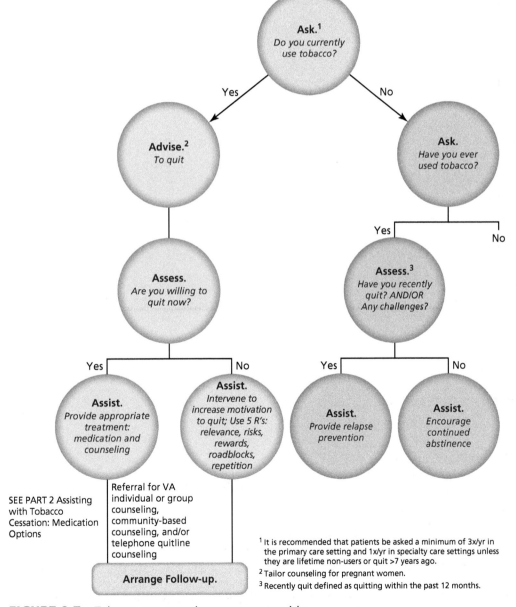

FIGURE 9-7 Tobacco use cessation treatment guide.

Source: U.S. Department of Veterans Affairs Office of Public Health and Environmental Hazards.

INTERNET CONNECTIONS

U.S. Department of Health and Human Services Strategic Plan 2010–2015

The US Department of Health and Human Services (DHHS), an agency of the federal government, also has to create a strategic plan. This is published on the Internet and available for download.

http://www.hhs.gov/secretary/about/priorities/strategicplan2010-2015.pdf

American Hospital Association Strategic Plan 2012/2013

The American Hospital Association has posted its strategic plan on this International Hospital Federation website. Read through their vision, mission, values, and goals.

http://www.ihf-fih.org/en/IHF-Newsletters/Articles/February-2011/Hospitals-and-Health-Services-Worldwide-News/Americas/American-Hospital-Association-Strategic-Plan-2011–2013

Practical Techniques for *Strategic Planning* in *Health Care*

An article from the Health Information Management Systems Society (HIMSS) in conjunction with the American College of Physician Executives created this 4-page summation of strategic planning for health care organizations.

http://www.himss.org/files/HIMSSorg/content/files/Code%2039-Practical%20Techniques%20for%20Strategic%20Planning_ACPE_2010.pdf

RISK MANAGEMENT

adverse outcome
cost-benefit analysis
harm
mitigation
proactive strategy
reactive strategy
risk
risk management

LEARNING OBJECTIVES

Upon completion of this chapter, you should be able to:

- Define commonly used terms, abbreviations, and acronyms.
- Identify the steps required to complete a risk assessment.
- Explain the benefits of performing a risk assessment.
- Enumerate the challenges to completing a risk assessment.
- Complete a cost-benefit analysis.

WHEN YOU ARE THE ADMINISTRATOR . . .

Your responsibility as a health care administrator includes doing everything you can to protect the facility, the patients, and your staff. Therefore, you will need to be able to:

- Research, analyze data, and determine the validity of recommendations for the addition, expansion, or reduction of specialized services currently provided by the organization.
- Create a balanced budget, along with a strategic plan, to maintain fiscal health for the organization.

INTRODUCTION

The community is clamoring for hospice care to be established, the emergency department needs expansion, and your chief of surgery claims robotic surgical equipment is *required* to properly care for patients. The smallest health care office to the largest hospital may seek to expand services and increase revenues. At the same time, you, as the administrator, will need to keep control over the **risk** and liability issues that accompany any improvements, such as upgrades to digital imaging equipment, expanding services. or investing in telemedicine. The financial issues are important in a decision of this magnitude; however, there is more to these decisions than money.

Laws that affect virtually every type of business mandate various levels of risk management. For example, the Occupational Safety and Health Administration (OSHA) has its rules and regulations to ensure that your facility provides a safe work environment for your staff. Health care laws, regulations, and ethical codes demand that you prevent negligence and substantiate that everything possible is done with regard to patient safety. This chapter will discuss these and other elements within your purview as an administrator that may present any type of risk to your organization.

RISK

The word risk indicates the likelihood that a piece of equipment or service will not perform according to expectations; that instead of benefit to a patient or the facility, **harm** may actually be the result. A risk assessment will include identification of what bad things *could* happen, the estimation of how serious the harm could be, and to whom. You need to evaluate what could possibly go wrong. The process of risk assessment will help you determine how strong a possibility this might be, thereby helping you to predict if the action will be one of more harm than benefit and, therefore, too risky.

Risk management is the creation and enactment of strategies determined to reduce the negative impact of risk. There are two ways you can reduce the effect of risk on the facility: proactive and reactive. A **proactive strategy** will work to diminish the opportunity for an **adverse outcome** (harm). These are policies, actions, and set-ups that will prevent or, at least, minimize the harm from transpiring. These strategies will, very often, support patient care quality improvement as well as compliance with health care legal and ethical requirements. A **reactive strategy** is the agreed-upon plan that instructs staff what to do after an adverse outcome has occurred. In addition, the reactive strategies should be studied to determine if a proactive strategy might be developed to prevent this specific outcome from happening again. Reviewing complete incident reports and investigating the origin of the incident will support improvement efforts (Figure 10-1 ■).

PROJECTS THAT POSE RISK

In addition to the standard risks associated with almost every medical procedure, service or treatment, there are projects that may be proposed for growing the facility. Let's begin with an overview of the types of proposals that may be presented to you, as the administrator, for evaluation of implementation. You may initiate a proposal yourself or a physician or other member of the staff may originate one. Ideas can come from anyone, however, the final decision to proceed, or not, will come from you and your board of directors. Some examples are:

- New equipment: The purchase of anything from a new brand of tongue depressors to a new robotic operating system
- New physical space: Expansion of the existing physical space or moving to a new location
- Additional staff: The hiring of clinical or administrative staff
- Additional services: The addition of services provided to your patients, such as an in-house pharmacy or imaging equipment.
- Expansion of population services: The addition of community outreach initiatives, such as flu shots provided at the local community center.
- Telemedicine: The use of robots or enabling physicians to access patient information from outside the facility so they can provide interpretation and consults.

risk
the statistical calculation that an adverse outcome might occur.

harm
physical or psychological injury.

risk management
the process by which an organization can reduce the opportunity for an adverse outcome, or harm, to result.

proactive strategy
a plan to prevent, or diminish the opportunity for an adverse outcome.

adverse outcome
an unexpected reaction (harm) from a procedure, service, or treatment, including medications; also known as adverse effect.

reactive strategy
a plan that specifies what actions staff members should take after an adverse outcome has occurred.

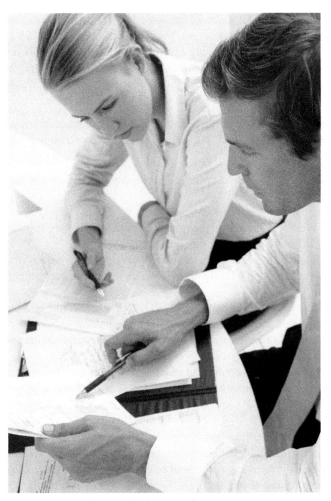

FIGURE 10-1   Incident reports can reveal unforeseen concerns.

Photo credit: Monkey Business Images/ Shutterstock.

STEPS OF A RISK ASSESSMENT

It is expected that the proposal itself will focus on the benefits, the contribution to the greater good, future profitability, as well as available tax deductions or credits. However, nothing is perfect; not humans, not machines. Therefore, everything has risk.

The complexity of the proposed project will govern how intense this assessment will become. However, even with the simplest idea, completing all of these steps diligently can only serve to protect your facility and your people.

Step 1: Identify the Harm That Could Be Caused

This step requires you and your team to look deeply into any proposal to determine what possible harm, *any* possible harm, could be caused. You may need to broaden your perspective—do not only think about physical harm. Some projects or actions may cause psychological harm, while others may result in financial harm.

Examples:

1. *The request for a security door into the back area of the emergency department was denied due to the cost. Annette wandered into the area while the receptionist was helping someone else. While looking for her husband who had been brought in earlier, she observed a car accident victim being brought in by paramedics. The victim's face had gone through the windshield; he was bloody and screaming in pain. Annette sued the hospital for psychological trauma because she has been having nightmares about that patient.*

2. *One of the physicians used his political influence to get approval for a telemedicine robot. The funds to pay for this were taken from the budget planned to pay for the expansion of the intensive care unit (ICU) including additional staff and beds. This action resulted in having to send patients to another facility, delaying their treatment, further endangering their lives as well as denying the facility future revenue from the additional patients that could have been cared for in the expanded unit.*

In addition to the potential physical, financial, and psychological harm, you must also evaluate the cost to the organization—not just the price tag on the equipment but the hidden costs (Figure 10-2 ■).

- Will implementation result in lost productivity of any member or members of the staff? If so, to what extent?
- How intense is the learning curve to train staff to use the new equipment or provide the new service? What will happen to their other job tasks while they learn? What is the cost for temporary fill-ins, overtime, or other costs?
- Will continued use of the equipment or service increase the overhead of the organization; utilities, staff, property and liability or malpractice insurance, support equipment? If so, to what extent?
- What is the expected return on investment (ROI)? In other words, how long will it take for the investment in this equipment or service to be profitable?
- Will any part of the implementation phase cause an interruption of current services to existing patients?
- Does the project require government or other agency authorization prior to implementation? If so, what is involved to apply for approval? How long does this approval process take?

Step 2: Identify Who May Be Potentially Harmed

As the administrator, you have three primary groups for whom you are responsible: staff, patients, and visitors. Investigate carefully to determine what might possibly go wrong with each aspect of the proposed equipment or service, and how it might cause physical, financial, or psychological harm to any member of any of these groups. Again, keep your perspective broad. For example, you might feel that patients could not be harmed by the implementation of an electronic health records system because only staff members use it. However, patients might be harmed if their

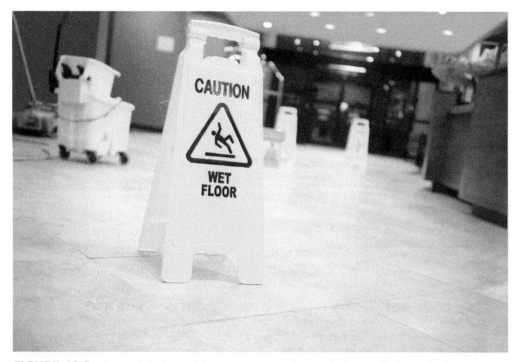

FIGURE 10-2 Potential physical hazards must be identified and eliminated whenever possible.

Photo credit: Martin Haas/Shutterstock.

records are not available during the transition from paper to digital and the physician cannot get the background data needed for accurate medical decision making.

Step 3: Determine the Risk Level

In order to accurately assess the level of risk, you will need to quantify it. The most precise method is to quantify each individual component and calculate an average rating. Begin with a definition of the various levels of risk determined by the degree of probability that harm could occur and how serious the consequences may be. The most common levels used are:

- Low risk = probability of any harm is unlikely (less than 10 percent); any harm caused could be minor or insignificant
- Medium risk = probability of harm is moderate (10 percent—50 percent); any harm caused could be moderate; preventive measures can reduce possibility; moderate limitations should be initiated
- High risk = probably of harm is likely or almost certain (over 50 percent); any harm caused could be major or catastrophic; preventive measures can somewhat reduce probability; strict limitations must be initiated

For example, the use of paper poses risk. A person can get a paper cut. A paper cut is minor physical harm and generally causes no psychological harm. However, consider this—if the paper cut is deep enough and is not properly cared for, this person can get an infection that could enter the blood stream, cause sepsis, and the patient could die. The probability of one of your staff dying (catastrophic harm) from a paper cut is very low.

Next, assign a numerical value for each, such as:

1 point = low risk
5 points = medium risk
10 points = high risk

Go through each and every element from steps 1 and 2. After you assign the risk level, list the item with the number of points for that level. When you have gone through every item on the list, add the points together, and divide the total by the number of items on the list to determine the average score. This will guide you back to a quantifiable indicator of the risk level. Table 10-1 ▪ and Figure 10-3 ▪ may help you.

Step 4: Identify Precautions That Are Already in Place

Unless you are working for a brand new facility, there are some safety measures and precautions already in place. This is an excellent time to review the organizational policies and procedures manual and evaluate how well those policies are working in reality. Review accident reports, incident reports, workers' compensation claims, and any complaints filed by staff, patients, or visitors. Interview those who work in that specific area of your facility and encourage them to suggest improvements or adjustments—or to tell you the current policy works very well. The current policies may be all you need to support the new proposal, or you may only need to make an adjustment to cover the new situation.

Step 5: Identify Additional Precautions Needed Prior to Implementation

When considering a new piece of equipment, begin by reading (actually reading, not scanning) the manufacturer's manual for proper use as well as the material safety data sheet (MSDS), if applicable. These instructions will often identify potential hazards and harm as well as provide ideas for preventive actions.

Local chapters of national trade organizations will give you access to those who work for other, similar health care facilities in your community. Discuss with them how they are supporting

TABLE 10-1 Quantifying Risk

	Minor Harm	Moderate Harm	Major Harm
UNLIKELY	Low risk	Medium risk	High risk
MODERATE	Medium risk	Medium/High risk	High risk
ALMOST CERTAIN	Medium/High risk	High risk	High risk

Risk Assessment Code Matrix (RAC)				
Probability Code / Severity Code	Frequent (A) Immediate danger to health and safety of the public, staff or property and resources.	Likely (B) Probably will occur in time if not corrected, or probably will occur one or more times.	Occasional (C) Possible to occur in time if not corrected.	Rarely (D) Unlikely to occur; may assume exposure, will not occur.
Catastrophic Imminent and immediate danger of death or permanent disability. — I	1 Critical	1	2	3
Critical Permanent partial disability, temporary total disability. — II	1	2 Serious	3	4
Significant Hospitalized minor injury, reversible illness. — III	2	3 Moderate	4 Minor	5
Minor First aid or minor medical treatment. — IV	3	4	5	5 Negligible

RAC levels are identified by a numerical scale 1–5, with RAC-1 being the most critical requiring immediate response, RAC-5 being the least critical. RACs are annotated by the RAC Number, followed by the Frequency and Severity. Examples of RAC annotations are 1(A)(I) for a RAC-1 that has catastrophic consequences and a immediate danger frequency. A 4(IV)(B) would be a low level risk, with a minor severity and a likely probability.

Risk Assessment Code (RAC)

Severity Code
Catastrophic (I)   Imminent and immediate danger of death or permanent disability.
Critical (II)   Permanent partial disability, temporary total disability.
Significant (III)   Hospitalized minor injury, reversible illness.
Minor (IV)   First aid or minor medical treatment.

Hazard Probability
Frequent (A)   Immediate danger to health and safety of the public, staff or property and resources.
Likely (B)   Probably will occur in time if not corrected, or probably will occur one or more times.
Occasional (C)   Possible to occur in time if not corrected.
Rarely (D)   Unlikely to occur; may assume exposure, will not occur.

Definitions
Probability   The likelihood that a hazard will result in a mishap or loss (Exposure in terms of time, proximity, and repetition).
Severity   The worst credible consequence that can occur as a result of a hazard.
Hazard   Any real or potential condition that can cause injury, illness or death of personnel, or loss and damage to equipment.
Risk   An expression of possible loss in terms of severity and probability (associated with human interaction).

FIGURE 10-3   Risk Assessment Code Matrix.
Source: U.S. Department of the Interior Indian Affairs.

the implementation of this same new equipment or service. This feedback can be invaluable to you and your team as you complete this assessment.

One more area might provide important information—a check on the Internet for any lawsuits or official complaints, citations, or investigations related to this specific equipment or service. Sites for the Federal Drug Administration (FDA), the agency that approves equipment and devices for medical use, as well as The Joint Commission, the Agency for Healthcare Research and Quality (AHRQ), and the Office of the Inspector General (OIG), amongst others, may be very helpful. For example, the FDA posts approvals, recalls, and communications regarding medical devices, as shown in Figure 10-4 ■. Previous legal issues can provide critical information on elements you might not have previously considered. You may also find adaptations made by other users that you might initiate from the beginning.

Medical Devices

FDA Safety Communication: Metal-on-Metal Hip Implants

Date Issued: Jan. 17,2013

Audience:

- Orthopaedic surgeons
- Health care providers responsible for the ongoing care of patients with metal-on-metal hip implants
- Patients who are considering or have received a metal-on-metal hip implant

Medical Specialties: Orthopaedics, General Medicine, Family Practice, Radiology, Radiologic Technology, Clinical Laboratory Managers and Directors

Device:

Metal-on-metal hip implants consist of a ball, stem and shell, all made from cobalt-chromium-molybdenum alloys.

There are two types of metal-on-metal hip implants:

- Traditional total hip replacement systems
- Resurfacing hip systems

Purpose: In February 2011, the FDA launched a metal-on-metal hip implant webpage. The FDA is providing updated safety information and recommendations to patients and health care providers. This new information is based on the FDA's current assessment of metal-on-metal hip implants, including the benefits and risks, the evaluation of the published literature, and the results of the June 2012 Orthopaedic and Rehabilitation Devices Advisory Panel meeting.

Summary of Problem and Scope:

Metal-on-metal hip implants have unique risks in addition to the general risks of all hip implants.

In metal-on-metal hip implants, the metal ball and the metal cup slide against each other during walking or running. Metal can also be released from other parts of the implant where two implant components connect. Metal release will cause some tiny metal particles to wear off of the device around the implant, which may cause damage to bone and/or soft tissue surrounding the implant and joint. This is sometimes referred to as an "adverse local tissue reaction (ALTR)" or an "adverse reaction to metal debris (ARMD)."

Soft tissue damage may lead to pain, implant loosening, device failure and the need for revision surgery (a surgical procedure where the implant is removed and another is put in its place). Some of the metal ions released will enter the bloodstream and travel to other parts of the body, where they may cause symptoms or illnesses elsewhere in the body (systemic reactions).

Presently, the FDA does not have enough scientific data to specify the concentration of metal ions in a patient's body or blood necessary to produce adverse systemic effects. In addition, the reaction seems to be specific to individual patients, with different patients having different reactions to the metal wear particles.

Recommendations for Orthopaedic Surgeons:

Before Surgery

- Select a metal-on-metal hip implant for your patient only after determining that the benefit-risk profile of using a metal-on-metal hip implant outweighs that of using an alternative hip system (metal-on-polyethylene, ceramic-on-polyethylene, ceramic-on-ceramic or ceramic-on-metal). Factors to consider include the patient's age, sex, weight, diagnosis, and activity level.
    - Note that a 2012 FDA advisory panel of experts identified young males with larger femoral heads as the best candidates for hip resurfacing systems.
- Inform patients about the benefits and risks of metal-on-metal hip implants, including the risk that the hip implant may need to be replaced. Also discuss the patient's expectations and review the potential complications of surgery with a metal-on-metal hip implant.
- Pay close attention to patient populations for which metal-on-metal hip systems are contraindicated. Be aware of the risk factors that may predispose a device to excess wear and early failure.

Additional information on the FDA's recommendations for orthopaedic surgeons before, during and immediately following metal-on-metal hip replacement surgery can be found in Information for Orthopaedic Surgeons

Patient Follow-Up

- Follow-up of asymptomatic patients with metal-on-metal hip implants, including physical examinations and routine radiographs, should occur periodically (typically every 1 to 2 years). If the hip is functioning properly, the FDA does not believe there is a clear need to routinely perform additional soft tissue imaging or assess metal ion levels in the blood.
- Be aware that there are certain patients who are at risk for increased device wear and/or adverse local tissue reactions (ALTR) and should be followed more closely. They may include:
    - Patients with bilateral implants
    - Patients with resurfacing systems with small femoral heads (44mm or smaller)
    - Female patients
    - Patients receiving high doses of corticosteroids
    - Patients with evidence of renal insufficiency
    - Patients with suppressed immune systems
    - Patients with suboptimal alignment of device components
    - Patients with suspected metal sensitivity (e.g. cobalt, chromium, nickel)
    - Patients who are severely overweight
    - Patients with high levels of physical activity.
- Pay close attention to signs and symptoms that may be associated with metal-on-metal hip implants. Please see the website for a list of common ALTRs and systemic symptoms/complications.

FIGURE 10-4 *(Continued)*

- Conduct a thorough evaluation if a patient with a metal-on-metal hip experiences local symptoms such as pain or swelling at or near the hip, a change in walking ability or a noise from the hip joint more than three months after metal-on-metal hip implant surgery.
- Follow symptomatic patients with metal-on-metal hip implants at least every 6 months.

Additional information on the FDA's recommendations for patient follow-up can be found in Information for Orthopaedic Surgeons.

For additional information regarding soft tissue imaging or assessing metal ion levels, please review the FDA's recommendations below.

Imaging

For some symptomatic patients with metal-on-metal hip implants, additional diagnostic imaging is required to assess and diagnose soft tissue findings surrounding the implant. Please be aware of the FDA's recommendations:

- Consider the benefits and risks of using different types of diagnostic imaging procedures (e.g. MRI with metal artifact reduction, CT, or ultrasound) as well as the availability of specialized radiology expertise when determining the most appropriate imaging modality for each patient.

If you determine that an MRI of a metal-on-metal hip implant patient is appropriate, the FDA recommends the following:

- Consult with the radiologist to evaluate the benefits and risks of utilizing MRI with metal artifact reduction;
- Review the available device-specific labeling from manufacturers for MRI Conditions; and
- Inform the MRI site that the patient has a metal-on-metal hip implant.

For additional information on the FDA's recommendations about imaging a patient with a metal-on-metal hip implant, please see Imaging Evaluation.

Assessing Metal Ion Levels

Some patients with a metal-on-metal hip implant may have elevated metal ion levels (e.g. cobalt and/or chromium) in their bloodstream. Several factors can impact the accuracy, reproducibility, and clinical interpretation of metal ion test results. Please be aware of the FDA's recommendations:

- The FDA does not believe there is a clear need to routinely check metal ion levels in the blood if the orthopaedic surgeon feels the hip is functioning properly and the patient is asymptomatic.
- Patients with metal-on-metal hip implants who develop any symptoms or physical findings that indicate their device may not be functioning properly, should be considered for metal ion testing.
- If measuring metal ions, consider obtaining and following serial measurements (using the same sample type, the same measurement method, and preferably the same laboratory) in determining metal ion levels in symptomatic patients.
- At this time, the FDA is not recommending a specific metal ion level as a trigger for revision or other medical intervention. The metal ion concentration values, including increases in metal ion levels over time, should be considered in addition to the overall clinical scenario including symptoms, physical findings, and other diagnostic results when determining further actions.

For additional information on the FDA's recommendations on metal ion test methods, selecting a test lab and interpreting test results, please see Metal Ion Testing.

Device Revision

The decision to revise a metal-on-metal hip implant should be made in response to the overall clinical scenario. In case of adverse local tissue reactions (ALTR), revision of a metal-on-metal hip implant may have a worse prognosis than revision of other types of bearing surfaces.

In selecting components for revision:

- Consider the benefits and risks of all bearing surfaces for each patient.
- Check the specific device labeling for compatibility of device components.
- If a patient is suspected to have developed metal sensitivity, carefully select the materials of the revision components (potentially avoiding materials with nickel or chromium).

For additional information, please review the FDA's considerations on device revisions, which includes our recommendation for a retrieval analysis of every failed metal-on-metal hip implant.

Summary of FDA Recommendations for Orthopaedic Surgeons

	Symptomatic Patients	Asymptomatic Patients
Regular Clinical Evaluation	At least every six months	Typically at least once every 1 to 2 years
Soft Tissue Imaging	Consider the benefits and risks of MRI, CT and ultrasound for each patient.	Not necessary if you feel the hip is functioning properly.
Metal Ion Testing	Consider monitoring serial metal ion levels. Currently, the most reliable test results are available for cobalt in EDTA-anticoagulated blood*. In repeat tests, use same sample type, measurement method and preferably the same laboratory.	Not necessary if you feel the hip is functioning properly,

*For chromium testing, a validated method that resolves potential interferences must be used. Please review FDA's recommendations for chromium testing.

Recommendations for Health Care Providers:

Metal-on-metal implant patients with systemic symptoms are more likely to visit their primary care practitioner than their orthopaedic surgeon, which makes it important for all health care providers to be aware of metal ion adverse events that may occur in metal-on-metal hip implant patients. Based on case reports, these events may include:

- General hypersensitivity reaction (skin rash)
- Cardiomyopathy
- Neurological changes including sensory changes (auditory, or visual impairments)
- Psychological status change (including depression)
- Renal function impairment
- Thyroid dysfunction (including neck discomfort, fatigue, weight gain or feeling cold.

Patients with systemic findings that are thought to be related to a metal-on-metal hip implant should be advised to follow-up with his or her orthopaedic surgeon to determine the appropriate course of action.

For additional information, please review the FDA's considerations to Health Care Professionals.

FIGURE 10-4 (Continued)

Recommendations for Patients Considering Hip Implants:

- Be aware that every hip implant has benefits and risks.
- Discuss your options for hip surgery with your surgeon.

A list of some questions to ask your orthopaedic surgeon can be found in Patients Considering a Metal-on-Metal Hip Implant.

Recommendations for Patients with Metal-on-Metal Hip Implants:

- If you are not having any symptoms and your orthopaedic surgeon believes your implant is functioning appropriately, you should continue to routinely follow-up with the surgeon every 1 to 2 years.
- If you develop new or worsening problems such as pain, swelling, numbness, noise (popping, grinding, clicking or squeaking of your hip), and/or change in your ability to walk, contact your orthopaedic surgeon right away.
- If you experience changes in your general health, including new or worsening symptoms outside your hip, let your physician know you have a metal-on-metal hip implant.

Additional information for patients with a metal-on-metal hip can be found in Patients who have a Metal-on-Metal Hip Implant.

FDA Activities:

The FDA is committed to providing reliable safety recommendations to patients and health care providers about the utilization of these devices. Recent activities include:

1. On May 6, 2011, the FDA instructed manufacturers of metal-on-metal total hip replacement (THR) systems to conduct postmarket surveillance study of these devices. Five manufacturers currently market metal-on-metal hip implants in the U.S. and all five have approved postmarket surveillance study plans. Data from these studies will provide patients and health care providers with additional information about the safety profiles of the implants, including the effect of metal ion concentrations in the bloodstream.
2. On June 27-28, 2012, the FDA convened the Orthopaedic and Rehabilitation Devices Panel of the Medical Devices Advisory Committee to seek expert scientific and clinical opinion on the benefits and risks of metal-on-metal hip systems. Information from this panel meeting has helped form these recommendations.
3. On January 17, 2013 the FDA issued a proposed order requiring manufacturers of metal-on-metal total hip replacement systems to submit premarket approval (PMA) applications. Metal-on-metal total hip replacement systems were evaluated under the 510(k) premarket notification program. Metal-on-metal total hip replacement systems were marketed in the U.S. prior to 1976 legislation that gave the agency premarket authority over medical devices. As "preamendment devices," they were designated as Class III (higher risk) devices but were regulated under the 510(k) premarket notification program.

Additional information on FDA ongoing activities are provided in FDA's Role and Activities.

Other Resources:

For additional resources, see Metal-on-Metal Hip Implants: Other Resources.

Reporting Problems to the FDA:

Prompt reporting of adverse events can help the FDA identify and better understand the risks associated with medical devices. If you suspect a problem with a metal-on-metal device, we encourage you to file a voluntary report through MedWatch, the FDA Safety Information and Adverse Event Reporting program Health care personnel employed by facilities that are subject to the FDA's user facility reporting requirements should follow the reporting procedures established by their facilities. Device manufacturers must comply with the Medical Device Reporting (MDR) regulations.

Reports to the FDA about adverse events related to metal-on-metal hip systems include, but are not limited to: pain, malposition, adverse local tissue reaction, metallosis, hypersensitivity (allergy), loosening, and dislocation.

To help us learn as much as possible about the adverse events associated with metal-on-metal hip implants, please include the following information in your reports, if available:

- Date of implantation
- Date of implant removal (if applicable)
- Clinical cause for revision (if available)
- System components affected by the adverse event.

FIGURE 10-4 Part of an FDA Safety Communication: Metal-on-Metal Hip Implants.

Source: U.S. Department of Health & Human Services.

Step 6: Consult with Those Involved or Affected By the Proposal

Before making a final determination, consult with those affected or involved in the proposal. Create an open discussion to determine the concerns and benefits perceived by your staff. Examine with them any questions or apprehensions uncovered by steps 1 through 5. Get their ideas about what may be done to reduce any perceived risks and make a sincere attempt to get a consensus. Obtaining mutual agreement on the proposal, along with any precautions or limitations, prior to implementation or denial of the project will encourage a better working relationship within the facility. In business management, this is known as *getting the buy-in*.

Step 7: Complete a Cost-Benefit Analysis

As you learned at the beginning of this chapter, risk assessment is not only about money. However, you are still responsible for doing everything possible to ensure every dollar is spent wisely. Therefore, every risk assessment should include a **cost-benefit analysis** to confirm that the investment in this new project will not cause a financial risk to the facility.

cost-benefit analysis
a mathematical process by which to evaluate whether or not the purchase of something has a value equal to or greater than the amount paid.

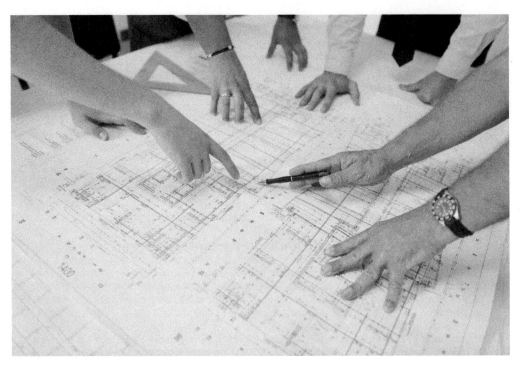

FIGURE 10-5   Costs of construction must be included in the cost-benefit analysis.
Photo credit: dotshock/Shutterstock.

Conducting a cost-benefit analysis will require the answers, in estimated dollars, to many of the questions listed in step one relating to the hidden costs of implementing the project, whether equipment or services. You will also need to factor in the estimated costs of implementing any additional policies or procedures (from step 5 and possibly step 6). In addition, you will need actual or estimated dollars for the out-of-pocket costs such as equipment, hiring temporary workers during training, and additional physical space (including construction) (Figure 10-5 ■).

A thorough analysis must also include data on the cost to the organization if the project is denied. Will the facility lose current staff or lose the ability to attract highly skilled professionals? Will the facility lose patient referrals to another facility that has this service or equipment? Are there any revenue streams, such as extensions of existing grants, which would not be available if the project is not implemented?

Now, you need to complete the other side of this analysis: income and other potential benefits. What additional patient population may be served? How much revenue could be generated from the new equipment or service? Are there additional revenue streams, such as potential grants, for which the facility would be eligible only with the new equipment or service?

The most challenging part of calculating the benefit side of this analysis is trying to determine the value (for this purpose only) of patients helped and lives saved. Of course, everyone feels that one life saved is worth any amount of money. However, that involves emotion, and this process must be limited to the business aspect of what health care professionals do. At the same time, no one can deny that patients helped and lives saved are benefits that have their place in a cost-*benefit* analysis. Figure 10-6 ■ shows you what a cost-benefit analysis may look like.

Step 8: Determine What to Do

Add it all up—the benefits and the risk—to support the decision to proceed, delay awaiting further information, or deny the proposal. Make a commitment to your choice or choices and begin the process of doing what needs to be done.

Step 9: Create the Official Document

Once the risk has been fully assessed and a final determination has been agreed upon, everything in the entire risk assessment should be documented, published, and disseminated to the board of governors, the administration, and those staff members involved. In addition, the document

COST-BENEFIT ANALYSIS—PURCHASE OF NEW X-RAY MACHINE

(Costs shown are per month and amortized over four years)

Purchase of Machine .... [including shipping, interest, and taxes]	−$55,000
Installation of Machine .... [including technician controls]	−7,338
Increased Revenue .... [net value of 3/day, 5 days/week]	+ 139,227
Material costs .... [e.g. patient shield, booties, etc.]	−375
New Technician............................. [salary plus overhead and training]	− 3,825
Utilities .... [power consumption increase for new machine]	− 250
Insurance .... [property/liability increase]	− 180
Construction .... [alter room to accommodate machine]	−500
Patient convenience, good will	+++
Net Revenue per Month	++$71,759+++

FIGURE 10-6 An example of a cost-benefit analysis.

should specify a length of time, such as six months or one year, after which a review should be performed to ensure that the process is working. In the case where a proposal has been denied, you might include a review for reconsideration, if applicable, in six months or one year due to the fact that health care changes rapidly and experimental procedures today are the standard of care tomorrow. Any necessary adjustments should be made to the document and implementation should begin.

Sometimes, the harm that can befall the organization is a lawsuit claiming the facility is liable for damages. A thorough risk assessment, including the effort to ensure that the facility has done everything possible to protect all individuals from harm, can provide evidence that you did enact preventive measures. At the least, this documentation may establish **mitigation** of liability and reduce the negative impact to your organization.

mitigation
an action taken that will lessen the severity of harm.

RISK MANAGEMENT TO-DO LIST

The Department of Health and Human Services (DHHS) published a list of suggestions for developing risk management strategies that you might use for your facility. Most of these focus on physician documentation and administrative actions. The elements may provide some ideas for you to create other strategies, as well. This is an adaptation of the DHHS list.

1. *Do maintain proper licensure, credentials, and privileges at all times.* Here, it reinforces the need to ensure these are ongoing checks maintained at least annually.
2. *Do maintain professional decorum at all times.* The provision of health care services can get very emotional for the patient and the patient's family. However, your staff must be taught methodologies to stay professional. Do not assume everyone is able to keep his or her composure when faced with another person's emotional outburst. Include this in your mandatory staff training.
3. *Do treat patients with dignity and respect.* The culture of your organization should be one that accepts nothing less than treating everyone with respect: staff, patients, and visitors. No one should ever be permitted to violate this policy—from the president and chief physician to housekeeping and reception.
4. *Do write legibly.* Electronic health records, e-mail, and other technological advancements should reduce the opportunity for handwritten notes to be illegible. However, teach your staff—if you need to write something, write it neatly.

5. *Do use only standard terminology.* Any abbreviations and acronyms should be provided in a list with agreed upon definitions to avoid miscommunication. It is not uncommon that some individuals use abbreviations and acronyms so fluidly they forget that not everyone knows what they mean. In addition, in health care, some abbreviations represent more than one phrase. For example, ROI stands for *release of information* AND *return on investment*. One printed document with approved abbreviations and acronyms, along with their accepted meanings in your facility, will eliminate any confusion and thereby eliminate the opportunity for an error.

6. *Do chart as soon after the encounter as possible.* Physicians must be trained to record their notes as soon after a patient encounter or procedure has concluded. The sooner it is all documented, the more accurate it will be. While the physician and nurse are the only creators of documentation, multiple other staff members use this documentation for coding, billing, patient referrals, statistical analysis, and more.

7. *Do chart comprehensively.* Ideally every detail should be included in the documentation.

8. *Do document any patient noncompliance.* This should include a patient refusing recommended treatment, failure to take prescribed medications or therapies, as well as failure to show up for appointments.

9. *Do initial and date all test results when reviewed.* The test results are documentation that the test was performed (lab or imaging). Ensure that the attending physician is instructed to initial and date those results to document he or she has seen this data.

10. *Do obtain proper written, informed consent prior to any non-emergency invasive procedure or any procedures not expected to be covered by insurance.* The patient must sign an informed consent document prior to the provision of many procedures or services. Make certain your documents fulfill the legal requirements and are used properly. For example, Medicare requires an advance beneficiary notice (ABN) (Figure 10-7 ■) when a procedure is to be provided for which Medicare is not expected to pay. This is an excellent policy to employ for all third-party payers. In addition, health care staff can be charged with battery—unlawful touching of an individual—should they provide a procedure or service on a patient without the patient's consent.

11. *Do ensure that patient records are clearly labeled to indicate drug sensitivities.* Include any other propensities for adverse reactions of any kind, such as an allergy to latex or penicillin.

12. *Do ensure that a suspected occurrence of malpractice or other liability is never documented in a patient's chart.* This is not the correct forum for these opinions. These suspicions should be reported as per your compliance plan reporting system.

13. *Do inform health care providers that they should never criticize another professional or staff member in the patient's chart.* Again, these complaints or issues should be presented and dealt with outside of the patient's record.

14. *Do educate all members of the staff on the proper way to change or correct chart entries.* Once something has been entered into a patient's chart, it cannot ever be obliterated, erased, or otherwise altered. Your electronic health record software should have a feature specifically for identifying an error along with entering in the correct data. On paper, a single line is to be drawn through the incorrect information and have the word "error" written above, along with the initials and date of the person making the correction. Then, the correct information should be noted, initialed, and dated.

15. *Do ensure that no part of any patient's record is destroyed without sufficient direction to do so by the administration.* There are legal requirements for the length of time documentation is to be secured. With digital files being so compact and easy to store, arrangements should be made whenever possible to keep all patient records indefinitely.

16. *Do instruct your staff never to promise a cure or guarantee results.* Every individual is different and no one can guarantee positive results. There may be a one in 100 chance something will not go as planned, but think about that one patient who is expecting a cure and ends up with a complication.

17. *Do clearly direct your staff to avoid communication with a plaintiff's family, friends, or attorney.* Once a lawsuit has been initiated, all communication between the facility and the plaintiff should be channeled through the organization's legal representative.

A. Notifier:

B. Patient Name: **C. Identification Number:**

Advance Beneficiary Notice of Noncoverage (ABN)

<u>NOTE:</u> If Medicare doesn't pay for D. _____ below, you may have to pay.

Medicare does not pay for everything, even some care that you or your health care provider have good reason to think you need. We expect Medicare may not pay for the **D.** _____ below.

D.	E. Reason Medicare May Not Pay:	F. Estimated Cost

WHAT YOU NEED TO DO NOW:

- Read this notice, so you can make an informed decision about your care.
- Ask us any questions that you may have after you finish reading.
- Choose an option below about whether to receive the **D.** _____ listed above.

    Note: If you choose Option 1 or 2, we may help you to use any other insurance that you might have, but Medicare cannot require us to do this.

G. OPTIONS: Check only one box. We cannot choose a box for you.
❏ **OPTION 1.** I want the **D.** listed above. You may ask to be paid now, but I also want Medicare billed for an official decision on payment, which is sent to me on a Medicare Summary Notice (MSN). I understand that if Medicare doesn't pay, I am responsible for payment, but **I can appeal to Medicare** by following the directions on the MSN. If Medicare does pay, you will refund any payments I made to you, less co-pays or deductibles.   ❏ **OPTION 2.** I want the **D.** _____ listed above, but do not bill Medicare. You may ask to be paid now as I am responsible for payment. **I cannot appeal if Medicare is not billed.**   ❏ **OPTION 3.** I don't want the **D.** _____ listed above. I understand with this choice I am **not**responsible for payment, and **I cannot appeal to see if Medicare would pay.**

H. Additional Information:

This notice gives our opinion, not an official Medicare decision. If you have other questions on this notice or Medicare billing, call **1-800-MEDICARE** (**1-800-633-4227/TTY: 1-877-486-2048**).

Signing below means that you have received and understand this notice. You also receive a copy.

I. Signature:	**J. Date:**

Form CMS-R-131 (03/11)   Form Approved OMB No. 0938-0566

FIGURE 10-7 Medicare ABN.

Source: CMS.gov, Form CMS R-131; http://www.cms.gov/Medicare/CMS-Forms/CMS-Forms/CMS-Forms-List.html

CHAPTER REVIEW

SUMMARY

The ability to perform an accurate risk assessment and cost-benefit analysis can enable you, as the administrator, the board of directors, and all others involved, to make decisions based on complete information. The decision may result in the alteration of existing policies and procedures, the creation of new polices and procedures, or the denial of a proposed project. Key to the process, and a part of your success as a health care administrator, is that decisions are not determined by emotion or influence but via logical and complete analysis of the facts. Completing each and every step of a risk assessment by thoroughly analyzing the potential benefits as well as the potential negative outcomes is an important process that will support projects intended to establish longstanding improvements to your facility and what it can do for its community. The vision to investigate, calculate, and prevent risk from impeding your facility's opportunities to help its patients is critical.

REVIEW QUESTIONS

MULTIPLE CHOICE

Choose the most accurate answer.

1. The word *risk* refers to the statistical calculation that a(n) _____ may occur.
   a. revenue increase
   b. adverse event
   c. funding
   d. mitigation

2. A _____ is a plan that instructs staff members what to do after an adverse outcome has occurred.
   a. proactive strategy
   b. cost-benefit analysis
   c. reactive strategy
   d. marketing

3. A _____ may be used to help decide whether or not to proceed with a proposal.
   a. staff assessment
   b. internal audit
   c. employee evaluation
   d. risk assessment

4. When assessing potential harm, consider only that which may cause
   a. physical harm.
   b. psychological harm.
   c. financial harm.
   d. all of the above.

5. Hidden costs to implementing a new piece of equipment or a new service would include
   a. lost productivity during training.
   b. taxes and delivery of the equipment.
   c. increased insurance premiums.
   d. installation.

6. In creating a risk assessment, the acronym ROI stands for
   a. reduction of income.
   b. revolutions on installation.
   c. return on investment.
   d. relative only investigation.

7. The acronym MSDS stands for
   a. material safety data sheet.
   b. manufacturers structural design strategy.
   c. medical security dental sensors.
   d. management of severe demolition sequences.

8. "Getting the buy-in" means
   a. staff must chip in to pay for the new item.
   b. budget will come from every department.
   c. mutual agreement has been reached.
   d. investment funds will come from the government.

9. A risk assessment process can be used
   a. only to determine liability.
   b. to evaluate medical treatments only.
   c. for virtually any decision making process.
   d. only when doing a cost-benefit analysis.

10. Proactive strategies are designed to
    a. diminish the cost of a project.
    b. diminish the negative publicity.
    c. increase the opportunity for an adverse outcome.
    d. reduce the opportunity for an adverse outcome.

SHORT ANSWER QUESTIONS

11. One of the physicians in your office requests a switch from wooden to plastic tongue depressors. What type of harm (physical, financial, or psychological) should be considered?

    a. Wooden sticks may result in a splinter, which is potentially a _____ harm.

    b. Plastic sticks cost more money, which is potentially a _____ harm.

12. Two new clinical trials have shown evidence that bariatric surgery considerably helped obese patients with type 2 diabetes mellitus (DM). List at least two questions to which your risk assessment will require the answers.

    a. _____

    b. _____

13. Since your hospital's pediatric emergency department opened three years ago, the number of patients coming in has increased 600 percent—doubling each year. Make a list of at least three things you will need to include in any expansion plan proposal.

    a. _____

    b. _____

    c. _____

14. Go to the website for the Federal Drug Administration, Medical Devices—News Items page...*http://www.fda.gov/MedicalDevices/NewsEvents/default.htm*

    Choose one item from the list, and then write a blog (approximately 150 words) about what you read. Focus on any risks or precautions available to avoid risk to the facility.

TRUE/FALSE

15. An adverse outcome is different than an adverse effect.

16. A mitigating circumstance is one that will lessen the severity of the harm caused.

17. When a risk assessment determines harm, it is only referring to physical harm, such as a broken leg or a laceration.

18. A proactive strategy is a plan to prevent or diminish the opportunity for an adverse outcome.

19. Risk management is the creation and enactment of strategies determined to reduce the negative impact of risk.

20. Hiring of additional staff can only help patients and never equate increased risk to the patients or the facility.

21. It is possible that patients could be harmed from the conversion from paper patient charts to electronic health records, if there is no attempt to reduce the risk.

22. Accident reports, incident reports, workers' compensation claims should be hidden and never accessed because of the risk of a lawsuit.

23. A cost-benefit analysis can help identify hidden costs to the organization of purchasing a new piece of equipment or initiating a new program.

24. A thorough cost-benefit analysis must also include data on the cost to the organization for a project that is denied.

WHEN YOU ARE THE ADMINISTRATOR . . .

Critical Thinking and Analysis

Case Study #1

Risk Identification

There are several ways that you, as the administrator, and your team can identify risks associated with your health care facility or an individual department. These methods include: brainstorming, interviewing members of the department, performing a SWOT (strengths, weaknesses, opportunities, threats) analysis, and/or diagramming.

First, choose a specific type of health care facility or specific department within a specific facility for whom you will perform a risk identification analysis. For example, choose the nurses' station in a skilled nursing facility (SNF) or a pediatrician's office.

Second, perform a risk identification analysis using one of the methods listed above to determine what environmental factors may present a risk to staff members and/or patients. Be certain to be very detailed in your analysis. Note that to really enhance the learning opportunity with this exercise, you can find a facility in your community and ask them for permission to perform a risk identification analysis in person. You might interview staff members at the facility you choose, or diagram out the physical location of any elements that could cause risk, along with any risk prevention components already in place. What improvements could you make?

Case Study #2

Risk Management and Medical Liability

Create or find a scenario that resulted in an adverse event or other unsafe occurrence for a patient or staff. Go through these steps: diagnosis, assessment, prognosis, and management for that situation and determine if there is a proactive policy or procedure that could be developed and

(Continued)

implemented. If so, describe it. If not, and this situation can only be responded to reactively, describe the steps you would take after it happens.

The Indian Health Service, of the Federal Health Program for American Indians and Alaska Natives, created this Risk Management Manual titled, "Manual for Indian Health Service and Tribal Health Care Professionals" and includes the following in section one:

"Risk management refers to strategies that reduce the possibility of a specific loss. The systematic gathering and utilization of data are essential to this concept and practice. Risk management programs consist of both proactive and reactive components. Proactive components include activities to prevent adverse occurrences (i.e., "losses"), and reactive components include actions in response to adverse occurrences. In both cases, the risk management process comprises:

- *Diagnosis—Identification of risk or potential risk.*
- *Assessment—Calculation of the probability of adverse effect from the risk situation.*
- *Prognosis—Estimation of the impact of the adverse effect.*
- *Management—Control of the risk."*

Source: Indian Health Service.

Case Study #3

U.S. Environmental Protection Agency (EPA) Risk Management Plan (RMP) Audit Program

There are several "exposures" that your facility must be prepared to deal with for the protection of your employees, such as having eyewash stations in case of an accidental splash into the eyes of a pathogen, infectious materials, or a chemical. Imagine that an accidental splash of bleach hit an employee's eyes. Create the documentation as required by the following two items that might be reviewed in an EPA audit. Itemize the required first-aid and emergency medical treatment, the emergency response protocols, and any other steps that must be taken during an exposure of this nature.

Section 112(r) of the Clean Air Act (CAA) requires EPA to publish rules and guidance for chemical accident prevention. The rules promulgating the list of regulated substances (published January 31, 1994) and the Risk Management Program provisions (published June 20, 1996) are found at 40 CFR Part 68. The Risk Management Program contains three elements: a hazard assessment, a prevention program, and an emergency response program. The entire program is to be described and documented in an RMP, which is submitted to EPA. RMP audits help ensure compliance with the Risk Management Program. EPA may require companies to modify their RMP to ensure that the RMP meets the requirements of the regulation.

A few of the elements required for compliance that will be reviewed during an audit are:

1. *Documentation of proper first-aid and emergency medical treatment necessary to treat accidental human exposures*
2. *Procedures and measures for emergency response after an accidental release of a regulated substance are documented*

Source: United States Environmental Protection Agency.

 ## INTERNET CONNECTIONS

Food and Drug Administration (FDA)

The Food and Drug Administration (FDA) is an agency of the US federal government that oversees drugs and medical devices for safety and efficacy.
http://www.fda.gov/default.htm

American Society for Healthcare Risk Management (ASHRM)

American Society for Healthcare Risk Management (ASHRM) is a national trade organization created to support risk management, patient safety, insurance, law, finance, and other related professions with an interest in risk management within the health care system.
http://www.ashrm.org/

Centers for Disease Control and Prevention (CDC)

This website contains interesting information from the Centers for Disease Control and Prevention (CDC) regarding cost-benefit analysis.
http://www.cdc.gov/owcd/eet/cba/PrintAll.html

CHAPTER 11

CRISIS MANAGEMENT

LEARNING OBJECTIVES

Upon completion of this chapter, you should be able to:

- Define commonly used terms, abbreviations, and acronyms.
- Identify the steps required to protect your facility from a crisis.
- Explain the benefits and challenges of preventive crisis management policies and procedures.
- Enumerate the various types of crises and potential impact of each.
- Complete a crisis management policy/procedure.

WHEN YOU ARE THE ADMINISTRATOR . . .

Your responsibility as a health care administrator includes doing everything possible to protect the facility, patients, and staff. Therefore, you will need to be able to:

- Design and implement crisis management plans for dealing with any extraordinary situation.

KEY TERMS

concurrent phase
crisis
endemic
epidemic
external crisis
internal crisis
medical malpractice
never event
pandemic
post-event analysis
preventive phase
recovery phase
sentinel event

INTRODUCTION

The meteorologist at the local television station has announced that a hurricane is headed directly for your city, and a tornado watch has been issued for the rural areas. Lightning has hit an electrical transformer near your facility, leaving you without electricity for seven hours, and the health department has alerted you to a possible outbreak of influenza. A physician showed up inebriated wanting to perform surgery, and the police are investigating a nurse for alleged pharmaceutical theft with the intent to distribute. You have just received notification that an ambulance is bringing a major movie star, who was involved in a car accident, into your emergency department (ED), and this must be kept absolutely confidential under the threat of major lawsuits. As the administrator, you are the one everyone will look to for direction and leadership and to keep the facility running as smoothly as any other day.

PREPARATION

The only way a good leader can handle any of these situations is to plan ahead and be prepared. This entire chapter is about preparation and will review what you may need to know, analyze, and do to ensure that your facility continues to function with only minor interference. A crisis management plan maps out, step by step, the policies and procedures that the individuals within your organization can effectively and efficiently, legally and ethically, prevent a crisis, whenever possible. In those cases where a crisis cannot be prevented, this plan will empower your staff to respond to the event and support recovery for the facility, as well as for patients and their families.

The Federal Emergency Management Agency (FEMA) created the checklist in Box 11-1 ■, which itemizes the components of a preparedness plan. It will help get you started.

BOX 11-1	**Preparedness Planning for Your Business**

The five steps in developing a preparedness program are:

1. Program Management
   1.1. Organize, develop and administer your preparedness program
   1.2. Identify regulations that establish minimum requirements for your program
2. Planning
   2.1. Gather information about hazards and assess risks
   2.2. Conduct a business impact analysis (BIA)
   2.3. Examine ways to prevent hazards and reduce risks
3. Implementation
   Write a preparedness plan addressing:
   3.1. Resource management
   3.2. Emergency response
   3.3. Crisis communications
   3.4. Business continuity
   3.5. Information technology
   3.6. Employee assistance
   3.7. Incident management
   3.8. Training
4. Testing and Exercises
   4.1. Test and evaluate your plan
   4.2. Define different types of exercises
   4.3. Learn how to conduct exercises
   4.4. Use exercise results to evaluate the effectiveness of the plan
5. Program Improvement
   5.1. Identify when the preparedness program needs to be reviewed
   5.2. Discover methods to evaluate the preparedness program
   5.3. Utilize the review to make necessary changes and plan improvements

Source: Federal Emergency Management Agency, U.S. Department of Homeland Security.

TYPES OF CRISES

Working in health care means that you and your staff (both administrative and clinical) will be involved, in some fashion, with virtually any type of **crisis** that may impact your facility, your neighborhood, your state, the nation, or possibly the world. There are many different types of crises for which you will need to be prepared.

The first step to categorizing a crisis is the determination of whether the event is internal or external.

An **internal crisis** is one that occurs within the facility and primarily effects only those within the organization. This might be a disgruntled former employee or the family member of a patient who did not survive who comes back to confront a physician, manager, or administrator. Or, this might be confrontation on a larger scale, such as a strike, picketing, or a boycott by a group that does not agree with certain organizational policies. The most well known issues that might motivate a group to picket or boycott a health care organization include anti-abortion groups and those against stem cell research. Another type of internal crisis may be the result of malevolence. For example, a criminal might enter the facility and threaten a staff member to get drugs. If you have ever seen the movie *John Q*, you will recall an example of criminal activity of this nature at a hospital. The character played by Denzel Washington held staff and patients hostage at gunpoint in the hospital's emergency room. Another type of internal crisis is organizational mismanagement. Accusations of fraudulent billing practices and a resulting investigation by the Office of the Inspector General (OIG) can cause quite an upheaval within the organization, especially between staff and patients and patients' families.

An **external crisis** is one that is focused outside of the organization. In these cases, a health care facility must be able to organize and be at the ready, as first responders or support to first responders. This category of crisis typically involves the facility doing what it does, every day, at a more intense level.

Both internal and external crises may be further classified, such as:

- *Natural Disasters*: hurricanes, tornados, earthquakes, flood, fire, lightening (Figure 11-1 ■)
- *Technological Disasters*: power failures, power surges, hackers (security breach)

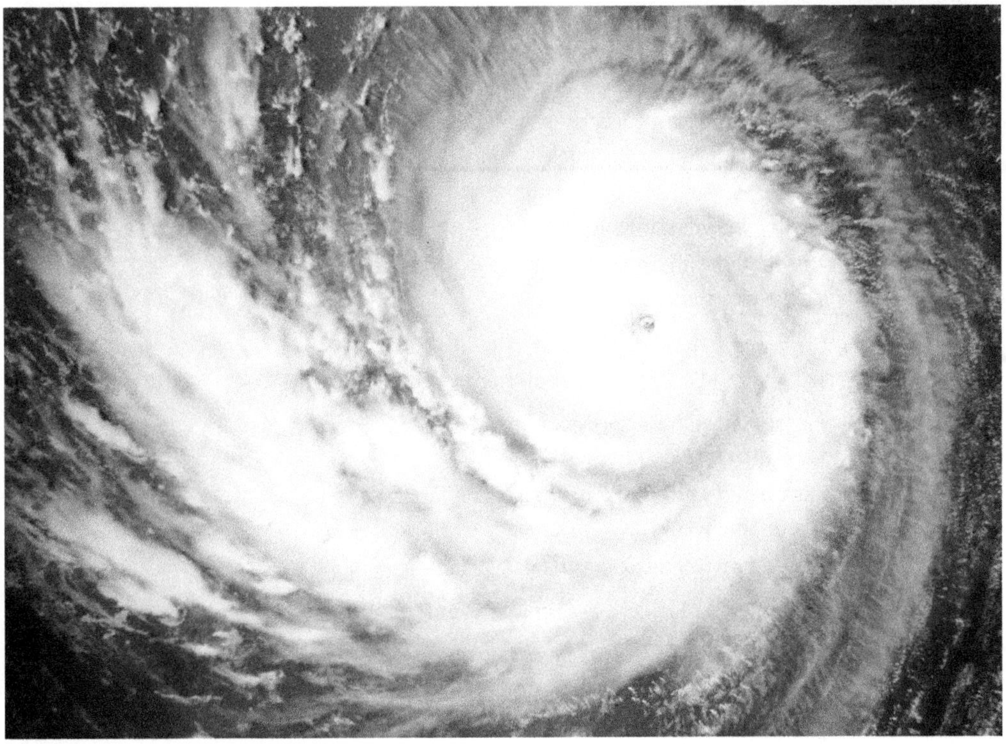

crisis
a circumstance or event that is expected to cause difficulty or danger.

internal crisis
an event that occurs within the facility and, primarily, affects only those within the organization.

external crisis
an event that is focused outside of the organization.

FIGURE 11-1 Weather events can directly affect health care facilities.
Photo credit: Vladislav Gurfinkel/Shutterstock.

medical malpractice
a legal concept that identifies negligence by a medical professional.

endemic
a disease that spreads throughout a small area, such as a community.

epidemic
a disease that spreads over a large area.

pandemic
an epidemic that occurs over a very large geographic area.

- *Human Disasters*: Staff error, **medical malpractice**, negligence, malfeasance, criminal activity, accidental injury
- *Health care Disasters*: **Endemic/epidemic/pandemic** pathogen/disease outbreak
- *Media Events and Community Relations*: celebrity patients, dealing with the media, working with law enforcement and regulating agencies such as the Federal Emergency Management Agency (FEMA)

In health care, there are certain situations relating to the quality of care provided to your patients that will require a crisis management protocol.

Medical error. All members of the staff are human and humans make mistakes. As careful as anyone may be, mistakes do happen. Following preexisting crisis management protocols in these

---

BOX 11-2 **Current NQF Serious Reportable Adverse Events**

Surgical Events

Surgery on wrong body part
Surgery on wrong patient

Wrong surgery on a patient
Foreign object left in patient after surgery

Post-operative death in normal health patient
Implantation of wrong egg

Product or Device Events

Death/disability associated with use of contaminated drugs

Death/disability associated with use of device other than as intended

Death/disability associated with intravascular air embolism

Patient Protection Events

Infant discharged to wrong person

Death/disability due to patient elopement

Patient suicide or attempted suicide resulting in disability

Care Management Events

Death/disability associated with medication error

Death/disability associated with incompatible blood

Maternal death/disability with low risk delivery

Death/disability associated with hypoglycemia

Death/disability associated with hyperbilirubinemia in neonates

Stage 3 or 4 pressure ulcers after admission

Death/disability due to spinal manipulative therapy

Environment Events

Death/disability associated with electric shock
Incident due to wrong oxygen or other gas

Death/disability associated with a burn incurred within facility
Death/disability associated with a fall within facility

Death/disability associated with use of restraints within facility

Criminal Events

Impersonating a heath care provider (*i.e.*, physician, nurse)

Abduction of a patient

Sexual assault of a patient within or on facility grounds

Source: Centers for Medicare & Medicaid Services.

cases can mitigate the impact of this error on the facility, the staff member responsible, as well as the patient and his or her family. There are many documented cases of further harm being averted because the facility handled the error in an ethical and legal manner.

Never event (also known as a **sentinel event**). A *never event* is one that *should* never happen. It *is not supposed to ever* happen; unfortunately, it happens anyway. As a result, a patient, or member of the staff, suffers serious injury or death. A *never event* is not the same thing as medical error or malpractice. Not all errors in health care qualify as a sentinel event, and not all sentinel events are the result of human error. Real life examples of never events include:

never event
an event that is not supposed to
ever happen; also known as a
sentinel event.

sentinel event
see *never event.*

- The staff was unsure which physician was assigned to a patient, resulting in delayed treatment to the patient's injury. Now, this patient's leg must be amputated because of that delay.
- A surgical instrument was left inside a patient after surgery
- Patient B was given patient D's dialysis treatment.

Your staff should have training on clearly identified policies and procedures that are specifically created to ensure these things never happen at your facility. CMS lists *never events* for which specific initiatives have been put into place shown in Box 11-2 ▨.

Malpractice. Malpractice is a legal term that requires evidence of professional negligence. This might be the failure to do something (omission of an act) required by the standard of care, such as not following up on abnormal test results, or doing something that should not be done (commission of an act) such as performing a surgical procedure while intoxicated. You, as the administrator, must be prepared to deal with the accusation of malpractice against one of your staff, whether or not the individual is actually guilty.

Inappropriate or inadequate care. An x-ray could have revealed the correct diagnosis much sooner saving the patient quite a bit of pain—but it was never done. The nurse never got back to administer that medication or the therapist never showed up, as per physician's orders. Things happen every day that result in the patient getting the wrong procedure or not getting a correct procedure. Your crisis management plan should provide the direction for staff so they will know how to handle these situations.

LEVELS OF HEALTH CARE CRISES

External crises that involve communicable diseases and their spread throughout an area can have a crisis-like impact on your facility. If you are the administrator for a hospital, your emergency department may be presented with an atypical overload of patients. All types of health care facilities, particularly physicians' offices, will be deluged with hundreds of phone calls from the community wanting to know what the signs and symptoms are and what to do. You, as an efficient administrator, need to have a plan in place to ensure a coordinated response. Which staff members should come into the facility, and which employees should stay home? Do staff members first need additional vaccinations or other method to prevent them from getting sick? Who will be in charge of triage? Who will be responsible for obtaining more medications and other necessary medical supplies? Who will answer the phones? What should they say or not say? What statements should be posted on the website? What should inquiring patients be told to do or not do? Your plan should be written to prepare in case of an endemic, epidemic, or pandemic that affects your patient population.

Endemic is identification of a disease that has spread throughout a small area, such as a community. In addition to caring for the patients as they require, you will also need to communicate with your state's health department and possibly the CDC. In addition, you will need to coordinate with the community, deal with massive numbers of phone calls, heightened traffic to your website, and potentially communicate with the media.

Epidemic is a disease that spreads over a large area, throughout your state, possibly to adjoining states. You and your staff will need to interact and follow directions from the state's health department as well as the CDC. You need to assign individuals to attend to the dramatic increase in the number of phone calls and website visitors.

Pandemic is an epidemic that occurs over a very large geographic area. While the CDC and your state's health department will provide specific direction for many of the things you will need to handle, you will still need to assign staff members to deal with all of the above. FEMA created

BOX 11-3 **Managing for a Pandemic**

Preparing for a Pandemic

- Store a two-week supply of water and food. During a pandemic, if you cannot get to a store, or if stores are out of supplies, it will be important for you to have extra supplies on hand. This can be useful in other types of emergencies, such as power outages and disasters.
- Periodically check your regular prescription drugs to ensure a continuous supply in your home.
- Have any nonprescription drugs and other health supplies on hand, including pain relievers, stomach remedies, cough and cold medicines, fluids with electrolytes, and vitamins.
- Talk with family members and loved ones about how they would be cared for if they got sick, or what will be needed to care for them in your home.
- Volunteer with local groups to prepare and assist with emergency response.
- Get involved in your community as it works to prepare for an influenza pandemic.

During a Pandemic

- *Avoid close contact* with people who are sick. When you are sick, keep your distance from others to protect them from getting sick too.
- If possible, *stay home* from work, school, and errands *when you are sick*. You will help prevent others from catching your illness.
- *Cover your mouth and nose* with a tissue when coughing or sneezing. It may prevent those around you from getting sick.
- *Washing your hands* often will help protect you from germs.
- *Avoid touching your eyes, nose or mouth*. Germs are often spread when a person touches something that is contaminated with germs and then touches his or her eyes, nose, or mouth.
- *Practice other good health habits*. Get plenty of sleep, be physically active, manage your stress, drink plenty of fluids, and eat nutritious food.

Source: Federal Emergency Management Agency, U.S. Department of Homeland Security.

a checklist of action items for patients should a pandemic be identified (Box 11-3 ■). When your staff has this information, they can pass it along to patients feeling confident they are imparting credible directions.

● THE CRISIS MANAGEMENT TRIAD

Interestingly, crisis management for a health care facility is similar to caring for a patient. There are three phases (the triad) to which you should attend: **preventive** (before the event); **concurrent** (during the event); and **recovery** (after the event) (Figure 11-2 ■). Whether starting from the beginning or reviewing an existing crisis management plan, it is imperative that the strategic thinking and analysis be completed prior to the crisis when cool, calm heads can prevail and every option can be considered and thoroughly evaluated.

It can be difficult sometimes to get members of the board and staff to take this process seriously as you may often hear, "I have been working here for ten years and there has never been a problem." It is true that preparation year after year for an event that has not yet occurred breeds

preventive phase
the opportunity to implement policies and procedures designed to avert a crisis.

concurrent phase
the time during the crisis.

recovery phase
the segment of time, after the crisis has passed, during which the organization, and all its members, must recoup and get back to a pre-crisis state.

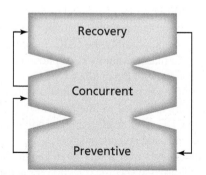

FIGURE 11-2 Crisis management triad.

complacency. This psychological problem is seen in areas such as Florida, where warnings are regularly issued to residents to prepare for hurricane season. Sometimes, years pass when no hurricanes hit land. People no longer want to pay money for preparations that go unused. They no longer want to experience the worry and anxiety—therefore, they decide that all preparations and instructions are a foolish waste of time and money. Unfortunately, the foolishness lies in the lack of preparation. A hurricane eventually hits and endangers those who have not made the necessary arrangements.

For some crises, such as a hurricane, you will be given advance notice, so you can carefully prepare for the onset of problems that may occur, such as a large influx of patients, damage to the building, or power outages. On the other hand, you will not be aware of some crises until afterward, such as when a *never event* has occurred.

What does this all mean to you, as the administrator? It means that you must attend to the need for the psychological aspects of crisis management as well as the physical and logistical, and you must prepare everyone for many more situations than just the arrival of a weather event.

Preventive Phase

Internal crises can be prevented with policies and procedures in place to ensure both patient and staff safety. Using checklists, for example, has been proven to be effective, in all clinical procedures as well as administrative tasks, for preventing errors. See Box 11-4 ■ for advice from AHRQ on the benefits of such policies. Training and reinforcement of specific patient safety protocols must be ongoing. A zero-tolerance policy should be in place so that the tiniest infraction is taken seriously. This organizational-based perspective will clearly communicate the importance

---

BOX 11-4   **Standard Written Checklists Can Improve Patient Safety During Surgical Crises.**

Patient Safety and Quality

When doctors, nurses, and other hospital operating room staff follow a written safety checklist to respond when a patient experiences cardiac arrest, severe allergic reaction, bleeding followed by an irregular heart beat or other crisis during surgery, they are nearly 75 percent less likely to miss a critical clinical step, according to a new study funded by the Agency for Healthcare Research and Quality (AHRQ). While the use of checklists is rapidly becoming a standard of surgical care, the impact of using them during a surgical crisis has been largely untested, according to the study published in the January 17 issue of the *New England Journal of Medicine*.

"We know that checklists work to improve safety during routine surgery," said AHRQ Director Carolyn M. Clancy, M.D. "Now, we have compelling evidence that checklists also can help surgical teams perform better during surgical emergencies." Surgical crises are high-risk events that can be life threatening if clinical teams do not respond appropriately. Failure to rescue surgical patients who experience life-threatening complications has been recognized as the biggest source of variability in surgical death rates among hospitals, the study authors noted. For this randomized controlled trial, investigators simulated multiple operating room crises and assessed the ability of 17 operating room teams from three Boston area hospitals—one teaching hospital and two community hospitals—to adhere to life-saving steps for each simulated crisis.

In half of the crisis scenarios, operating room teams were provided with evidence-based, written checklists. In the other half of crisis scenarios, the teams worked from memory alone. When a checklist was used during a surgical crisis, teams were able to reduce the chances of missing a life-saving step, such as calling for help within 1 minute of a patient experiencing abnormal heart rhythm, by nearly 75 percent, the researchers said.

Examples of simulated surgical emergencies used in the study were air embolism (gas bubbles in the bloodstream), severe allergic reaction, irregular heart rhythms associated with bleeding, or an unexplained drop in blood pressure. Each surgical team consisted of anesthesia staff, operating room nurses, surgical technologists, and a mock surgeon or practicing surgeon "For decades, we in surgery have believed that surgical crisis situations are too complex for simple checklists to be helpful. This work shows that assumption is wrong," said Atul Gawande, M.D., senior author of the paper, a surgeon at Brigham and Women's Hospital and professor at the Harvard School of Public Health. "Four years ago, we showed that completing a routine checklist before surgery can substantially reduce the likelihood of a major complication. This new work shows that use of a set of carefully crafted checklists during an operating room crisis also has the potential to markedly improve care and safety." Hospital staff who participated in the study said the checklists were easy to use, helped them feel more prepared, and that they would use the checklists during actual surgical emergencies. In addition, 97 percent of participants said they would want checklists to be used for them if a crisis occurred during their own surgery. The practice of using checklists is borrowed from high-risk industries such as aviation and nuclear power, where checklists have been tested in simulated settings and shown to improve performance during unpredictable crisis events.

Current as of March 2013

Internet Citation: Standard written checklists can improve patient safety during surgical crises: Patient Safety and Quality. March 2013. Agency for Health care Research and Quality, Rockville, MD. http://www.ahrq.gov/news/newsletters/research-activities/13mar/0313RA4.html

Source: U.S. Department of Health & Human Services.

of these policies and procedures. Does this seem harsh? When small infractions go without consequences, the gray areas of acceptable rule breaking becomes wider and wider until there are hardly any rules with consequences left. You and your staff must find methods for properly caring for patients in a speedy and efficient manner that maintains patient safety protocols. No excuses. Listen carefully to staff complaints so they can be addressed to gain understanding and ultimate agreement to policies. When your staff members understand the reasoning, it is easier for them to comply.

Some disasters are easy to plan for, as long as the money is available, such as the installation of power generators to keep electrical equipment working, computer software backup systems with off-site storage to ensure patient records are always safe, as well as updating virus protection and firewalls to fend off hackers. The bottom line is that action must be taken to protect the massive infrastructure of the organization. As expensive as this all may be, regardless of the size of your organization, all of these elements must be in place and working at all times.

Due to the massive need that health care organizations have for electricity and technology, having a technical professional on-site with up-to-date skills and knowledge is essential. Many smaller facilities use an outside vendor for technical services; however, if you are presented with a disaster, you will only be one of their many clients begging for assistance. At the very least, one member of your regular staff should have foundational knowledge of software and hardware systems so someone is capable of troubleshooting (Figure 11-3 ■).

Emergency systems (i.e., generators, fire extinguishers, alarms) need to be tested on a set schedule. You don't want to lose power and engage a generator to find a component has burnt out. The data on the backup computers should be checked to ensure it is viable. If you need to use the backup patient records, you don't want to find the files have been corrupted.

As per policies and procedures, human resources personnel should review staff rosters to ensure that everyone has a preassigned role in case of a crisis. They also need to confirm that each individual knows for what specific tasks they are responsible and how to accomplish those tasks. For example, it may be preparing patients in rooms 1 through 5 for transportation, grabbing files from drawers 15 through 17, or switching on the automatic voice mail message to answer the phone. Prepare a "What to Do Should *This* Happen" binder containing your crisis management plan—the viable solutions you have established for all of the types

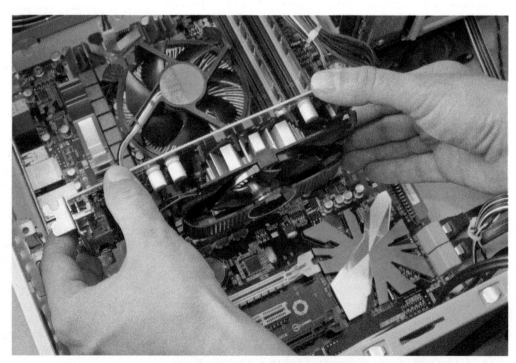

FIGURE 11-3 Someone on staff should be able to troubleshoot computers.
Photo credit: Mny-Jhee/Shutterstock.

of crises mentioned earlier. Yes, the binder should be paper (hard copies) because the information needs to be available even when power goes out. You need to ensure clearly marked copies of these crisis management binders are readily available throughout the facility and are updated as needed. The viable solutions should be enumerated steps that can be followed easily. For example, if a tornado or hurricane is approaching, close blinds and drapes, move patients away from windows, and get extra blankets to protect them. If a celebrity is coming into your facility and the media starts to call, everyone should forward the calls or direct the individual to the designated media liaison. Every facility must have one. If the health department sends an alert about a potential outbreak, get all staff members vaccinated or confirm their shots are up to date.

Your human resources personnel should be instructed to maintain an emergency personnel roster that can be called in to work should your facility get hit with an overload of patients or if an environmental disaster prevents current staff from getting to work. This list may include retired, part-time, and locum tenens (physicians who temporarily fill in for other physicians). In addition, you might call upon community health workers (CHW) to plan and publicize information to specific at-risk patient populations during an emergency. The CDC identifies these trained individuals and identifies what they can be expected to add to the effort to support at-risk populations in an emergency (Box 11-5 ■).

Of course, emergency exit routes should be mapped out in advance, in case staff and patients must evacuate the building. These routes should be checked several times a year. Confirm that boxes or furniture have not been placed in front of that emergency exit door; confirm the fire escape is not rusted through; and ensure that all automatic doors have a manual opener that works and that several employees know how to use it. Confirm that there is at least one phone in the office (or at least one on each floor) that can work without electricity. Many phone systems are digital and will not work during a power failure. Depending upon the disaster, cell phones may or may not be functional. If there is an elevator in the building, someone should be designated to check for anyone who might get stuck during a power outage. You may think getting stuck in an elevator is not cause for immediate concern; however, that person may have a health condition, such as asthma, making this a life or death situation.

Someone in your office, no matter how large or small, should be responsible for responding to internal reports of potential hazards (i.e., people, equipment) as well as failing emergency backup systems. Don't panic, but take everything seriously. A broken doorknob on the emergency door or no batteries for the emergency flashlight seems like no big deal—until you can't

---

BOX 11-5 **Community Health Workers Can Help Support the Community During an Emergency**

Community Health Workers (CHWs)

- CHWs play a pivotal role in meeting the health care needs of rural communities.
- They might work under many labels, including CHW, community health advisor (CHA), promotora, ayudante, and other locality-specific titles.
- CHWs help increase access to health services (particularly among racial and ethnic minority groups).
- They contribute to broader social and community development.
- According to the National Rural Health Association, "the most significant commonalities of CHA programs are that: they are focused on reaching at-risk populations; the workers usually are indigenous to the target population; their expertise is in knowing their communities rather than formal education" (National Rural Health Association, 2000).
- As "in-between people," CHWs draw on their insider status and understanding to act as culture and language brokers between their own community and systems of care.
- Although not always accepted by the medical establishment, a number of key organizations support the development of CHW programs, including The American Public Health Association (2002), the CDC (2005), and the National Rural Health Association (2000).
- The Pew Health Professions Commission recommended in its 1998 report, *Recreating Health Professional Practice for a New Century*, that public health schools, programs and departments focus some of their resources on training lay health workers and community residents to understand the mission of public health and equip them in basic competence to achieve this mission.
- CHWs might be paid or unpaid/volunteer and could have varying levels of job-related education or training.
- As isolated populations increase, their dependence on these multitasking and frequently overburdened health care workers also increases.

Source: Centers for Disease Control and Prevention.

use the emergency door to get out, or the power fails and that flashlight doesn't work. That is no time to go to the store for batteries.

You may be working at a facility that has a specific obligation to its community and patient population. In these circumstances, it is important to identify your at-risk patient population so that you will know, before an emergency occurs, who might need your help. Categorizing them by issue will enable you to set up specific protocols to support their safety quickly and smoothly in a crisis situation (Box 11-6 ■). For example, for those who do not speak English, you can find and document which staff members may be able and willing to interpret.

BOX 11-6 **Categories of At-Risk Members of the Community**

The Categories Checklist

Economic Disadvantage
- Living at or under the poverty line, including those who have been in poverty for at least two generations
- Homeless
- Medicaid recipients
- Working poor with limited resources, often working multiple jobs
- Single mothers and sole caregivers
- Low-wage workers in multiple jobs
- Ethnic and racial minorities

Language and Literacy (limited English proficiency, low literacy or non-English speaking groups):
- Spanish
- Asian and Pacific Island languages (Chinese, Korean, Japanese, Vietnamese, Hmong, Khmer, Lao, Thai, Tagalog, Dravidian, Polynesian, and Micronesian languages)
- Other Indo-European languages (Germanic, Scandinavian, Slavic, Romance French, Italian), Indic, Celtic, Baltic, Iranian, and Greek languages)
- All other languages (Uralic and Semitic languages, as well as indigenous languages of the Americas)
- Sign Languages/American Sign Language (ASL)
- Limited language proficiency (read, write) in native language
- Foreign visitors
- Illegal/undocumented immigrants
- Immigrants/refugees

Medical Issues and Disability
- Blind and visually impaired
- Deaf and hard of hearing
- Developmentally disabled
- Mobility impaired
- Medically dependent (life support/medical equipment)
- Chronic disease/infirm
- Diagnosed with HIV/AIDS
- Immunocompromised
- Drug and/or alcohol dependent (perhaps not in treatment)
- Diagnosed with mental illness and substance abuse
- Mentally ill or having brain disorders/injuries
- Chronic pain
- Non-hospitalized patients: require renal dialysis; require supplemental oxygen; require daily medication (e.g., insulin, antihypertensive agents, narcotics, antipsychotics); receiving chemotherapy for cancer treatment; clinically depressed individuals who may be unable to follow directions; stroke patients with limited mobility and additional care requirements
- Pregnant women

- People recuperating at home from acute injury (e.g., broken bones, recent surgery, back injury, burns)
- Individuals who do not identify as visually impaired, but would be impaired if they were to lose their glasses during an emergency.

Isolation (cultural, geographic, or social)
- Homebound elderly
- Homeless people
- People living alone
- Sole caregivers
- Single individuals without extended family
- Low-income people
- People living in remote rural areas with spotty or no reception of mass media
- People living in shelters, for example, homeless people, runaways, or battered persons
- Undocumented immigrants
- People dependent on public transportation
- Rural and urban ethnic groups
- Religious communities (e.g., Amish, Mennonite)
- Seasonal or temporary populations and those in temporary locations
- Commuters
- People displaced by a disaster
- Schools; students, teachers, administrators, and employees at schools, universities, and boarding schools
- Seasonal migrant workers
- Seasonal tourists, residents, and workers
- People isolated by recreational activity (e.g., primitive campers or backpackers)
- Truckers, pilots, railroad engineers, and other transportation workers
- Military personnel
- Campers and staff at residential summer camps

Age
- Elderly with limited strength, but not disabled
- Senior citizens
- Infants
- Mothers with newborns
- Teens, school-age children, latchkey children
- Families with children who have health care needs
- Grandparents who are guardians of grandchildren

Source: Centers for Disease Control and Prevention.

From the beginning, and every day thereafter, the administration of the organization should consistently communicate the ethical and moral culture of the facility—from the top down—and ensure that each and every individual is held accountable for behaving according to the highest standards of care for patients.

Concurrent Phase

As you learned earlier in this chapter, there are numerous sorts of crises. No two celebrity patient situations are the same, nor are two hurricanes. Therefore, the minute you have been alerted to a situation, do not trust your memory; pull out the crisis management plan. It will help everyone to stay focused and it will provide clear direction for what to do. All members of the management team should be onsite, so wherever they may be at the time, everyone needs to come in.

During an environmental or community disaster, such as a hurricane hitting the area, everyone on your staff will be torn between two strong loyalties: their patients and their family. Your staff members are worried about their families and homes in addition to wanting to be on the job to care for patients. You cannot ignore this need by ordering them to stay on the job when they want to check on their spouses and children. This shortsightedness is going to simply add resentment to the stress of the situation with no benefit to your facility or your patients. Therefore, you must find a way to permit them to be people as well as health care staff.

Depending upon the situation, try to find a way to allow each employee to, at least, contact family to confirm they are safe. In addition, you may create a rotating leave of one hour so staff members can actually go home to secure their physical belongings. If there is a large room, such as an auditorium or cafeteria, encourage staff to invite or bring immediate family on site to keep them safe. You might even engage some of the adults and teenagers to volunteer providing support to other health care staff. There is plenty they can do, and it would be a great experience. Requesting their help will give them something to keep them busy so they don't panic as well as provide them the opportunity to do something good in the middle of this crisis by providing assistance to the facility—freeing up experienced staff to do more critical work. Now, with their families safe and secure, your staff can focus all of their energy on patient care.

The most important thing that an administrator can do during the crisis is to keep things organized and calm. You have a crisis management plan in place and now is the time to follow it—step by step. Including an Incident Command System in your plan, as explained by the Agency for Healthcare Research and Quality (AHRQ) in Box 11-7 ■, will help everyone involved know exactly who is in charge and identify individual responsibilities.

Things often don't go according to plan, so you will most likely be required to think on your feet. Delegate to those you trust, and even if you are scared inside, stay strong on the outside. Have only the media liaison communicate with the media and agree upon, in advance, the message that will be delivered (Figure 11-4 ■) .

Communications are critical—not just with the media—but with your staff, too. Treat your employees with respect and let them know, as much as possible, what is going on during this time. Some managers believe that telling people details about a crisis will cause panic. However, your staff members are adults and if you don't provide accurate details, they will use their imaginations. What they imagine is always worse than reality. Be honest and open with them. They will be able to sense if you are lying or hiding anything. Along with the details of the crisis, share

---

BOX 11-7 | **Incident Command Systems**

Incident command systems (ICS) use a consistent organizational structure that includes individual positions for overall management of emergency situations. ICS systems are designed to facilitate interagency coordination (because each agency has organized their response on the same model). This is one of the system's most important advantages. ICS can also expand and contract to meet the needs of the particular emergency situation at hand.

 ICS structure is hierarchical. For example, there will be one incident commander, three key assistants (safety officer, liaison officer, and public information officer), and four subordinate managers who report directly to the incident commander (operations, logistics, planning, and finance).

Source: Agency for Healthcare Research and Quality, U.S. Department of Health & Human Services.

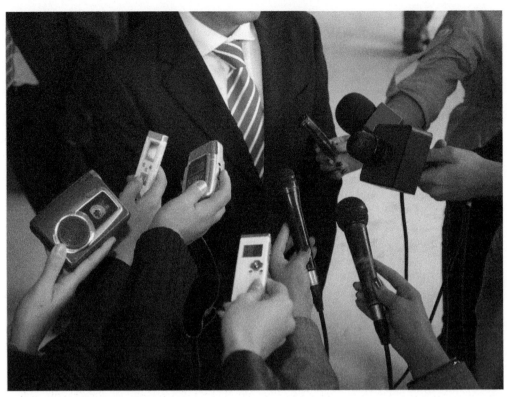

FIGURE 11-4 Sometimes a hospital representative must talk with the media.
Photo credit: Picsfive/Shutterstock.

with them your calm confirmation that everyone is properly prepared to handle the event and all will be fine. If you have concern for an injured individual or group, express this empathy. It will not make you look weak; it will make you look human. If you don't know the answer to a question, be honest and state that you will look into this and return with an accurate response. This is no time for assumptions or premature conclusions. As new information or details emerge, keep your staff members updated. This will build trust and confidence, enabling them to do their jobs without worrying.

If the crisis is legal in nature (such as a medical misadventure), do not handle it without the advice of the facility's attorney. Don't talk to the staff or the media without consulting with legal representation first. This is not intended to cover anything up, but to ensure that you do not break any laws in the process of managing the situation.

Recovery Phase

post-event analysis
an evaluation of how the organization handled each aspect of the crisis.

The storm has cleared. Whether a literal windstorm, a storm of media attention, or the occurrence of a *never event*—the crisis is over. However, your work is not complete because a **post-event analysis** must be performed. Exactly what this will entail, of course, will be determined by the specific event. Following an external disaster, you might need to request that a Community Assessment for Public Health Emergency Response (CASPER) be performed. This is alternately known as a Rapid Need Assessment (RNA) or Rapid Health Assessment (RHA). The CDC recommends that, when at least one of these conditions exist, a CASPER should be considered:

- The impact of the disaster on the community or patient population is unknown
- The health status and basic needs of the affected population are unknown
- There are reasonable, general concerns about specific groups or individuals (such as your at-risk members of the population) (See Box 11-6 on page 194).
- When response and recovery efforts need to be evaluated

If a CASPER is deemed necessary, it should be started as soon as possible, and certainly within seventy-two hours.

Whichever type of post-event analysis needs to be completed, everyone should remember that this is an investigation to find the truth—the reality of the event and its impact—not to determine fault and not to hide anything. Some concepts that you should consider:

1. All members of the team should focus on the procedures, processes, and organizational aspects of the event. This will not provide true value to the facility if everyone is merely seeking someone to blame.
2. Every step leading up to the event, during the event, and immediately after the event should be documented and evaluated. Again, the protocol itself should be analyzed, as well as how individuals performed their tasks.
3. When a disruption to the organizational protocols is identified, be certain to ferret out the reasons why this disruption occurred, in addition to when and who was involved. Research has proven that some common causes include: poor communication processes between physicians, staff, and administration; unclear or confusing labeling; and insufficient patient monitoring.
4. Include all levels of personnel involved in the event, as well as those who were not involved as they may provide an objective viewpoint. Gather input from everyone, not only to amass the details of the event but also to understand what people were doing, thinking, and feeling at the time. Ask for their suggestions as to how this event may be prevented from happening again.
5. Evaluate all statements and accounts of the event, including all incident reports (Figure 11-5 ■), before determining what to do next. Highlight opportunities for the initiation of additional preventive measures, adjustments or additions to current policies or procedures, or other action to reduce the opportunity for a repeat of those things that went awry.
6. Be certain to praise those individuals who did the right things, perhaps lessened the negative outcome of the event, or supported the reporting and investigation so the event could be addressed.
7. Implement any corrective action determined to be necessary for educational and preventive benefits, and punitive actions.

As you analyze the physical aftermath of the crisis, do not ignore its emotional and psychological impact. Mental health professionals should be made available to deal with the emotional effects of virtually any type of emergency—for staff as well as patients or community members.

CREATING A PLAN

You don't have to use much imagination to come up with crisis situations and scenarios upon which to build a crisis management plan. The daily newspaper, as well as industry journals, can provide many real stories. Here are some synopses from true events that you can use to practice developing management strategies.

If you were the administrator of this facility, how would you handle this situation? What is the first thing you would do? What would you say to the media? What would you say to your staff? What preventive measures could have been taken to avoid or lessen the impact of this event on your facility?

Never Event

Scenario:

Surgeon amputated wrong leg of patient at your facility

However. . .both legs were acutely affected by disease, the patient's operative schedule documented the wrong leg for removal, and the hospital's computer system noted the wrong leg for surgery. The operative team nurses had draped and sterilized the wrong leg for surgery prior to the surgeon entering the operating room (OR).

Analysis:

It is easy to jump to the conclusion that this surgeon should lose his license and be blamed entirely for amputating the wrong leg of this patient. Once the investigation reveals the details above, is he really to blame at all? Is he the only one to blame? What processes could you implement to prevent this from ever happening again?

➤ A P P E N D I X ~ A

Example Incident Report

Below is a reproduction of an incident report we received during data collection. We redacted all patient and hospital information.

Incident Info: Patient Fall	People Involved:
Incident Number: 8726	(Reporting Employee Name)
Log Date: 10/01/2008 2:25:21 PM	**Other People Involved:**
Incident Date: 10/01/2008 2:20:00 PM	Witness
Location: BATHROOM	(Attending Physician Name)
Primary Person Involved: (Patient Name)	(Employee Reviewer Name)
Account Number:	(Employee Reviewer Name)
Birth Date:	(Employee Reviewer Name)

Comments/Incident Description/Additional Details
Review Comment *Made by: (Employee Name)*
RN and LPN had walked patient to bathroom several times. Patient used call light and or they checked in with her and walked her back from bathroom. At the time of this fall, the patient unexpectedly got up unassisted and fell. C/o rib pain, physician notified, no injury confirmed per radiology. The plan of care was updated with communication regarding nature of fall.

Details		
Falls		**Patient Outcomes**
Type of Fall	-To/In bathroom	
		Were the healthcare personnel caring for the patient notified? -Yes
Injury Type	-Other: *LT RIB DISCOMFORT* -Abrasion/ Laceration/ Bruise	
Restraints/Siderails	-Mattress sensor -SR up x2	**Was additional treatment provided to the patient?** -No
Physician	-Physician was notified	**Patient Outcomes** -14 Other: PAIN LT RIB -03 Abrasion/Bruise
Was equipment involved?	-No	**Severity of Injury**
Mental status at time of fall	-Other: *FORGETFUL* -Alert and oriented ×3	**Severity of Injury:** -MINOR-NO TREATMENT REQUIRED OR MINIMAL TREATMENT (FIRST AID)
		Level 1 Review
Current Documented Risk Assessment Level Prior to this Fall	-High	**Contributing Factors** -N/A
Could medication have been factor in fall?	-No	**Follow Up Actions** -Additional Data Collection
		Level 2 Review
		Was the bill adjusted? -N/A
		Level 3 Review
		Has a memo been drafted to Medical Staff Leadership? -N/A

FIGURE 11-5 Example Incident Reporting Form.

Source: Office of the Inspector General, U.S. Department of Health & Human Services.

New Policy: Patient is asked to mark his or her own anatomical site for treatment with a special marker.

New Policy: Supervisor or another professional must approve all entries into the operative schedule to double check accuracy of details.

Community Crisis

Scenario:

Plane crashes into supermarket

A small plane lost power and crashed into a local supermarket, injuring five people. The pilot and his passenger, along with three customers of the store, were burned and taken to your hospital for care of their injuries. Law enforcement officers and reporters are seeking information on the injured.

Analysis:

Your emergency department (ED) is about to get five injured patients, some requiring very specialized care (burns) at one time. This will cause a tremendous overload on the current staff and there may not be enough available rooms or equipment. What do you, as the administrator, need to do?

1. Contact the ED chief and get an assessment of what the staff will need to handle this situation.
2. Authorize the human resources department to call in off-duty or locum tenens, physicians, nurses, and so on.
3. If there are not sufficient rooms and/or equipment, contact your peers at other area facilities to see if some patients can be transferred there.

Criminal Activity

Scenario:

Hospice audited by Medicare for questionable billing practices

Medicare notified your hospice that the facility's records would be included in a widespread review of billing practices. The audit found an error rate of 18 percent. The government-allowed error rate is 15 percent. As a result, a second audit was automatically triggered. The second review revealed a 77 percent problem rate believed to be the result of improper claims creation.

Media trucks are parked outside the building trying to get an interview with anyone on staff. The staff members are distracted and anxious, afraid this will put the hospice out of business and they will lose their jobs. Patients and their families have been calling trying to find out if their bills are those that were overcharged and fraudulent.

Analysis:

This is certainly a complex situation. The best way to deal with everything is to break it down into pieces and deal with one piece at a time.

- This is a legal matter, so contact your facility's attorney.
- Gather all staff and volunteers and tell them that you are taking this seriously and that no determinations can be made—human error or criminal activity—until after an investigation has been completed. Until then, everyone should continue as usual. Request that anyone with factual information about this situation contact you privately.
- Identify the individual who will act as the media liaison and meet with the attorney to ensure any public statements do not endanger the facility or its patients. There should be no perception of a cover-up, and no assumptions should be expressed, just known facts.
- Channel all patient and family contact through the media liaison.

Celebrity

Scenario:

Hospital workers punished for peeking at celebrity's file

You are notified that an ambulance is bringing a famous movie actor into your ED. What do you do first? What do you say to the media? What do you say to your staff? After the actor has been discharged and has left the hospital, you receive a report, via your computer system, documenting that twenty-seven staff members looked at his records even though they had no valid professional reason to do this. This is a violation of HIPAA—a federal patient privacy law—because, although these staff members had clearance to view patient records, that permission is only valid when there is a job-related necessity to do so. Gossip and curiosity is not valid under the law.

Analysis:

- First, remind all staff members that celebrities are entitled to the same patient confidentiality—ethically and legally—as every other patient of the facility.
- Create an official statement regarding patient confidentiality to present to the media.
- These curious staff members have put your facility in danger with the federal government, potentially making the entire organization liable for fines and penalties, unless you take corrective action immediately. You may understand their desire to learn more about this celebrity, however, your actions must convey to everyone, including the federal government, that you take this violation seriously. What should you do—suspend with pay, suspend without pay, terminate their employment? (This scenario is based on an actual event. In that case, the employees were suspended without pay for 30 days.)

Endemic/Pandemic

Scenario:

Shigella outbreak causing severe stomach ailments at child care centers, preschools

Health officials are reporting a Shigella outbreak and say the diarrhea-causing germ is spreading through child care centers and preschools. This bacterium can be very serious, causing diarrhea, bloody diarrhea, as well as fever, stomach cramps, nausea, and vomiting. Most cases are mild, lasting several days to weeks, but severe complications, such as dehydration, can occur. There have been 78 reported cases of Shigella so far this year. Last year at this time, only four cases were reported.

Five children, patients at your pediatrics office, have been diagnosed during the last week. Parents of all your patients are afraid and clamoring for appointments to get their children checked. They are yelling at whomever answers the phone and some have camped out on the doorstep, showing up without an appointment demanding to be seen, causing virtually every member of your staff to feel stressed and anxious. The media has been calling trying to get an interview with Dr. Pearson, one of the pediatricians in your group practice.

Analysis:

Patient confidentiality is absolute, so no information about the five specific patients can be released. Therefore, Dr. Pearson can speak with the media about the disease, signs and symptoms, as well as precautions that parents might take, in a general manner only. He can do the same with patients' parents and guardians. Consider including a message about the outbreak on the phone's automatic answering system, Include suggestions for parents, as well. Sending out letters from the doctor to the entire patient list (via e-mail or postal mail) might also be an excellent way to subdue the panic.

CHAPTER REVIEW

SUMMARY

Some crises provide advance notice, enabling proper preparation ahead of time. Others happen in an instant, and you must know what to do immediately. Creating a crisis management plan ahead of any and all potential disasters, using reports of events that have happened at other facilities, will support management and secure their ability—and your ability as the administrator—to guide everyone through the crisis under the best possible circumstances.

The process of writing, or updating, a crisis management plan can empower you as a leader by giving you the information needed to actually prevent some crises from happening at all. In addition, you will be properly prepared to be a calm and organized adviser during a crisis, directing staff and patients to safety. After the event is over, you will know how to properly complete a post-event analysis so that, should this ever happen again, you and your staff will handle things even more effectively and efficiently.

 ## REVIEW QUESTIONS

MULTIPLE CHOICE

Choose the most accurate answer.

1. Performing a procedure on the wrong patient is known as a
   a. natural disaster.
   b. never event.
   c. preventive management plan.
   d. locum tenens.

2. The crisis management triad includes all of the following EXCEPT
   a. what happens during the event.
   b. prevention.
   c. education.
   d. recovery.

3. The Department of Health has notified you of a meningitis outbreak. This is a
   a. technological disaster.
   b. natural disaster.
   c. human disaster.
   d. health care disaster.

4. Your facility should adopt a _____ policy when it comes to patient safety protocols.
   a. zero-tolerance
   b. don't ask/don't tell
   c. locum tenens
   d. no harm/no foul

5. Which of the following is an example of a sentinel event?
   a. Hurricane
   b. Celebrity patient
   c. Power outage
   d. Surgical sponge left inside patient

6. Notification of which of the following situations should be attended to immediately?
   a. Broken doorknob on emergency exit door
   b. Patient fell out of bed
   c. Flashlights need batteries
   d. All of the above

7. The best way to prevent a power outage from becoming a major crisis is to
   a. install backup generators.
   b. close the facility.
   c. train staff to see in the dark.
   d. call a press conference.

8. The most important thing that an administrator can do during a crisis is to
   a. send everyone home.
   b. keep things organized and calm.
   c. make everyone work overtime.
   d. call the police.

9. After the crisis has passed, you, as the administrator, should
   a. get back to normal.
   b. construct a compliance plan.
   c. go home and rest.
   d. complete a post-event analysis.

10. During a crisis, administrators should always
    a. keep details to themselves.
    b. communicate openly with staff.
    c. call their lawyer.
    d. wait and see what happens.

FILL-IN-THE-BLANK

Fill in the blank with the accurate answer.

11. A _____ is an event that should never happen.

12. A legal term that requires evidence of negligence is _____.

13. A disease that has spread through a community is called _____.

14. Individuals in three countries have been diagnosed with influenza. This is now a _____.

15. The phase of a crisis situation that occurs after the crisis has passed is known as the _____ phase.

16. The most important thing that an administrator can do during the crisis is to keep things _____ and calm.

17. Once the storm has cleared and the crisis itself is over, you, as the administrator should perform a _____.

18. When a disruption to the organizational protocols is identified, be certain to ferret out the _____ why this disruption occurred.

19. Emergency _____ should be mapped out in advance.

20. Human resources should maintain an emergency _____ roster of individuals who can be called in to work should your facility get hit with a patient overload.

TRUE/FALSE

Determine whether the statement is true or false.

21. Medical error is always termed as a sentinel event.

22. Once in place, an emergency generator should be left untouched until needed.

23. You, as an administrator, should attend to the physical and psychological needs of your staff and patients.

24. Post-event analysis is only required after major problems have arisen.

25. Health care administrators will only have to deal with crises such as outbreaks of communicable diseases.

26. A specific individual in your facility should be responsible for responding to internal reports of potential hazards.

27. Staff error, malpractice, and negligence are examples of human disasters.

28. Crisis management is not necessary when a top movie actor is brought into your facility.

29. Lightning hitting an electrical transformer near your facility, causing your organization to totally lose power, is an example of a technological disaster.

30. The best way to handle a crisis is to plan ahead.

WHEN YOU ARE THE ADMINISTRATOR . . .

Critical Thinking and Analysis

For each of the following case studies, create at least one policy or design a procedure to handle the following circumstances. These situations are all true events.
    What is your plan to deal with the staff and the media when this happens at your facility? What preventive plans can be put into place to avoid this happening again? How would you handle this situation during the event?

Case Study #1

DoJ joins lawsuit against hospital for violating Stark

The Department of Justice (DoJ) alleged that your hospital had improper contracts with nine physicians. The lawsuit claimed that the hospital overbilled Medicare by tens of millions of dollars over

several years and that there was an improper financial relationship between the hospital, the staffing company, and the physicians. If true, this is a violation of the Stark law (The Physician Self-Referral Act), a federal law that forbids referrals by physicians to those facilities in which they have a financial interest. This is intended to avoid a patient being sent to a facility or being provided services for the financial reward to the physician rather than on the basis of the best interests of the patient.

Case Study #2

Apartment building fire

More than ten people were hurt when fire raged through their apartment building. Fire fighters stated that three individuals jumped from the second floor to escape the flames, while several others were able to escape via a first floor window. Residents of the building were taken to your emergency department (ED) with smoke inhalation, a couple of fractures resulting from those who jumped from the second floor, cuts from glass, and some minor injuries. Due to the size of the fire and the injuries, the media has swarmed your ED attempting to interview survivors as well as hospital staff who are treating the victims.

Case Study #3

Man dies of massive heart attack after being sent home from ED

A seventy-three-year-old man and his wife walked into the ED at 3:00 A.M. He told the nurse at the desk that he was having chest pain and tingling in his arm. The nurse phoned the physician on duty who was upstairs. The nurse spoke with the doctor, handed the phone to the patient who spoke with the physician for several minutes, then, handed the phone back to the nurse. The nurse spoke with the physician again, then hung up and told the man and his wife to go home and call his personal physician in the morning. She explained that his insurance did not cover treatment at their facility and that the pain and tingling was probably nothing—just old age. The couple left the hospital and walked the three blocks back to their home and up the four flights to their apartment. While taking his shirt off to get into bed, the man had a massive heart attack and died instantly.

 INTERNET CONNECTIONS

Emergency Planning: Health Care Sector

Federal Communications Commission

This website provided clear bulleted lists to support the creation of a crisis management plan for any type of health care facility.
http://transition.fcc.gov/pshs/emergency-information/guidelines/health-care.html

Response to Grief Crisis Management Plan

Department of Human Services

Sadly, when some crises occur, death is involved. This crisis management plan specifically guides professionals with handling the survivors.
http://dhs.sd.gov/ddc/documents/griefplan.pdf

A Crisis Communication Primer for Hospital CEOs

This article covers a list of questions that should be asked and answered, within a health care facility to ensure proper emergency preparation.
http://www.aha.org/advocacy-issues/emergreadiness/crisiscomprimer.shtml

CHAPTER 12

PERFORMANCE IMPROVEMENT

KEY TERMS

accountable care
  organization (ACO)
continuing education
cross-training
employee retention
extrinsic motivation
intellectual capital
intrinsic motivation
motivation
patient-centered care
performance improvement
  plan (PIP)
staff satisfaction

LEARNING OBJECTIVES

Upon completion of this chapter, you should be able to:

- Define the commonly used terms, abbreviations, and acronyms.
- Explain the importance of a performance improvement process.
- Develop a performance improvement plan.
- Integrate employee support into patient-centered care.
- Enumerate the elements of accountable care organizations.

WHEN YOU ARE THE ADMINISTRATOR . . .

Your responsibility as a health care administrator includes doing everything you can to protect the facility, the patients, and your staff. Therefore, you will need to be able to:

- Provide leadership and promote effective and efficient integration of services in a worker-friendly environment.
- Coordinate organization-wide performance improvement activities, including the maintenance of performance improvement documentation to support credentialing.
- Analyze data for trends of improvement and provide a plan to identify and follow up on areas of concern.

INTRODUCTION

A majority of discussions about health care focus on technology and innovation—robotic surgery, new drugs with fewer side effects, new prosthetics, and more. Any organization might purchase the latest software or prescribe the up-to-date drug protocol in an attempt to establish themselves as a leader in the community. However, the level of performance of your facility and the quality of care provided to your patients are distinctions that go beyond the caliber of your equipment. It is about your people. The true variance in the quality of care lies with the providers themselves. Therefore, as the administrator of any size health care facility, you must find the best possible individuals to hire and do everything possible to keep them. Note that, despite what many people think—this does not begin and end with salary negotiations. You need to create a work environment that encourages the best from every staff member.

IMPROVING STAFF PERFORMANCE

The assets of your organization show up on a balance sheet as furnishings and cash in the bank. However, your staff members are the most valuable asset you have. This is known as **intellectual capital**—the value of everything your people provide to your patients. There is much involved in the provision of excellent care: knowledge, skill, and personal attributes. Knowledge can be confirmed by licensing or certification exams. However, skill sets and personal attributes are more difficult to identify during a thirty-minute interview. Therefore, once you have evidence, over time, that an employee is one who performs with excellence, you must do everything possible to keep him or her. Human resources professionals refer to this concept as **employee retention**.

There is a cost for hiring the less competent. Known as *bad hires*, the cost of advertising, interviewing, orientating, and lost productivity is money virtually impossible to recoup. In health care, there are additional liability factors involved with *any* employee (administrative or clinical) not doing his or her job properly. That's right; doctors or nurses are not the only members of the team who can increase your liability. Consider the negative impact on your facility if a member of your administrative staff committed fraud (whether intentional or because they are not capable), if an employee failed to obtain proper patient documentation (e.g., failure to get proper consent), or a member of your environmental services staff enabled the spread of infection by failing to use adequate cleaning methods.

Some managers think that getting and keeping quality people on staff is only about money—how high a salary can be offered. They mistakenly believe that if they cannot compete with top area salaries they have no hope of attracting the best personnel. However, this is not true. Successful health care professionals are emotionally invested in their careers. They are passionate about what they do; they are happy to come to work every day, especially when they work in an environment where administration appreciates the importance of **staff satisfaction**. There are specific things you can do to cultivate an organization for which the best staff members in the industry want to work.

Enhancing the performance of each of your staff members can be a daunting task, especially because you will need to include personalized attention at least part of the time, and it is a continuous process. The U.S. Office of Personnel Management (OPM) describes the process as having five parts, as illustrated in Figure 12-1 ■: planning, monitoring, developing, rating, and rewarding. The OPM further defines these stages as:

- Planning work in advance so that expectations and goals can be set;
- Monitoring progress and performance continually;
- Developing the employee's ability to perform through training and work assignments;
- Rating periodically to summarize performance; and,
- Rewarding good performance.

Improve the Attitude about Employees

Attitudes, the air of your organization, must begin with you, the administrator, setting a tone of quality care for patients that begins with the way the facility cares for its staff.

1. *Create a culture of caring*. Care for the patients *and* for every member of the staff. Organizational culture is a set of attitudes, behaviors, and emotions that are the foundation

---

intellectual capital
the assets provided to an organization by the staff: ideas, innovations, energies, and efforts.

employee retention
the ability of an organization to ensure that high quality staff continue working for their company.

staff satisfaction
employees who feel appreciated and valued for their job performance.

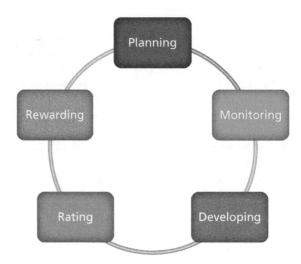

FIGURE 12-1 Employee performance improvement is a continuous cycle.
Source: U.S. Office of Personnel Management.

for virtually all actions, behaviors, policies, and procedures. Establish employee policies that are fair and reasonable, taking into consideration that your staff members have personal lives, families, and outside obligations. The salary you pay them is in exchange for the knowledge and skill they share; it is not ownership. When an organization truly cares for its staff members as people, this attitude flows smoothly to true caring for the patients.

2. *Clear, timely communications.* Communicate clearly and openly with everyone. Some managers keep secrets from the staff only to find out later the staff already knows, suspects, or has imagined worse things. No matter how small or large the organization, it is just foolish to think a closed-door meeting is protecting confidentiality about business matters. Whether you use the facility intranet, e-mail, or have an in-person staff meeting, let employees know what is going on. When new policies and procedures are introduced, remember that not everyone was at the meeting. They did not get to hear the rationale or the discussion of pros and cons. Share the understanding, and listen as they voice their concerns. Then, explain and get their support for the new policy.

3. *Begin with clear expectations.* The hiring process should include specific information about what is expected from the staff member and what will be given to them in return. On their first day (or earlier), each individual should be given a written list of expectations and have the opportunity to review these with their supervisor. When anything changes, such as reorganization or a promotion, update these expectations. You do not want an employee to waste time and energy wondering what you want or the company wants.

4. *Provide staff with what they need to do their jobs well.* Equipment, supplies, and education must be available to the staff members as they need these things to do their jobs at the highest level. As a health care facility administrator, you would not approve of one of your people bandaging a patient's wound with a paper napkin and a rubber band, would you? Of course not. You must ensure that proper supplies are available. In addition, there should be a process for thorough consideration to be given to the adoption of new innovation.

   Health care is an ever-changing field, and many of your staff members will be required, by licensing or certification authorities, to participate in some type of **continuing education**. Your staff—both administrative and clinical—must be encouraged to keep their knowledge and skills up to date. You can arrange for training on site, pay for employees to go to seminars and conferences, provide quiet rooms so they can attend online webinars, or offer tuition reimbursement (full or partial). If this is not in the budget, at least provide them with the time to attend these events. Sometimes, all it takes is encouragement from the administration of the facility to get individuals to understand the importance of continuing education, and they will go on their own.

5. *Encourage cross-training.* When you are successful at employee retention, you may also need to permit longstanding staff to change departments or foci (Figure 12-2 ■).

continuing education
educational events required for the maintenance of a professional license or certification.

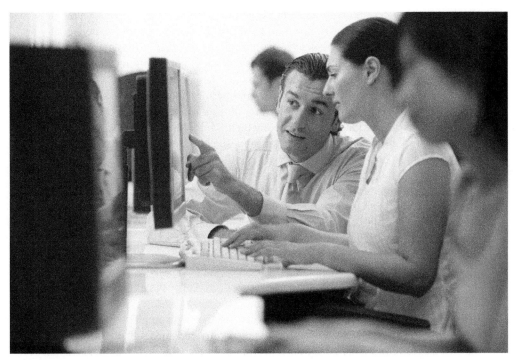

FIGURE 12-2   Cross-training keeps employees fresh and able to multi-task.

Photo credit: Monkey Business Images/Shutterstock.

For example, Joan has been with your facility for ten years and is the best neonatal nurse you have ever seen. When she begins to show signs of being burned out or outwardly states a desire to move to an administrative role, encourage her, share the cost of her new training, and do whatever it takes to keep her on your payroll. She has already proven herself to be a valuable asset to the facility. Show her you value her as a person not only for her skill in neonatology but for all of her professional skills. Hiring from within is another way to retain quality staff members. However, keep in mind, department member and department manager are two very different jobs. One requires the ability to do the work, while being a manager requires the skill to supervise those who do the work. The individual needs to have the ability to create/review budgets, handle various personalities, and successfully complete other administrative tasks. Therefore, in addition to a promotion, provide the cross-training necessary for this individual to be successful as a manager.

6. *Establish an environment of open communication.* You must do everything possible to ensure your staff members that they can come to talk with you. If they need to vent their opinions about the color of their uniforms, make time to listen and respond. You do not need to agree with everything, but you do need to show them the respect of taking them seriously. The main purpose of establishing an open-door policy is to create a habit, so if staff can come to you about the small things, they will feel confident that they can come to you with the big things such as: Dr. Maxwell showing up inebriated again, Sara yelling at a patient, or Henry coming in late and leaving early. Some things may not matter, but others can potentially be serious liability issues about which you need to know. They are not tattling; they are providing the information you need from the front line perspective. You can't be everywhere all the time, yet you are responsible for it all.

7. *Always show everyone respect.* You can give your staff members more money, gifts, and employee-of-the-month awards. However, the most important thing to give them is *respect.* You don't have to agree with them all the time (how absurd), but you do need to help them understand why they need to do something; don't just bark orders, never threaten their job, hours, or salary level; offer a compromise whenever possible; ask them for their ideas for compromise; and most of all, be honest—let them see that, even if you don't give them what they want, they can still trust you.

8. *Perform random acts of kindness.* Surprise employees with a pizza party or a basket of muffins in the break room. Arrange for a local dry cleaner to pick up and deliver at your offices or for a physical therapist to come in and provide chair or foot massages. This does not have to be a huge expenditure. This is a small act of appreciation that reinforces that you are glad they are part of your team.

9. *Do not reward poor performance.* Reward poor performance—who would do that? Actually, when you pay someone a salary for doing a bad job, showing up late, leaving early, taking two hour lunches, not meeting their job responsibilities as expected, you are rewarding this individual. Very often, you are also punishing the good workers who must pick up the slack and are becoming more resentful every day. You think you need to wait until you can find the time to replace him or her, but chances are, everyone on staff as well as the patients would be better off without this person. Make certain the details are documented, and terminate their employment. Like that one bad apple, keeping this less-than-capable person on staff can contaminate your environment and infect your good employees until they become slackers themselves or they quit.

10. *Nurture future staff.* Participate in internship/externship programs with a college or university near your facility. Whether a one-physician practice or a large hospital or assisted living facility, the experience is priceless to the student. At the same time, you can scout out attitudes of excellence and hire a future star.

11. *Implement personal improvement plans.* Work together with employees to help them identify and achieve their career goals. This will generally encompass many of the things in this list such as continuing education and cross-training. However, you may also uncover potential obstacles to this individual's ability to reach peak performance—a need for child care or elderly parent care, or a divorce in progress. You can make referrals available by informing staff members of resources to help them with personal crises. No, you are not a social worker; however, directing an employee in personal crisis to legal aid or other community-based services can provide critical support that will come back to your organization in a less distracted, higher quality, more productive staff member. You will read more about these plans in the next section.

Improve the Way You Motivate Employees

Ordinary companies, and even those that are so bad they are only referred to in whispers, expect their employees to be motivated to do their jobs by the salary they pay. Organizations of excellence, and the individuals within them that make them excellent, have an inner drive to act in a specific manner, and the facility is involved with fanning the flames of **motivation**. There are two types of motivators: intrinsic and extrinsic.

Intrinsic motivation relates to internal drives that are powered by an individual's pleasure center. He or she has an interest in the activity and gets pleasure from participation. Whether they have wanted to work in health care since childhood, or are engaging in a second career, these individuals wake up in the morning excited about going to work each day. They love their jobs, and getting to do them is the reward. Employers with intrinsically motivated staff members are very fortunate because they will work constantly to improve their skills and are first to volunteer for additional assignments. The best way to keep these employees at their best is to let them do their jobs. Support their desire for continuing education or **cross-training**. Listen to their ideas, and give real consideration to their proposals. There is no need for false praise. They just need to feel that you are as happy to have them working for you as they are.

Extrinsic motivation is a drive fueled by external forces. These individuals are empowered by rewards, prizes, and public acknowledgment, such as a mention in the facility newsletter. A competition between two departments will provide an incredible charge to these staff members, as will a certificate of appreciation or employee-of-the-month award. These staff members will also take notice of punitive action, or the threat of any type of punishment, very seriously.

Improve the Way You Manage the Staff

There are several methodologies used by companies to improve the way managers interact with staff. Two such systems are: Total Quality Management (TQM), a set of fourteen key principles for effective managers created by William E. Deming; and Continuous Quality Improvement (CQI), a structured system to guide the evaluation of outcomes, understanding expectations, and a never-ending study to seek performance improvements in all aspects of the business.

motivation
reason to act; forces beneath behavior.

intrinsic motivation
incentive derived from one's own desire or enthusiasm for doing a specific job or completing a task.

cross-training
orientation and education about job responsibilities in a different role or department.

extrinsic motivation
inspirational elements derived from outside forces, such as a reward or acknowledgement.

As a manager, your job is to ensure that your staff members do their jobs efficiently, effectively, and empathetically. You need to help them maintain focus on the reasons you are all there. This goes beyond just a philosophy of bandaging a wound or getting approval from the third-party payer so the patient can have the necessary procedure. The collective purpose you all share is the caring, and you must keep this thread constant throughout the hustle and bustle of each day.

A part of the managing process includes the need to nurture the talent with whom you work. **Performance improvement plans (PIPs)**, which you will learn more about in the next section, permit you to provide each individual in your department or your division, the feedback they need to continue to improve, to grow professionally, and to enhance their contribution to the organization as a whole. Their individual improvement is a joint function; both of you working together. Some business models teach managers how to coach. This perspective makes sense, as you, the manager, encourage, motivate, and empower your staff to success. This can have a side advantage in health care. You must remember that there are times when all the right things are done and yet something bad happens—a patient doesn't make it. Being a part of this environment, a part of the team that provided care even in the smallest manner can take an emotional toll. You must be there to help them through it.

Many studies on all types of businesses, including those in health care, have proven that staff satisfaction is key to employee retention. The leadership of your organization is not about its hierarchy; it is about the guidance and direction that is provided to everyone in the facility—the support, the respect, all of the things you have already learned about earlier in this chapter. Everyone working together is more than just a banner about teamwork. To actually be managing for excellence, all employees must work together like the pieces of a puzzle—interlocking, each providing his or her own skills and knowledge, to create a big picture of good health—inside and out.

The bottom line is that you need to do what you can. Creating a culture of positive attitudes and striving for excellence is easier said than done in some facilities. You may not have the ability or the authority to cleanse the air throughout. This is not an "all or nothing" situation. Do what you can. Whether it is your office, your department, or your division, treat your co-workers properly, and try to lessen the impact of corporate policies that breed bad will.

> **performance improvement plan (PIP)**
> documentation of a staff member's current skills as well as a list of those skills which need to be improved and what action(s) should be taken to ensure that improvement.

PERFORMANCE IMPROVEMENT PLANS (PIPs)

As mentioned in step 11 earlier, individualized performance improvement plans should be created and maintained. These should be done in writing at least once a year with one copy given to the staff member, one copy to the manager, and another to the human resources department to be placed in the employee's personnel file. Using a template can ensure uniformity and prevent an item from being forgotten. Remember that each category of job (clinical or administrative) may require alterations to the template. Let's go over some components of an effective performance improvement plan:

- *Name, employee number, hire date*: Put this in the header of the document so it appears on every page.
- *Job title, job description, and list of expectations*: These elements should be entered and be the same as that provided to the employee when hired. Amendments should be attached to document any changes over the course of the staff member's employment.
- *Professional development/continuing education*: Provide an opportunity for the employee to submit documentation of what he or she has accomplished in the past year and what is planned for the coming year. This should include *everyone* on staff and all activities should relate to their specific job improvement or a future opportunity with your facility. The receptionist may take typing courses to improve input accuracy, while those in environmental services might read an article or attend a seminar on antibacterial cleaners that leave no toxic residue.
- *Employee stated goals*: Does this individual want to become a manager someday? Is there a desire to cross over from administrative to clinical or vice versa? Does he or she want to go back to school? You need to coax these desires from the staff member and do whatever possible to support this dream. You might find that, in their current position, this person's performance is "good" but in a different position, he or she excels. This can provide the organization an opportunity to save a trusted but mediocre staff member and turn him or her into a trusted, excellent staff member.

- *Overall statement of performance*: Based on the established criteria, there should be an overall statement of performance using a five-point Likert-type scale (Excellent, Good, Acceptable, Improvement Required, Unacceptable). A more detailed evaluation should be attached with an itemized list (from the *List of Expectations*) evaluated individually using the same five-point Likert-type scale.
- *Plan of action*: For any performance assessed with a rating of *Good* or lower, a plan of action for improvement should be detailed, crafted by the supervisor together with the employee including deadlines for completion prior to the annual review date. Should the staff member need any assistance to complete this plan, such as help to pay course fees or time off to study, this should also be itemized. Teamwork is an important part of showing support for employees so they know they are not alone. In addition, specific consequences for failing to complete this plan of action for improvement should be listed. Both the staff member and the manager would then sign this plan to document agreement. When a *plan of action* is created, the manager should plan appointments with the staff member to follow up on progress, provided in a supportive manner rather than to scrutinize.

Employee Name: _____   Employee ID# _____
Job Title: _____

Job Description (or items from List of Expectations)	Current Level of Performance [1 to 5]	Action Items for Improvement	Employee Initial for Agreement to Actions

Employee: Itemize any specific assistance you may need (e.g., training, education, etc.) to achieve expected level of performance. Manager: Initial agreement to assist employee to obtain all resources available from the organization.

Specific Assistance	Mgr Initial

Professional Development/Continuing Education

Activity (Course, Webinar, Conference, etc.)	Expected Date of Completion	Completed [Yes/No] Documentation attached

Employee Goals

Goal	Action(s) required to accomplish goal	Expected Date of Completion

Overall measure of current performance: Rank___on scale of 1 to 5
Date of next assessment:_____

Employee Signature and Date	Manager Signature and Date

FIGURE 12-3   Performance improvement plan template.

When creating a performance improvement plan for an employee, you might use the template shown in Figure 12-3 ▪ or a similar form created by your company. Using a preexisting template can help you ensure that all plans are created equally for each and every staff member, and that nothing is accidentally omitted.

IMPROVING PATIENT CARE

Once you have established that your facility truly respects and cares for the people who work with you, you will find that they will be freer and better prepared to concentrate their complete attention on the patients. By improving themselves, administrative and clinical staff members can improve the provision of care to your patients. Although some lament that health care is no longer about caring for patients because so much time and energy must be invested in dealing with the government and third-party payers, the truth is that the entire package revolves around the best care possible for the patients.

When coders and billers are educated properly, claims to third-party payers are paid, not denied, enabling the patient to get the care they need. When compliance with legal issues is accomplished, these elements ensure that the patient is protected—as well as the facility and all its staff members. When clinical staff members are trained in the latest, least-invasive procedural methods, the patient will pay less and have a shorter recovery time. The bottom line is that every administrator of every health care facility should consistently focus on the team approach—a team including clinical staff, administrative staff, and the patient. Working toward the ultimate goal is a win-win-win situation.

Currently, there are two organizational concepts in the forefront of health care. Analysis of these approaches has shown improvement of patient outcomes and a simultaneous reduction in health care costs.

Patient-Centered Care

Patient-centered care is a 360-degree health care circle, with the patient in the middle and in full control of the process. Procedures, services, and treatments should be provided in a manner that attends to the patient's emotional and psychological needs as well as their physical requirements.

patient-centered care
a full-circle approach to health care, with the patient in the middle, in full control of the process.

- *Respect*: Patients should not be ordered to have procedures; they should be consulted and included in all decision making.
- *Inclusion*: When individuals are ill or injured, often they feel powerless and helpless. However, they can be empowered if they are included in the coordination of processes dealing with their treatment. Involving them in even small decisions, like scheduling an x-ray, can help them feel more in control.
- *Inform*: Fear about the unknown is exacerbated when patients feel that their providers are withholding details, especially when the mystery of it all affects them so personally. There is no need to pull out medical textbooks; however, the essential details of the information can all be delivered in a manner that can be understood. There are websites, such as *MedlinePlus* and *WebMD* to which the patient can be referred and there are organizations, such as the American Cancer Society, that can support patient education. They can help educate patients about their diagnoses, procedures, alternative treatments, potential adverse reactions, as well as how the prognosis may change when the option for no treatment is taken.
- *Comfort*: Patients' physical comfort is important to the overall psychological well-being of the care process. If the patient is complaining of the temperature (feeling too hot or too cold), offer a fan or a blanket; don't permit anyone to discount the complaint. When a patient states they are in pain, ensure that attention will be paid and provide some relief. Labeling a patient as having a low tolerance or as being a whiner is unfair. No one can feel what this patient is feeling. Respect them enough to take them at their word. Psychological comfort is important, as well. You may have performed or assisted with this procedure a hundred times and know it is no big deal. However, this is the patient's first experience and to them it is monumental. They are scared, anxious, and nervous. Again, everyone should be empathic and understanding, not dismissive.
- *Support*: Involve the patient's family and friends and encourage their support. You should obtain the patient's permission, of course—some family members may invoke more stress

than calm. Find a place for this extended support group to wait, involve them in decision making whenever possible, and realize these people care about the patient and may need emotional support and information, too.

- *Transition*: Once you have empowered the patient and supported their physical and emotional comfort levels, at some point, the time may come for change. Events such as a discharge, a transfer to another facility, or transfer of care from physician to therapist—all signify progress to you and your staff but may invoke fears of change and abandonment in the patient, especially after a long treatment period. Printed, easy-to-understand follow-up information, directions for medications, physical or dietary restrictions, and access to care (i.e., the weekend phone number or the address of the nearest clinic) will help the patient feel more confident about the separation. If the patient will require an appointment in the future or with another facility, it helps when the patient can have the schedule set prior to leaving. "Transfer of care" is more than just paperwork. You are handing off the care and comfort of this patient to the patient him or herself or to another health care professional. Take a minute to ensure a smooth transition.

Accountable Care Organizations (ACOs)

accountable care organization (ACO)
a voluntarily created team of health care providers who will care for a patient together, sharing responsibility.

An **accountable care organization (ACO)** is a voluntarily created team of health care providers who will care for a patient together, sharing responsibility for all of the health care needs of the individual (Figure 12-4 ■). Physicians, hospitals, and other providers work collectively, communicating with each other, creating a network of coordination that results in a higher level of quality of care. In addition, this communication will reduce the performance of duplicate tests and services and is shown to reduce the potential for medical errors. This results in more effective and efficient expenditures of health care dollars, whether from a third-party payer or the patient himself. There is a provision for the providers to benefit by receiving a portion of the monies saved, as well.

The ACO concept is not new. Many manufacturers have been using this system for years. The fabric manufacturer, the zipper company, the clothing designer, and the seamstress all work together as a team, in coordination, to ultimately produce a jacket. Using this same principle, the primary care physician, the specialist, the physical therapist, home health care, and the hospital all work together using a connective communication system to care for the same patients. They fit their knowledge, skills, and personal attributes together like puzzle pieces, creating a complete picture for the patient.

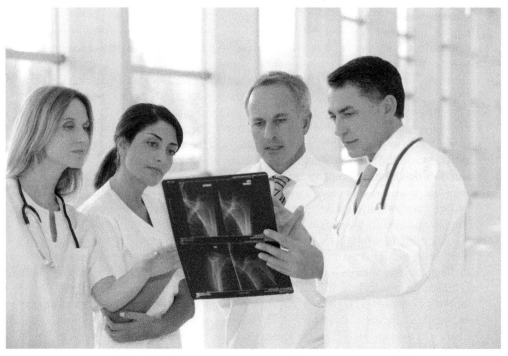

FIGURE 12-4 Physicians, administrators, therapists—all working as a team.
Photo credit: Goodluz/Shutterstock.

You may recognize features from the ACO concept that emulate HMO (health care maintenance organizations). However, in an ACO there is more freedom for the patients. Medicare patients who chose providers that have created an ACO (approved by Medicare) retain all of their benefits and coverage. This includes the right to seek services from health care professionals who are not part of the ACO without paying more.

Providers who would like to participate in or create an ACO have lots of guidance available. Centers for Medicare and Medicaid Services (CMS) have established the *Medicare Shared Savings Program*, the *Advance Payment Initiative*, and the *Pioneer ACO Model*. In addition, other options supported by CMS include: *Comprehensive Primary Care initiative*, *Bundled Payments for Care Improvement Initiative*, and the *Community Based Care Transition Program*. Many hospitals and health care organizations have already begun setting up ACOs throughout the country, improving the way patients are cared for.

CHAPTER REVIEW

SUMMARY

If you were working in the management of a factory, you would constantly make every effort to ensure the quality of the product you manufacture. As an administrator of a health care facility, you have the same obligation—to ensure the quality of your product. However, in health care, the product begins with your staff members and ends with the patient. You must do everything possible to provide the proper environment for your employees to thrive and improve, which in turn will enable them to provide excellence in patient care. These things would include providing them with personalized performance improvement plans, encouraging continuing education, and permitting cross-training when desired.

Patient care can also be improved by creating programs within your facility or your community to establish patient centered care organizations or accountable care organizations, as described by CMS. Very often, the team approach helps everyone involved, not only the patients.

REVIEW QUESTIONS

MULTIPLE CHOICE

Choose the most accurate answer.

1. The cumulative knowledge and skill provided by staff members are known as
   a. patient-centered care.
   b. intellectual capital.
   c. accountable care.
   d. personal improvement.

2. An excellent employee who is burned out in his or her department may benefit from
   a. a pizza party.
   b. a raise.
   c. cross-training.
   d. continuing education.

3. Doing everything to keep good employees is known as
   a. bad hires.
   b. open communications.
   c. advanced training.
   d. employee retention.

4. When a statement of performance is anything except excellent, the facility and the employee may benefit from a
   a. plan of action.
   b. list of expectations.
   c. muffin basket.
   d. keeping their review a secret.

5. When a patient is completing a long treatment and is ready for discharge, the patient may experience a
    a. sense of well-being.
    b. feeling of powerlessness.
    c. fear of abandonment.
    d. low tolerance for pain.

6. Motivating staff members to strive for excellence begins with
    a. a big raise.
    b. creating a culture of caring.
    c. paid vacations.
    d. pizza parties.

7. Participating with local colleges to cultivate student interns can enable you to
    a. provide a comfort level.
    b. extend education to your staff.
    c. nurture future staff members.
    d. get free employees.

8. Support for a patient throughout their treatment should be provided by
    a. the physician.
    b. all staff members.
    c. patient family and friends.
    d. all of the above.

9. A voluntarily created team of health care providers who share responsibility for the needs of the patient may be
    a. an accountable care organization.
    b. a patient-centered facility.
    c. part of a performance improvement plan.
    d. cross-training.

10. Excellent professionals want to work in an environment that
    a. pays for continuing education.
    b. rewards poor performance.
    c. appreciates staff satisfaction.
    d. provides extra supplies.

FILL-IN-THE-BLANK

Fill in the blank with the accurate answer.

11. The value of everything your employees provide to your patients is known as _____ capital.

12. An organization must work to keep good employees satisfied so they will stay with the company. This is known as _____.

13. There is a great cost to hiring the less-competent, known as _____.

14. Organizational _____ is a set of attitudes, behaviors, and emotions that are the foundation for virtually all actions, behaviors, policies, and procedures.

15. The most important thing an administrator can give to a staff member is _____.

16. Motivation that is derived from an employee's personal love of the job is known as _____ motivation.

17. There is a distinct improvement in productivity and quality of care when the hospital has its annual competition between departments. These staff members are being encouraged using _____ motivational elements.

18. William E. Deming developed fourteen principles for improvement, known as _____.

19. Many studies have proven that staff satisfaction is key to employee _____.

20. By improving themselves, administrative and clinical staff members can improve the provision of _____ to your patients.

TRUE/FALSE

Determine if each of the following statements is true or false.

21. With patient-centered care, the primary care provider is at the center of the care circle, in full control of the process.

22. Patients should be included in coordination and decision making about their own health in an effort to empower them.

23. When a primary care physician, a specialist, a physical therapist, home health care agency, and a hospital all work together, in sync, to share responsibility for a patient's care, this is known as an Accountable Care Organization (ACO).

24. HMOs and ACOs provide equal freedom for patients to choose specific providers.

25. Performing random acts of kindness will support feelings that the organization and management care about their employees.

26. Working an environment where administration shows their appreciation for their staff is not going to make any difference to the care patients receive in a facility.

27. Establishing an open-door policy will help staff members to come to management with concerns of wrongdoing.

28. Continuing to pay individuals who have proven themselves to be less than competent in their job performance is actually rewarding poor work quality.

29. Participating with local colleges and universities in their internship/externship programs can enable a facility to nurture future staff members.

30. Each month, the department rewards the employee of the month with a certificate and a little party. This is an example of intrinsic motivation.

WHEN YOU ARE THE ADMINISTRATOR. . .

Critical Thinking and Analysis

Case Study #1

Performance Improvement Plan

Find a classmate, friend, or relative for whom you can create a performance improvement plan, or create a plan for yourself. Write up the plan using the form provided in Figure 12-3, and once you have completed it, submit it to your instructor. Be certain to address every item on the list and include specific action items.

Case Study #2

Continuing Education Opportunities

Research continuing education opportunities in health care administration. You can try the Healthcare Finance Management Association (www.hfma.org), American Hospital Association (www.aha.org), American Association of Healthcare Administrative Management (www.aaham. org), American Health Information Management Association (www.ahima.org), Healthcare Information and Management Systems Society (www.himss.org) or another credible organization in this sector of the health care industry. Find an upcoming educational event, such as a convention, conference, or webinar. Write a proposal to your *supervisor* to request financial support to attend the educational event. Be certain to include all of the reasons why you should be permitted to attend, as well as an explanation of what benefit to your job and the facility may result.

Case Study #3

Performance Improvement Plan Monitoring

As you learned earlier in this chapter, it is not enough to create a plan of improvement for each employee; the plan must be monitored so you can work together with each staff member to ensure his or her optimal achievements. The U.S. Office of Personnel Management (OPM) states that monitoring is a critical stage in the success of this process.

"The regulatory requirements for monitoring performance include conducting progress reviews with employees where their performance is compared against their elements and standards. Ongoing monitoring provides the supervisor the opportunity to check how well employees are meeting predetermined standards and to make changes to unrealistic or problematic standards. By monitoring continually, supervisors can identify unacceptable performance at any time during the appraisal period and provide assistance to address such performance rather than wait until the end of the period when summary rating levels are assigned."

Create a schedule for monitoring your employees' progress in accomplishing those action items listed in their performance improvement plans. What tools can you find or develop to make this process work to the best possible level while not becoming a burden that will interfere with fulfilling their job responsibilities? Use the performance improvement plan you created in Case Study 1, if you like, as a basis for this schedule.

Source: Performance Appraisal Assessment Tool (PAAT), U.S. Office of Personnel Management.

 ## INTERNET CONNECTIONS

AAFP Quality Improvement Tools and Resources (American Academy of Family Physicians)

The American Academy of Family Physicians (AAFP) offers several different Quality Improvement (QI) Tools and Resources on topics such as Performance Measurement and Pay for Performance, including a video, to assist physicians in improving their practices.
http://www.aafp.org/online/en/home/practicemgt/quality/qitools.html

The Joint Commission (TJC)

The Joint Commission's website offers several performance measurement initiatives that can be used by any health care facility, especially hospitals and ambulatory care facilities, to support performance improvement efforts.
http://www.jointcommission.org/performance_measurement.aspx

Performance Management and Measurement

U.S. Department of Health and Human Services, Health Resources and Services Administration (HRSA)
HRSA has included several tools for health care administrators and managers to use to enhance the quality of work provided by each staff member.
http://www.hrsa.gov/quality/toolbox/508pdfs/performancemanagementand-measurement.pdf

CHAPTER 13

AUDITS AND INSPECTIONS

KEY TERMS

audit
comprehensive audit
concurrent audit
covert problem
current
external audit
extrapolation
internal audit
occult problem
overt problem
redetermination
retrospective audit
sampling audit
subpoena ad testificandum
subpoena duces tecum
trend analysis
upcoding

LEARNING OBJECTIVES

Upon completion of this chapter, you should be able to:

- Define commonly used terms, abbreviations, and acronyms.
- Identify the administrator's role in the internal and external auditing processes.
- Interpret the parameters of the various types of audits.
- Evaluate the impact of governmental audits on any size facility.
- Comprehend the appeals processes to be implemented, as necessary.

WHEN YOU ARE THE ADMINISTRATOR . . .

When you are the administrator overseeing a health care facility, you must take into account your responsibility to:

- Cooperate with external auditors by assigning an audit liaison and providing all documentation as requested.
- Develop and implement policies and procedures to successfully conduct internal audits to enable corrective measures to be completed.
- Understand and utilize the appeals processes.

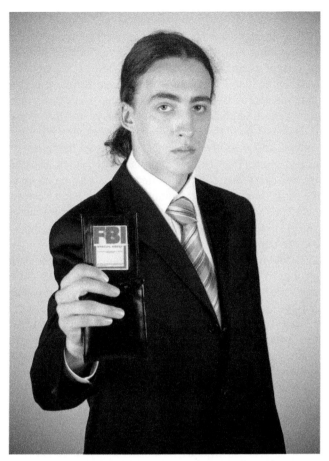

FIGURE 13-1 Once the auditors arrive, it is too late to improve performance.

Photo credit: Brocorwin/Shutterstock.

INTRODUCTION

At any time, an agent or investigator may show up at your office with a notification that you are being audited by any one of a number of government agencies or private third-party payers (Figure 13-1 ■). An **audit** is an assessment of specified data points to determine compliance with previously identified standards and can be performed in virtually every department within your facility: from food service to medical services; from medication inventories to patient discharges.

In real life, the first few phases of an **external audit** is completed electronically. Private insurance companies, the state government, the federal government, and multiple agencies within each have the authority to audit your facility. Being prepared for an external audit actually begins by performing an internal audit.

audit
an assessment of specified data points to determine compliance with previously identified standards.

external audit
an assessment to determine compliance performed by an authorized agency or organization.

TYPES OF PROBLEMS

Essentially, there are three categories of problems that, as the administrator, you need to uncover and address—the sooner the better: overt problems, covert problems, and occult problems. An entire book could be filled with the actual cases of audits resulting in the payment of millions of dollars in restitution, fines, and penalties, in addition to jail or prison sentences. Without question, it is better for you and your staff members to uncover and correct these issues than to be notified by a report from the Office of the Inspector General (OIG), the Department of Justice (DoJ), or other investigative agency. (Appendix A has twenty cases for you to review.)

overt problem
a noncompliant event that is obvious or easily seen.

Overt Problems

Some problems existing throughout your facility are **overt** (obvious) once you actually look for them. Virtually everything that goes on in a physician's office or hospital is done electronically, and built in reports are an excellent side benefit. It is important that you review these reports and use them to identify potential problem areas. When any are evident, you can investigate, determine the source of the problem, and find ways to correct the situation. For example, a problem with getting claims paid is NOT always the third-party payer refusing to pay their fair share. This may be indicative of poor documentation by clinical staff, untrained or poorly trained coders, staff members ignoring queries from the third-party payer for additional information, and more. Take patient complaints seriously, especially when there is a pattern. Generally, for every one complaint filed, there may be as many as 100 unhappy patients thinking the same thing. These complaints can point you to a void in your organization's compliance, such as with patient privacy, billing, or clinical competence. It is your obligation to find out if these actions are insights into the inner workings of your facility or simply disgruntled customers.

   Would you rather find out that two medical assistants gossip about patients within earshot of the waiting room from a patient or from the Office of Civil Rights (OCR) investigating a HIPAA Privacy Rule violation? For example, there is a case about a celebrity patient's record being viewed by unauthorized hospital personnel. In this real life case, the hospital administrator, in his regular review of internal reports, realized that several employees had accessed the celebrity's file when they had no valid reason to do so. The administrator investigated and this resulted in those staff members being either suspended or fired. Your first reaction may be that suspension or termination is harsh for an understandable curiosity. If a complaint had been filed with the OCR and the hospital had not taken action on its own, the hospital could have been liable for thousands and thousands of dollars in fines and penalties. Had the OCR investigated and found that the hospital did take swift action on its own, to make it known there are consequences to noncompliance with federal law, any fines and penalties assessed would have been greatly reduced—in some cases, by as much as a 70% reduction.

covert problem
a noncompliant event that is not obvious or easily seen.

trend analysis
the review and assessment of data taken over a period of time with the intention of identifying patterns.

Covert Problems

Unlike the look-and-you-will-see clarity of overt problems, **covert** problems are concealed and more challenging to uncover. These may be behaviors that can only be revealed by reviewing data over a period of time. This is known as **trend analysis**. For example, only by comparing the statistics of paid/rejected/denied claims over the last six months or one year, might a pattern show itself that, over the last three months, the number of denied claims has risen dramatically. This alerts you to a problem in your coding/billing department that began in the last 90 to 120 days, giving you a specific problem and a specific time period to investigate further. These analyses over a period of time can also reveal statistical creep. This means that something is skewing slightly off very slowly and only when you look at the statistical overview can you see the problem. For example, in your monthly budget meetings with department heads, the manager of food service reports a 1 percent food cost increase. On its face, this does not seem alarming. However, when a trend analysis is completed, you might see that food costs have increased by 1 percent every single month for the last six months. Now, you don't have a 1 percent increase but rather a 6 percent increase over a short time. A trend analysis comparison with the prior year may reveal that last year, food costs actually fluctuated every month, and over the last five years, there has not previously been a steady increase such that which is identified here. The cause of this anomaly can only become evident after an investigation. The key point here is, without the original analysis of the reports, you, as the administrator, would never have known there was a problem to investigate.

occult problem
a noncompliant event that is deeply hidden and cannot be identified without an in-depth investigation.

Occult Problems

Occult problems are deeply hidden behaviors and actions that may be difficult to discover but can put your facility is serious danger when (yes, *when* and not *if*) this comes to light. This may be a physician or other clinician who is a functioning alcoholic or drug addict, a staff member syphoning and selling drugs or other supplies, or violating patient privacy by selling patient rosters (punishable by fines of up to $50,000 per name). Whether it is unethical, negligent, or criminal behavior, believing that "no one in my facility would ever behave this way" is a belief, not fact. If you really believe that they are all good, honest people, then an audit will only prove this fact. Think of the old adage, "Trust, but verify." If your belief is wrong, you need to uncover this immediately. A continuous program of rolling internal audits (audits of different areas or departments randomly chosen) will help to reveal these activities and enable you and your organization to remedy the root cause.

AUDITS

An audit is an investigation focused on analyzing and evaluating certain amounts of data (Box 13-1 ■). Once you determine that an audit, or series of audits, will occur, you will need to decide what the scope of the audit will be to provide the most useful information.

BOX 13-1 **OIG Audit of a Hospital**

Objective
Our objective was to determine whether the Hospital complied with Medicare requirements for billing inpatient and outpatient services on selected claims.

Scope
Our audit covered $2,675,038 in Medicare payments to the Hospital for 293 claims that we judgmentally selected as potentially at risk for billing errors. These 293 claims consisted of 188 inpatient and 105 claims. Of these 293 claims, 285 had dates of service in CYs 2009 and 2010. Eight of the 293 claims (involving replacement medical devices) had dates of service in CY 2008.

We focused our review on the risk areas that we had identified during and as a result of prior OIG reviews at other hospitals. We evaluated compliance with selected billing requirements and subjected only a limited number of claims to focused medical review to determine whether the services were medically necessary.

We limited our review of the Hospital's internal controls to those applicable to the inpatient and outpatient areas of review because our objective did not require an understanding of all internal 4 controls over the submission and processing of claims. Our review enabled us to establish reasonable assurance of the authenticity and accuracy of the data obtained from the National Claims History file, but we did not assess the completeness of the file.

This report focuses on selected risk areas and does not represent an overall assessment of all claims submitted by the Hospital for Medicare reimbursement. We conducted our fieldwork at the Hospital during January and February 2012.

Methodology
To accomplish our objective, we:
- reviewed applicable Federal laws, regulations, and guidance;
- extracted the Hospital's inpatient and outpatient paid claim data from CMS's National Claims History file for CYs 2009 and 2010;
- obtained information on known credits for replacement cardiac medical devices from the device manufacturers for CYs 2008 through 2010;
- used computer matching, data mining, and analysis techniques to identify claims potentially at risk for noncompliance with selected Medicare billing requirements;
- selected a judgmental sample of 293 claims (188 inpatient and 105 outpatient) for detailed review;
- reviewed available data from CMS's Common Working File for the sampled claims to determine whether the claims had been cancelled or adjusted;
- reviewed the itemized bills and medical record documentation provided by the Hospital to support the sampled claims;
- requested that the Hospital conduct its own review of the sampled claims to determine whether the services were billed correctly;
- used CMS's Medicare contractor medical review staff to determine whether a limited selection of sampled claims met medical necessity requirements;
- reviewed the Hospital's procedures for assigning HCPCS codes and submitting Medicare claims;
- discussed the incorrectly billed claims with Hospital personnel to determine the underlying causes of noncompliance with Medicare requirements;
- calculated the correct payments for those claims requiring adjustments; and
- discussed the results of our review with Hospital officials.

We conducted this performance audit in accordance with generally accepted government auditing standards. Those standards require that we plan and perform the audit to obtain sufficient, appropriate evidence to provide a reasonable basis for our findings and conclusions based on our audit objectives. We believe that the evidence obtained provides a reasonable basis for our findings and conclusions based on our audit objective.

Source: Office of the Inspector General, U.S. Department of Health & Human Services.

sampling audit
an assessment conducted on a statistically valid portion of the entire body of data.

comprehensive audit
an assessment of the entire body of data to determine compliance with previously identified standards.

concurrent audit
an assessment conducted at the same time with the creation of data or the performance of the activity.

retrospective audit
an assessment conducted on activities or events that have occurred in the past.

internal audit
an assessment to determine compliance performed by, or initiated by, the organization or facility itself, to look for improprieties, errors, and other wrongdoing.

current
the present time.

SCOPE OF THE AUDIT   The two most common methods of choosing specifically what data to audit are:

1. *Quantity of data to be analyzed*: A **sampling audit** is a method of performing an audit by randomly choosing a small percentage of the overall group. A **comprehensive audit** is to evaluate all units (people, records, etc.) within a particular section. For example: (a) you want to complete an internal audit to check the accuracy of coding, so you tell your auditors to review every seventh patient record. This would be a sampling audit that randomly selects the charts to inspect; (b) you have established a zero-tolerance policy for staff with regard to the use of drugs and alcohol. You order every employee in the radiation oncology department to submit to a drug test. This is a comprehensive audit because 100 percent of a subsector will be reviewed. Almost all external audits use sampling to determine which patient records to check.

   In Box 13-1, the OIG chose their sampling audit based on the results of previous audits performed by computers upon submission of claims. Those claims that were determined to be suspicious or selected as potentially at risk for billing errors formed the basis of this audit.

2. *Time frame from which data will be drawn*: With technology providing instantaneous access to data, an audit can actually be performed **concurrently** with the creation of the data or the performance of the activity. Not precisely simultaneously; a concurrent audit may analyze actions that happened yesterday or last week. When evaluating the claims process, this would indicate that the coding and claim form data is audited prior to submission to the third party. When auditing the pharmacy and the administration of drugs, for example, the audit would be performed before the medication is dispensed to a patient. The alternative is called retrospective. A **retrospective audit** will examine data from the past. This may be the past six months or the year prior. Almost all external audits are done retrospectively, sometimes from last year or the year before that. Recall the audit described in Box 13-1. This audit occurred in late 2012/early 2013 and was adjudicated in March 2013. However, you can see that the claims that were reviewed in this audit were from 2008, 2009, and 2010. Very often, these large investigations performed by the OIG and similar federal agencies are performed retrospectively as they are investigating a continuing pattern of criminal behavior.

Internal Audits

The best way to prepare for, or avoid, an external audit is to perform **internal audits** so you can identify *and correct* issues before any private, state, or federal agency discovers them. Whether a one-physician office or a huge hospital conglomerate, internal auditing should be woven into the regular course of doing business. At some point throughout the year, every corner, every nook and cranny of both administrative and clinical processes should be audited. An internal audit is one that is initiated by the organization itself. You might have **current** staff members perform the audit or hire an outside auditing company to come in and complete the mechanics of the assessment. Using employees to conduct an audit may save money. Consider that you still have to pay them their salaries and perhaps hire temporary workers to fill in their regular tasks during the audit period. In addition, employees may be uncomfortable about revealing a co-worker's incompetence or may even be tempted to cover it up. The motivation may be loyalty, fear of being ostracized, or other misguided attempts to protect someone else or themselves. This is not to state that an audit conducted by staff has no value. These are just potential obstacles to quality results.

With this in mind, you might choose an audit team to perform internal audits in another department. If possible, you might hire a dedicated internal audit team and have them attend a class or two to learn how to properly conduct an audit. This could be very valuable. You can be certain that the members of any external auditing team have been formally educated in auditing processes.

The following steps are involved in performing a valid internal audit:

1. *Identify the specific elements to audit.* While a general or overall audit of the workings of a department is not a bad idea, most audits provide better quality results when focused on one or two specific issues to investigate.

2. *Decide the scope of the audit.* Concurrent or retrospective, and sampling or comprehensive.
3. *Select the audit team.* Determine who will be responsible for performing the audit, processing the data, and creating the report. Interview and select an outside auditing company or choose current employees.
4. *Provide quiet, secure space.* The team should be given a conference room or other location where they can work uninterrupted and an area with lockable doors to secure the files being analyzed.
5. *Specify the length of time during which the audit will occur.* The audit team should not be given an open-ended time frame in which to complete their work.
6. *Designate the format of the audit report and to whom the report should be given.* You will want someone with authority to review the report prior to distribution to the board of directors, the full administration, and/or the staff.

Remember that, in order for the audit to have any value, follow-up action must be taken (Figure 13-2 ■). Within every organization, there is always room for improvement. If the audit provides no opportunities for improvement, then the audit should be questioned and possibly considered invalid.

One of the reasons that many external audits are done retrospectively is that they go beyond finding errors; they look at the ongoing repetition of the same error. While they track your data over a period of a year or so, they are giving you the opportunity to discover and correct the error yourself. It is quite common for an initial watch investigation to be halted, without ever going further, because the errors (the bad behavior) stopped. In those cases where the investigation continues to an audit, the proof that the facility implemented corrective behavior to prevent the error from continuing may result in lessened fines and penalties.

External Audits

As mentioned earlier, an external audit is one that is originated by an outside organization. Some of agencies and departments that are sanctioned to perform an audit at your facility includes, but are not limited to:

- Recovery Audit Contractors (RAC)
- Comprehensive Error Rate Testing (CERT)
- Occupational Safety and Health Administration (OSHA)

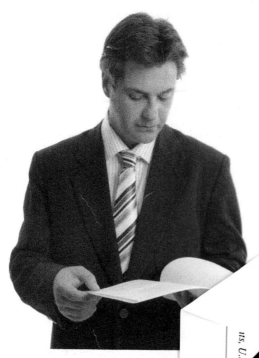

FIGURE 13-2 For the audit to have value, results

Photo credit: Thompson/Shutterstock.

- Department of Justice (DoJ)
- Office of the Inspector General (OIG)
- Health Care Fraud Prevention and Enforcement Action Team (HEAT)
- Medicare Administrative Contractors (MAC)
- The Joint Commission (TJC) (formerly the Joint Commission of Accredited Healthcare Organizations)

An audit of your facility may be a matter of random selection of all those within the scope of authority for the agency, a prescheduled annual or semi-annual event, or triggered by specific activity that has been deemed questionable, as mentioned in the previous section. This activity is most often monitored electronically and, therefore, the result of repeated or continuous issues. Most agencies use software specifically programmed to send out an alert based on their selected criteria. Again, these auditors may be from a state or federal agency or any other organization with whom your facility works, such as a private insurance carrier (e.g., Aetna, Prudential, or Humana) or The Joint Commission (TJC).

As stated earlier, external audits are most often sampling audits done retrospectively. An approved, credentialed statistician determines the sample size, selection method, and sampling method. Based on this guidance, a documentation request is issued. In virtually every case, a failure to respond to the request can have serious consequences. Therefore, as soon as notification is received, your team needs to move into action.

1. *Verify* from whom the request has come and that the request is authentic. Whether the documentation is being asked for electronically or by certified mail, hackers and other criminals might forge a request with the intent to commit identity theft. Make certain your organization does not contribute to this.
2. *Confirm* the names of those staff members who will be included in the audit process and identify the individual acting as your facility's audit liaison. Depending upon the situation, you might find that outside consultants, such as an attorney and/or certified public accountant, should be asked to participate.
3. *Review* the organizational policies (both your facility's policies as well as those governing the auditors). Ensure that everyone on your team working with this audit knows the limits and the level of compliance required by law and/or contract. Every audit will have its own protocol. See Box 13-2 ■ from the OCR about their audit protocols, for an example.
4. *Identify* the various types of record requests, time frames in which you must comply, and the specific individuals within your facility responsible for this activity. Emphasize that the request is complied with in total, and that originals are never sent—only copies. Originals must stay in your organization's possession. Ensure that, when documentation is sent, it is sent in a traceable manner. If hard copies are sent, they should be submitted via Federal Express, United Parcel Service, or another trackable method.

BOX 13-2   **OCR HIPAA Audit Program Analysis Protocols**

The OCR HIPAA Audit program analyzes processes, controls, and policies of selected covered entities pursuant to the HITECH Act audit mandate. OCR established a comprehensive audit protocol that contains the requirements to be assessed through these performance audits. The entire audit protocol is organized around modules, representing separate elements of privacy, security, and breach notification. The combination of these multiple requirements may vary based on the type of covered entity selected review.

he audit protocol covers Privacy Rule requirements for (1) notice of privacy practices for PHI, ghts to request privacy protection for PHI, (3) access of individuals to PHI, (4) administra- uirements, (5) uses and disclosures of PHI, (6) amendment of PHI, and (7) accounting of

overs Security Rule requirements for administrative, physical, and technical

requirements for the Breach Notification Rule.

Department of Health & Human Services.

5. *Prepare* information and documentation—separately from the above—that may be required for the appeals process, should it become necessary. Again, identify the parameters and processes for appeals with the specific auditing organization. Each one is different and most have multi-layered appeal processes.

After the results of the audit have been determined, a report is sent to the facility along with an outline of the specific methods used and if an error is revealed, the amount of money owed. Most often, **extrapolation** is used to determine the total amount due.

Extrapolation is a method of multiplying the sample to represent the whole. For example: The sample size is 10 percent of the total number of patient records, and the audit determined that, in this 10 percent, a $500 overpayment was made due to errors in claims submitted. This number ($500) is extrapolated to represent the same error rate for the total number of records: $500 \times 10 = $5,000 [10\% \times 10 = 100]$. Any applicable repayments, fines, and penalties are based on the extrapolated amount not the specific amount found in the audit.

extrapolation
a determination made by projecting existing experience or known data.

APPEALS

Your facility has received the results of an external audit containing a *notice of errors* and an order for payment. Once you and your team review the report, you might find an error in their determination or a conclusion with which you do not agree. When this occurs, the appeals process should be initiated.

- Confirm the auditing entity's appeals process steps.
- Gather the supporting documentation needed to prove your position. Remember, this entire process is about evidence, not opinion.
- Confirm appeals deadlines and ensure that your facility sets a schedule for this appeal that meets all of those requirements. It would be terrible if your facility had a valid appeal that would have reversed the penalties and you lost this opportunity because an appeal deadline was not met. In that case, your facility would be required to pay the penalties and files anyway.

If you completed step number 5 while cooperating with the external auditors, you are already prepared to this point. Many times, you or a member of your staff can accomplish the first level of appeals without the need for legal counsel. This should be individually determined based on the situation and the accusation. That is, if the *notice of error* alleges improper payment received due to **upcoding** (reporting a higher level of service than that which was actually performed), this can probably be handled with a letter of explanation and the supporting documentation to justify the codes reported. However, if there is an accusation of criminal activity or reckless disregard for the law, hiring an attorney immediately would be wise.

upcoding
an illegal practice of reporting a code for a higher level of service than that which was actually performed.

Medicare's first level of five levels of appeals begins with a request for a redetermination (Table 13-1 ■). **Redetermination** is CMS's (Centers for Medicare and Medicaid Services) term for a review of a claim. For example, you disagree with the original determination of denial, rejection, or *notification of error*. In addition to a letter explaining your rationale for disagreeing with the auditors, the documentation for the patient/incident, and a completed form is all that is required. The deadline for filing this appeal is 120 days (four months) after receipt of the original determination (*notification of error*).

redetermination
a term used by the Centers for Medicare and Medicaid Services for a review of a claim.

Occupational Safety and Health Administration (OSHA) permits an employer only fifteen days (approximately 2 weeks) to appeal a citation and notice of proposed penalty. This must be done in writing and is called a "Notice of Contest" that must clearly explain the employer's report of the situation along with supporting documentation. (See Box 13-3 ■.)

The Office of Civil Rights (OCR) provides thirty days (from receipt of notice) for the covered entity to appeal by providing written notification that you disagree with the Citation of Violation (Box 13-4 ■). This notification should include the supporting documentation that provides evidence that a violation did not occur.

As you can see here, with just these three organizations, all of whom have the authority to order an audit of your health care facility, you may have anywhere from 15 days to 30 days to 120 days to appeal. If you confuse the length of your window, your organization will lose its right to appeal. This could be a very costly mistake.

TABLE 13-1 The Procedures for Appealing a Determination for Original Medicare (Medicare Parts A&B)

Level of Appeal	File Request For Review Within	Claim Reviewer	Minimum Amount in Controversy	Request Format
1. Redetermination	120 days	CMS contractor (carrier, FI or MAC)	None	Form CMS-20027 or letter
2. Reconsideration	180 days	Qualified Independent Contractor (QIC)	None	Form CMS-20033 or letter
3. Administrative Law Judge (ALJ) hearing	60 days	ALJ	$130.00	Form CMS-20033 or letter
4. Appeals Council review	60 days	Appeals Council	None	As per the ALJ decision notice
5. Judicial Review in U.S. District Court	60 days	U.S. District court judge	$1,350.00	As per the Appeals Council decision notice

Source: Centers for Medicare & Medicaid Services.

BOX 13-3 **The Process for Appealing OSHA Citations and Penalties**

Appeals by employees and employers: If a complaint from an employee prompted the inspection, the employee or authorized employee representative may request an informal review of any decision not to issue a citation.

Employees may not contest citations, amendments to citations, penalties, or lack of penalties. They may contest the time allowed in the citation for abatement of a hazardous condition. They also may contest an employer's Petition for Modification of Abatement (PMA), which requests an extension of the abatement period. Employees who wish to contest the PMA must do so within 10 ten working days of its posting or within 10 ten working days after an authorized employee representative has received a copy.

Within 15 fifteen working days of the employer's receipt of the citation, the employer may submit a written objection to OSHA. If the PMA requests an abatement date that is two years or less from the issuance date of the citation, the Area Director has the authority to approve or object to the petition.

Any PMA requesting an abatement date that is more than two years from the issuance date of the citation requires the approval of the Regional Administrator as well as the Area Director. If the PMA is approved, the Area Director shall notify the employer and the employee representatives by letter.

The Area Director or Regional Administrator (as appropriate), after consultation with the RSOL, shall object to a PMA where the evidence supports non-approval (e.g., employer has taken no meaningful abatement action at all or has otherwise exhibited bad faith). In such cases, all relevant documentation shall be sent to the Review Commission in accordance with §1903.14a(d). Both the employer and the employee representatives shall be notified of this action by letter, with return receipt requested. Letters notifying the employer or employee representative of the objection shall be mailed on the same date that the agency objection to the PMA is sent to the Review Commission.

Employees may request an informal conference with OSHA to discuss any issues raised by an inspection, citation, notice of proposed penalty, or the employer's notice of intention to contest.

Source: United States Department of Labor.

BOX 13-4 **Appealing a Citation of a HIPAA Violation**

Development of the Record on Appeal

(a) The notice of appeal is referred to a panel of three Board members, one of whom presides over the development of the record on appeal. The Presiding Board Member is assisted by a staff attorney whom the parties may contact if they have questions about case status or procedures.

(b) The opponent of the party that filed the notice of appeal may submit a response, which may also raise any relevant issue not addressed in the notice of appeal. The response must be filed within 30 days after the opposing party receives a copy of the notice of appeal.

(c) The party that filed the notice of appeal may request permission from the Board to file a reply brief.

(d) The Board expects any party needing an extension for filing the response (or any additional submissions permitted or required by the Board) to file a request for an extension before the original due date, to include a statement about whether the opposing party objects to the requested extension, and to state the reasons for the request. The Board will grant an extension only for good cause shown.

(e) On rare occasions, the Board may grant a request for oral argument if the Board determines that oral argument would facilitate its decision-making. A party wishing to appear before the Board to present oral argument should request such an opportunity in the notice of appeal or the response and should state the purpose of the requested appearance. Generally, any oral proceeding will be conducted by the Presiding Board Member by telephone conference rather than in person.

Source: Department of Health and Human Services.

LEGAL INVESTIGATIONS

There are some investigations that may involve your staff or your facility in a legal action that does not have anything to do with any suspicion of wrongdoing by your organization. One of your patients may have been in a car accident or a slip-and-fall, resulting in his or her attorney wanting a copy of the patient's medical record. There may have been accusations of malpractice against one of your clinicians or a patient is suing a former spouse for full custody of a child.

In any of these, and other, situations, you may receive a **subpoena duces tecum**. A subpoena duces tecum is an order from a court of law requiring the delivery of specific documents to the court. This is not a request; you must comply or chance being found in contempt of court—an act against the law, making you subject to fines and/or incarceration. Another type of subpoena is a **subpoena ad testificandum**. This subpoena is an order for a person to come to court to provide sworn testimony (Figure 13-3 ■).

As a matter of organizational protocol based upon federal law, your staff should get a written *Release of Information* from the patient whose records have been requested by the court. This will expressly comply with HIPAA's Privacy Rule. If not, HIPAA's Privacy Rule, *"Permitted Uses and Disclosures: Number 5: Public Interest and Benefit Activities"* allows the health care professional and/or facility to use their own judgment as to whether or not to release the protected health information.

> "**Required by Law.** Covered entities may use and disclose protected health information without individual authorization as *required by law* (including by statute, regulation, or court orders)."

> "**Judicial and Administrative Proceedings.** Covered entities may disclose protected health information in a judicial or administrative proceeding if the request for the information is through an order from a court or administrative tribunal. Such information may also be disclosed in response to a subpoena or other lawful process if certain assurances regarding notice to the individual or a protective order are provided."

> "**Victims of Abuse, Neglect or Domestic Violence.** In certain circumstances, covered entities may disclose protected health information to appropriate government authorities regarding victims of abuse, neglect, or domestic violence."

Source: Summary of the HIPAA Privacy Rule, U.S. Department of Health & Human Services, Office of Civil Rights.

An example of an Authorization to Release Confidential Information is shown in Figure 13-4 ■. This example is used by the U.S. Department of Indian Affairs.

subpoena duces tecum
a court order for specified documents to be delivered to the authorities.

subpoena ad testificandum
a court order for an individual to testify under oath.

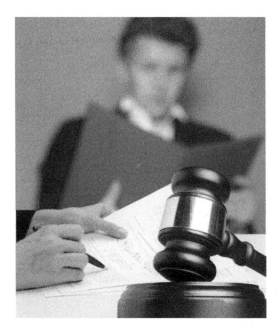

FIGURE 13-3 You may be called to testify.
Photo credit: Burkamin/Shutterstock.

IHS-810 (4/09)   DEPARTMENT OF HEALTH AND HUMAN SERVICES   FORM APPROVED: OMB NO. 0917-0030
FRONT   Indian Health Service   Expiration Date: 1/31/2013
                                                                        See OMB Statement on Reverse.

AUTHORIZATION FOR USE OR DISCLOSURE OF PROTECTED HEALTH INFORMATION

COMPLETE ALL SECTIONS, DATE, AND SIGN

I. I, _____ , hereby voluntarily authorize the disclosure of information from my

health record.   *(Name of Patient)*

II. The information is to be disclosed by: **And is to be provided to:**

NAME OF FACILITY	NAME OF PERSON/ORGANIZATION/FACILITY
ADDRESS	ADDRESS
CITY/STATE	CITY/STATE

III. The purpose or need for this disclosure is:

☐ Further Medical Care   ☐ Attorney   ☐ School   ☐ Research

☐ Personal Use   ☐ Insurance   ☐ Disability   ☐ Other *(Specify)* _____

IV. The information to be disclosed from my health record: *(check appropriate box(es))*

☐ Only information related to *(specify)* _____

_____

☐ Only the period of events from _____ to _____

☐ Other *(specify) (CHS, Billing, etc.)* _____

☐ Entire Record

If you would like any of the following sensitive information disclosed, check the applicable box(es) below:

☐ Alcohol/Drug Abuse Treatment/Referral   ☐ HIV/AIDS-related Treatment

☐ Sexually Transmitted Diseases   ☐ Mental Health *(Other than Psychotherapy Notes)*

☐ Psychotherapy Notes ONLY (by checking this box, I am waiving any psychotherapist-patient privilege)

V. I understand that I may revoke this authorization in writing submitted at any time to the Health Information Management Department, except to the extent that action has been taken in reliance on this authorization. If this authorization was obtained as a condition of obtaining insurance coverage or a policy of insurance, other law may provide the insurer with the right to contest a claim under the policy. If this authorization has not been revoked, it will terminate one year from the date of my signature unless a different expiration date or *expiration event* is stated.

_____
(Specify new date)

I understand that IHS will not condition treatment or eligibility for care on my providing this authorization except if such care is: (1) research related or (2) provided solely for the purpose of creating Protected Health Information for disclosure to a third party.

I understand that information disclosed by this authorization, except for Alcohol and Drug Abuse as defined in 42 CFR Part 2, may be subject to redisclosure by the recipient and may no longer be protected by the Health Insurance Portability and Accountability Act Privacy Rule [45 CFR Part 164] , and the Privacy Act of 1974 [5 USC 552a].

SIGNATURE OF PATIENT OR PERSONAL REPRESENTATIVE *(State relationship to patient)*	DATE
SIGNATURE OF WITNESS *(If signature of patient is a thumbprint or mark)*	DATE

This information is to be released for the purpose stated above and may not be used by the recipient for any other purpose. Any person who knowingly and willfully requests or obtains any record concerning an individual from a Federal agency under false pretenses shall be guilty of a misdemeanor (5 USC 552a(i)(3)).

PATIENT IDENTIFICATION	NAME *(Last, First, MI)*	RECORD NUMBER
	ADDRESS	
	CITY/STATE	DATE OF BIRTH

PSC Graphics (301) 443-1090   EF

FIGURE 13-4 Authorization to Release Confidential Information.

Source: Authorization for Use or Disclosure of Protected Health Information, Indian Health Service, Department Of Health And Human Services.

CHAPTER REVIEW

SUMMARY

Audits are one of the few ways that you can confirm your staff members are doing what they need to do—accurately and effectively. Every health care organization is filled with humans who can make errors innocently or due to lack of training or ability. Whichever the root cause, you as an effective administrator must discover these inconsistencies, mistakes, and illegal actions. It is best to uncover these instances so you can correct them prior to an audit being initiated by a government agency or other outside authority, therefore, conducting internal audits is a very effective way to uncover potential ethical and legal liabilities.

There are several government agencies, on both the federal and state levels as well as the private sector (private third-party payers) that can investigate your facility and its personnel to ensure compliance. However, when these agencies find problems, your organization may have to pay thousands or millions of dollars and individuals can be incarcerated. The bottom line is that no facility, of any size, should need to worry about an audit or prepare for an upcoming external audit. Instead day-to-day activities should be performed every day as though an audit was impending—because it probably is.

REVIEW QUESTIONS

MULTIPLE CHOICE

Choose the most accurate answer.

1. A subpoena duces tecum directs you to
   a. prepare to testify in court.
   b. deliver the requested documents to court.
   c. write an appeal letter.
   d. discharge a patient refusing treatment.

2. An overt problem is one that is
   a. deeply hidden.
   b. challenging to uncover.
   c. impossible to confirm.
   d. obvious.

3. An audit performed by randomly reviewing a percentage of the overall group is a(n)
   a. sampling audit.
   b. internal audit.
   c. concurrent audit.
   d. retrospective audit.

4. Your facility just received a request for documentation as part of an external audit. The first step to take is
   a. confirm your facility's audit liaison.
   b. send all the original documents.
   c. verify the request is authentic.
   d. mail the records via USPS.

5. You complete an internal audit on all of Dr. Ryan's patients' medical records. This is known as a
   a. sampling audit.
   b. comprehensive audit.
   c. physician Extrapolation.
   d. covert audit.

6. A problem that is concealed and more challenging to uncover is known as a(an)
   a. overt problem.
   b. occult problem.
   c. covert problem.
   d. inverted problem.

7. You begin an audit of all of the claims sent to Blue Cross Blue Shield during the first quarter of this year. This is a
   a. retrospective audit.
   b. concurrent audit.
   c. inverted audit.
   d. fiscal audit.

8. All of the following agencies have the authority to audit a health care facility EXCEPT
   a. OIG.
   b. RAC.
   c. MAC.
   d. DMV.

9. Internal audit teams should always have
   a. an unlimited budget.
   b. an open area in which to work.
   c. a specific length of time to conduct the audit.
   d. instructions to not tattle on co-workers.

10. A method of multiplying the sample to represent the whole is known as
    a. extrapolation.
    b. concurrency.
    c. reciprocity.
    d. subpoena duces tecum.

FILL-IN-THE-BLANK

Fill in the blank with the accurate answer.

11. An _____ problem is one that can easily be seen.

12. A method of performing an audit by randomly choosing a small percentage of the overall group is known as a _____ audit.

13. A _____ audit will examine data from the past.

14. A _____ problem is one that may only be revealed by reviewing data over a period of time, such as a trend analysis.

15. A _____ audit evaluates all units within a particular section or department.

16. The Office of the Inspector General informed City Nursing Home that they will be conducting an audit of their medication distribution records. This is an _____ audit.

17. A problem that is deeply hidden and can only be seen after a thorough investigation is known as an _____ problem.

18. Today's audit will review claims as they are being created before they are sent to the third-party payer. This is a _____ audit.

19. Susan Jones, vice president of the food service operation for City Hospital, assigned one of her managers to do an audit of the department to identify any evidence of noncompliance. This is an _____ audit.

20. A method of multiplying the sample results to represent the whole is known as _____.

TRUE/FALSE

Determine if each of the following statements is true or false.

21. External auditors must, by law, give you 120 days notice prior to an external audit.

22. To file a first-level appeal, you must have an attorney file a response with the court.

23. Performing internal audits may help you avoid an external audit being initiated.

24. Most external audits are sampling and retrospective.

25. Your organization is not required to comply with a subpoena unless the patient agrees to release of his or her records.

26. In order for an internal audit to have value, you must pay an outside company to perform it.

27. When you are notified that an agency is auditing your patient records, you should first verify the request for records is authentic.

28. The results of an external audit may be delivered in a document known as a notice of errors.

29. Receiving a subpoena duces tecum means that you will personally have to appear in court and testify.

30. Using current employees to conduct internal audits means this process will not cost the facility any money.

WHEN YOU ARE THE ADMINISTRATOR . . .

Critical Thinking and Analysis

Review each of the actual case studies below and analyze the situation. **If you were the administrator of the organization, how could you use internal audits to uncover the fraud before an external audit occurred? What type of internal audit would you use? Be certain to include a clear description of the scope of your audit.**

Case Study #1

On January 6, 2012, in El Paso, Texas, Anthony Valdez was sentenced to 300 months in prison, three years of supervised release, and ordered to pay $13,356,645 in restitution and to forfeit more than $1.7 million for health care fraud and money laundering. The judge also handed down a monetary judgment against Valdez of $9,741,649. According to court documents, Valdez, a former physician, was the owner of the Institute of Pain Management with clinics in El Paso and San Antonio. On July 1, 2011, Valdez was convicted by a jury of one count conspiracy to commit health care fraud, six counts of health care fraud, six counts of false statements related to health care matters and three counts of money laundering. Evidence during trial revealed that beginning in January 2005 and continuing through December 2009, Valdez caused fraudulent claims to be submitted to Medicare, Medicaid, and TRICARE for procedures which he did not perform or were non-reimbursable.

Source: Internal Revenue Service.

Case Study #2

Lee R. Rocamora, M.D., North Carolina, agreed to pay $106,600 to resolve his liability for allegedly violating the Civil Monetary Penalties Law. The OIG alleged that the practitioner requested payments from Medicare beneficiaries in violation of his assignment agreement. Specifically, the practitioner allegedly asked his patients to enter into a membership agreement for his patient care program, under which the patients paid an annual fee. In exchange for the fee, the membership agreement specified that the practitioner would provide members with: (1) an annual comprehensive physical examination; (2) same day or next day appointments; (3) support personnel dedicated exclusively to members; (4) 24 hours a day and 7 days a week physician availability; (5) prescription facilitation; (6) coordination of referrals and expedited referrals, if medically necessary; and (7) other service amenities as determined by the practitioner.

Source: U.S. Department of Health & Human Services.

Case Study #3

An indictment was unsealed today charging Penn Choice Ambulance Inc., operating from Philadelphia, PA, Huntington Valley, PA and Camp Hill, PA, its owner, Anna Mudrova, and operators Yury Gerasyuk, Mikhail Vasserman, Irina Vasserman, Aleksandr Vasserman, Valeriy Davydchik, and Khusen Akhmedov, with conspiracy to commit health care fraud. The alleged scheme involved more than $3.6 million in fraudulent claims submitted to Medicare.

The defendants were also charged with related crimes including making false statements in connection with health care matters, aggravated identity theft, paying kickbacks to patients, and money laundering, announced United States Attorney Zane David Memeger.

Valeriy Davydchik, 58, and Khusen Akhmedov, 22, Mikhail and Irina Vasserman, both 50, and Aleksandr Vasserman, 29, all of Philadelphia, were arrested this morning. Mudrova, 40, Gerasyuk, 41, also of Philadelphia, will make a court appearance tomorrow. According to the indictment, the defendants conspired to defraud Medicare by recruiting patients who were able to walk and could travel safely by means other than ambulance and who therefore were not eligible for ambulance transportation under Medicare requirements. It is alleged that the defendants, and others acting on their behalf, falsified reports to make it appear that the patients needed to be transported by ambulance when the defendants knew that the patients could be transported safely by other means and that many of them walked to the ambulance for transport. It is further alleged that the defendants themselves, or through others, paid illegal kickbacks to the patients as part of scheme. The defendants allegedly billed Medicare for these ambulance services as if those services were medically necessary and, as a result of the allegedly fraudulent billing, the Medicare program sustained losses of more than $1.5 million for this medically unnecessary method of transportation.

Source: United States Attorney's Office.

 INTERNET CONNECTIONS

Office of Audit Services (OAS), The Office of the Inspector General

The Office of the Inspector General's OAS audits virtually all facilities and organizations that do business with CMS. This includes hospitals, nursing homes, and physician's offices.

https://oig.hhs.gov/about-oig/about-us/office-of-audit-services.asp

Agency for Health Care Administration Monitoring of Hospital and Nursing Home Food Service Operations

The Agency for Health Care Administration is a Florida state agency that oversees all facilities that provide health care in the state. This document explains the steps included in their investigations of food operations within hospitals and nursing homes.

http://www.myfloridaeh.com/community/food/pdf/AHCA_MonitoringHospital
NursingHomeFoodServiceOperation.pdf

Health Information Privacy: Breaches Affecting 500 or More Individuals Office for Civil Rights, Department of Health and Human Services

The OCR maintains a database, available at this website, of the health care facilities that have been found in violation of HIPAA's Privacy Rule, and how the breach was accomplished: hacking/IT incident, theft, unauthorized access/disclosure, and so on.

http://www.hhs.gov/ocr/privacy/hipaa/administrative/breachnotificationrule/
breachtool.html

CHAPTER 14

LEGAL AND ETHICAL ISSUES

KEY TERMS

Affordable Care Act
(ACA)
Americans with Disabilities Act
(ADA)
Anti-Kickback Law
deontological
doctrine of corporate
negligence
Emergency Medical Treatment
and Active Labor Act
(EMTALA)
Equal Employment Opportunity
(EEO) Act
ethics
False Claims Act
Family and Medical Leave Act
(FMLA)
Health Insurance Portability
and Accountability Act
(HIPAA)
Hill-Burton Act
OSHA
Stark
teleological
wage and hour

LEARNING OBJECTIVES

Upon completion of this chapter, you should be able to:

- Define commonly used terms, abbreviations, and acronyms.
- Identify the laws, regulations, and statutes affecting health care.
- Interpret the laws into policies and procedures necessary to comply.
- Evaluate the impact of failure to comply.
- Enumerate the steps used in ethical decision making.

WHEN YOU ARE THE ADMINISTRATOR . . .

When you are the administrator overseeing a health care facility, you must take into account your responsibility to:

- Create and implement plans for compliance with all federal and state regulations and laws ensuring the participation of all staff and all departments.

INTRODUCTION

There can be no doubt that, when asked, every individual would state that they want to work for a legal and ethical organization. Sadly, this is not always a reality. An organizational culture of honesty and integrity, also known as legal and ethical behaviors, is one that originates at the top, with the administrators, and filters down to every staff member. To ensure you are working with, and reinforcing, a culture of this nature, you must become familiar with the parameters.

LEGAL CONCEPTS

There are some legal concepts that affect health care professionals—some of which you may not be aware of. As a health care administrator, you should know about:

- *Battery*: Health care professionals can be charged with battery—the illegal intentional touching of another person without his or her consent—if a procedure is performed without the patient's agreement. This is why it is critical to obtain a written *consent to treat* from all patients prior to treatment (Figure 14-1 ■).
- *Fraud*: Individuals, in addition to the organization as a whole, can be charged with fraud— willful and intentional misrepresentation that may cause harm, loss, or collection of monies not legitimately due. Your coding and billing department is particularly susceptible to these charges if they are not trained properly.
- *Failure to Report*: Virtually all states have laws directing health care professionals to report certain situations with patients. Circumstances such as suspected child abuse, domestic abuse, and cases of confirmed infectious disease are the most common of these mandatory

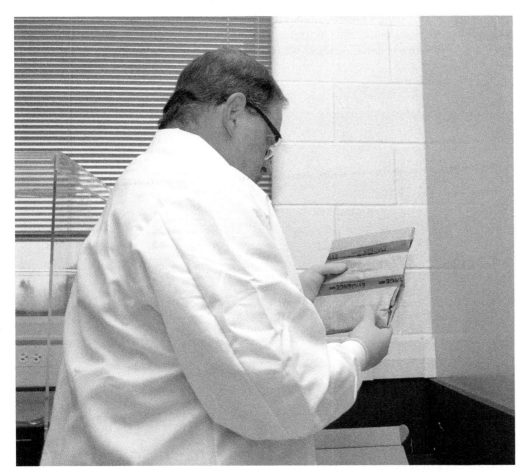

FIGURE 14-1   Police may investigate certain unlawful acts within your facility.

Photo credit: Kevin L. Chesson/Shutterstock.

situations that have legal obligations to report. Failure to report as required may be a chargeable offense.

- *Falsification of records*: Health care records are deemed legal documents and cannot be altered. When an error is found, specific protocols are approved for amending the documentation; however, nothing can ever be deleted or erased. Altered documents can be grounds for criminal prosecution.
- *Respondeat superior*: Also referred to as *vicarious liability*, this legal doctrine holds employers responsible for the actions of employees, in certain cases. Therefore, an employee's act of negligence can expose the facility to civil and/or criminal charges.
- *Malpractice*: In legal terms, this is professional negligence. This might be the failure to do something (omission of an act) required by the standard of care, such as not following up on abnormal test results, or doing something that should not be done (commission of an act) such as amputating the wrong limb.

PATIENT CARE LAWS AND REGULATIONS

Let's review a few of the many laws that directly relate to the care of your patients.

The Emergency Medical Treatment and Active Labor Act (EMTALA)

Emergency Medical Treatment and Active Labor Act (EMTALA)
a federal law binding on only those hospitals who are participating providers with CMS, directing them to care for anyone in an emergency situation without deference to the patient's ability to pay.

The **Emergency Medical Treatment and Active Labor Act (EMTALA)** was passed in 1986 to compel those hospitals that are participating providers for CMS to provide emergency services without regard to a patient's ability to pay. The law requires that any patient arriving at the facility must receive a medical screening exam along with any necessary emergency treatments needed to stabilize the patient so he or she can be safely discharged or transferred to another facility. This includes a woman in active labor (Figure 14-2 ■).

Not only is complying with this law the ethical and honorable thing to do, but failure to comply can result in tremendous liability as well as lawsuits and possible criminal charges. Therefore, if you are faced with a board of directors who recoil at the thought of providing uncompensated

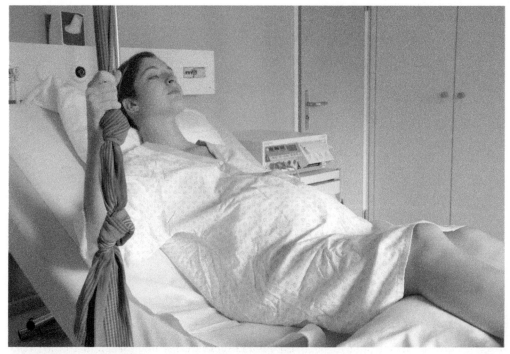

FIGURE 14-2   EMTALA requires care be given under certain circumstances, such as when a woman is in active labor.

Photo credit: ollyy/Shutterstock.

health care because the patient cannot pay, remind them that, not only is it a federal law, it will cost the facility less in the long run.

Stark

The **Stark** law, also known as the *Physician Self-Referral Act*, makes it illegal for a physician to refer a patient for treatment, services, or procedures to another facility or health care business in which that physician has a financial interest. The three versions of this law (Stark I, Stark II, and Stark III) were enacted to prevent any question of a situation where a physician referring a patient for tests or procedures did so for the physician's benefit rather than solely for the benefit of the patient. This law is related to the **Anti-Kickback Law** that prohibits facilities from paying referral fees to physicians.

Hill-Burton Act

Congress passed the **Hill-Burton Act** in 1946 so that health care facilities of all types and sizes could get loans and federal grants to fund construction for updating their facilities. In exchange for these grants, the health care facilities agreed to provide health care to those individuals unable to pay for those services who live in their communities. In 1975, an amendment to the program was passed that required all these health care facilities (that received financial assistance through this program) to provide that uncompensated care forever. The offering of the monies stopped in 1997, leaving just under 170 health care facilities around the country still obligated to provide free or reduced-cost care.

From 1946 through 1997, $6.1 billion was distributed ($4.6 billion in grants and $1.5 billion in loans) to 6,800 health care facilities located in over 4,000 communities within the United States through this program. It has been calculated that, just since 1980, over $6 billion worth of uncompensated services have been provided through this program to those individuals deemed eligible.

As of March 28, 2013, 167 facilities throughout the United States are still obligated to provide free or reduced-cost health care services to those individuals who are eligible. There are no obligated facilities in Alaska, Indiana, Minnesota, Nebraska, Nevada, North Dakota, Rhode Island, South Dakota, Utah, Wyoming, or any of the U.S. territories except Puerto Rico. The list of the participating facilities can be found at: http://www.hrsa.gov/gethealthcare/affordable/hillburton/facilities.html

🛡 BUSINESS OF HEALTH CARE LAWS AND REGULATIONS

It can be difficult to remember that, whether it is a physician's office or hospital, walk-in clinic or assisted living facility, this is a business. A few of the many laws that govern the business of health care are discussed in the following sections.

Health Insurance Portability and Accountability Act (HIPAA)

The **Health Insurance Portability and Accountability Act (HIPAA)** has two essential parts of note: the Privacy Rule and the Security Rule.

The Privacy Rule focuses on the obligation of all health care professionals to protect a patient's confidentiality. The law was written to ensure that patient information is available as required for optimum care of the patient while protecting those details from individuals who have no authority or honorable reason to view them.

The Security Rule addresses methodologies that must be in effect to protect patient data from technical breaches.

False Claims Act

The **False Claims Act** is a federal law that prohibits the submission of any claim to Medicare or Medicaid with the intention of obtaining reimbursement using information that is not true. Repayment, fines, penalties, and possible jail or prison time may be assessed on any individual involved in creating and submitting a claim with false information if this individual knows, or should know, that the information is untrue. This covers coding improprieties, including upcoding,

---

Stark
a federal law that prohibits physicians from making referrals to any facility or other health-related item in which that physician has a financial interest.

Anti-Kickback Law
a federal law that prohibits facilities from paying referral fees to physicians.

Hill-Burton Act
a federal act that provided loans and federal grants to fund construction for updating of health care facilities in exchange for the free provision of health care to those individuals unable to pay for those services who live in the facility's communities.

Health Insurance Portability and Accountability Act (HIPAA)
a federal law protecting patient confidentiality.

False Claims Act
a federal law, with individual states enacting their own versions, making it illegal to submit a claim form to a third-party payer containing information that is untrue.

unbundling, reporting the provision of services that were never provided, and submitting claims for ghost patients (patients who were never seen). Note that virtually all states have enacted their own versions of this law, making this same action—submitting claims requesting reimbursement under false pretenses—illegal with private and state third-party payers. This means that being found guilty of the federal law will often have state charges following closely.

Affordable Care Act (ACA)

Affordable Care Act (ACA)
a federal law that provides stronger protections for patients in their acquisition of health care insurance.

Signed into law in March 2010, the **Affordable Care Act (ACA)** provides stronger protections for patients in their acquisition of health care insurance on the federal level. The health insurance reforms phase in over a four-year period (Box 14-1 ■) and include protections such as the elimination of preexisting condition exclusions in health care insurance policies. Affordable health insurance is extended to more than 30 million Americans who had no insurance previously. This specific benefit is also a benefit to health care providers, including physicians and hospitals, because it reduces the number of individuals for whom health care services would have been provided without reimbursement. This act also continues to advance the adoption of electronic health record systems, supporting a goal to reduce the time necessary for physicians to fulfill administrative obligations thereby increasing the amount of time available for direct patient care.

The Comprehensive Primary Care (CPC) Initiative, created by a section within the Affordable Care Act, seeks to strengthen the provision of primary care services by having public and private health care payers collaborate. Those primary care providers (PCPs) who opt to participate in this initiative will be given access to special resources that will support improved coordination, as well as provide bonus payments.

The Community-Based Care Transitions Program (CCTP), also created by a section within the Affordable Care Act, was created to improve the processes involved in transfer of care for Medicare and Medicaid beneficiaries upon discharge from an inpatient hospital setting to other care settings, including a nursing home, the patient's private residence, or long-term care facility. The goals are to reduce the propensity for reasons for readmissions, especially for those who are at high risk, as well as an overall goal to improve quality of care.

ACA also contains additional incentives for companies of all types to establish and promote wellness programs and to ensure healthier workplaces. This section of the law underscores the importance and value of both participatory and health-contingent wellness programs. As stated on the Department of Labor website (www.dol.gov/ebsa/newsroom/fswellnessprogram.html):

> *"Evidence shows that workplace health programs have the potential to promote healthy behaviors; improve employees' health knowledge and skills; help employees get necessary health screenings, immunizations, and follow-up care; and reduce workplace exposure to substances and hazards that can cause diseases and injury. The proposed rules would not specify the types of wellness programs employers can offer, and invite comments on additional standards for wellness programs to protect consumers."**

BOX 14-1   **Affordable Care Act Timeline**

On March 23, 2010, President Barack Obama signed the Affordable Care Act. The law puts in place comprehensive health insurance reforms that will roll out over four years and beyond. The Affordable Care Act puts in place strong consumer protections, provides new coverage options and gives you the tools you need to make informed choices about your health. In this section, learn about how the law affects you.

Effective in 2013: The Health Insurance   Marketplace Individuals and small businesses can buy affordable and qualified health benefit plans in this new transparent and competitive insurance marketplace.

Effective in 2014: Tax Credits for Families   Tax credits to help the middle class afford insurance will become available for those with income between 100 percent and 400 percent of the poverty line who are not eligible for other affordable coverage.

Source: U.S. Department of Health & Human Services.

---

*United States Department of Labor.

EMPLOYMENT LAWS AND REGULATIONS

Where there are employees, there are laws guiding the relationship between the organization (the employer) and the staff. The Doctrine of Corporate Negligence, Equal Employment Opportunity Act, OSHA, ADA, Wage and Hour, and FMLA are several of the laws with which you, as the administrator, should become familiar.

Doctrine of Corporate Negligence

The courts have upheld that hospitals can be held liable for the competence of their staff under the **doctrine of corporate negligence**. The definition of *staff* in this legal covenant includes malpractice (negligent conduct by a professional) caused by independent physicians and surgeons (who are not employees but have privileges—the rights to practice medicine within the facility). As the administrator, you must do what you can to ensure the quality of your staff, as well as to ensure these quality people are doing quality work.

doctrine of corporate negligence
a law that states that hospitals can be held liable for the competence of their staff.

Equal Employment Opportunity Act (EEO)

You may have seen the **Equal Employment Opportunity Act (EEO)** mentioned in classified ads, but do you know what it really means? The law bars employers (private, federal government, state government, and local governments) from discriminating against a potential employee or against the promotion of a current employee, based on the applicant's age, color, religion, race, sex, or country of national origin. An exemption can be made if the organization can prove that this characteristic of the individual is a requirement of the job. For example, not hiring a qualified applicant who is male as a rape counselor because there is evidence that female victims feel more comfortable with female counselors is a justifiable situation.

Equal Employment Opportunity Act (EEO)
a federal law regulating hiring and firing individuals based on race, gender, or age.

OCCUPATIONAL SAFETY AND HEALTH ACT (OSHA)

The **Occupational Safety and Health Act (OSHA)** requires employers to develop and implement whatever necessary to ensure a safe and healthy place of employment for all staff (Figure 14-3 ■). This covers equipment, supplies, and training to prevent injury and illness to those doing their jobs.

Occupational Safety and Health Act (OSHA)
a federal law that requires employers to develop and implement whatever necessary to ensure a safe and healthy place of employment for all staff.

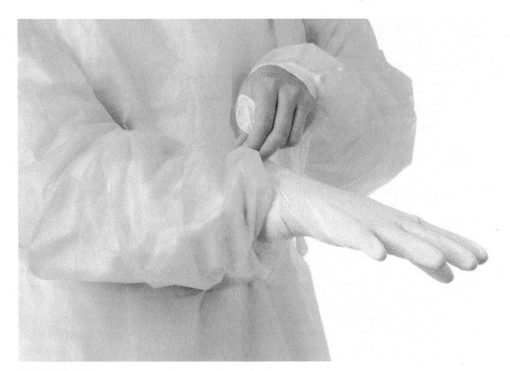

FIGURE 14-3 OSHA requires a safe workplace.
Photo credit: carlo dapino/Shutterstock.

In health care, examples of this include providing gloves, antibacterial wipes, and sharps disposal containers (boxes for the safe discarding of used syringes).

Americans with Disabilities Act (ADA)

Americans with Disabilities Act (ADA)

a federal law that offers protection from prejudice in employment for individuals documented with a disability.

The **Americans with Disabilities Act (ADA)**, updated in 2008, forbids any employer from discriminating against a potential employee on the basis that the individual is disabled (as defined by the law). Similar to the EEO Act prohibiting age, color, sex, and the like as the determining factor when deciding to hire or promote, the ADA prohibits disability from being the deciding factor.

Wage and Hour Laws

wage and hour

regulations that govern how much you pay your staff members (wages) and how that amount is calculated (hours).

You will find that **wage and hour** laws exist on both state and federal levels. These regulations govern how much you pay your staff members (wages) and how that amount is calculated (hours). These laws will guide you with consideration to employee compensation including: minimum wage, overtime pay, and recordkeeping.

Family and Medical Leave Act (FMLA)

Family and Medical Leave Act (FMLA)

a federal law directing companies to provide unpaid leave to employees with a personal or family health care crisis.

The **Family and Medical Leave Act (FMLA)** directs you, as an employer, to enable an employee to take unpaid leave when certain family or medical circumstances require time away from their job and ensure the staff member of having a job of equal or greater stature upon their return.

AN ADMINISTRATOR'S RESPONSIBILITIES

The legal responsibilities of the facility's administration go beyond the straightforward bulleted job description. Virtually everyone has a supervisor, and that includes the administrator of a facility who may be directed by the owner or a board of directors. In any event, you should understand that, if you are instructed to do something that you know, or should know, may present a risk of harm or creates a danger to staff or patients, and you proceed with this activity anyway, you might be held personally liable for any injury that might occur. You are responsible for informing your supervisor or board of directors of the ensuing danger and to educate them so the activity is not carried out. With access to the Internet and the availability of websites for virtually every governmental agency, you can do the research to support a more effective presentation of risks and consequences. This is part of your job.

While you may not be personally liable for the negligent acts of others (as long as you had no part in the event), you are responsible for ensuring that due diligence was done and that your staff has the proper credentials and skills to perform the tasks. For example, while performing a liver biopsy, the physician accidentally cut into the patient's kidney. The administrator cannot be found personally liable for this unless the investigation uncovers the fact that this physician does not have a current license to practice medicine in your state. This makes you, the administrator, culpable because if you had done your job correctly, this physician would not have been performing this surgery and could not have damaged the patient's kidney. In addition, under the doctrine of *corporate negligence* and the doctrine of *respondeat superior*, as mentioned earlier, the facility may be held liable, as well.

ETHICAL CONCEPTS

ethics

a previously determined set of correct, or right, conducts or behaviors.

Health care organizations are unique when it comes to ethics because they must constantly and consistently be guided by both clinical ethics and corporate ethics. Generically, the word **ethics** refers to a previously determined set of correct, or right, conducts or behaviors. It is understandable that this prescribed set of correct behaviors would require different variations of considerations if one were trying to determine the ethically correct action to take regarding a seriously ill child verses an ethical obligation to comply with legal requirements.

The 2011 Federal Sentencing Guidelines Manual states, "To have an effective compliance and ethics program . . . an organization shall (1) exercise due diligence to prevent and detect criminal conduct; and (2) otherwise promote an organizational culture that encourages ethical conduct and a commitment to compliance with the law."* [http://www.ussc.gov/

---

*United States Sentencing Commission.

Guidelines/2011_Guidelines/Manual_HTML/8b2_1.htm]. This statement seems to blur the lines of definition between ethical behavior and legal behavior.

Most often, professionals in many subsections of the industry agree that legal compliance typically comes from the legislature while ethical compliance comes from one's heart. As professionals in health care, it is important to distinguish between these two components and work to ensure they coexist in harmony. For example, the obligation to provide quality of care for our patients is one goal that does not cause conflict; therefore, the line between ethics and legal correctness is blurred—they are virtually one and the same.

There are some situations, however, within a health care facility when the line between ethics and legal compliance is clear and solid. Common hot buttons, such as abortion or stem cell research, are examples of times when the law has decreed one set of compliant behaviors while some individuals' ethics (or heartfelt feelings) direct them in the opposite direction. What is your obligation as the administrator? Most health care facilities have an institutional ethics committee or ethics advisory committee to assist with those decisions that are based in an extreme divergence between law and personal ethics. Virtually all ethics committees are comprised of professionals, representing the multiple disciplines throughout the facility including doctors, nurses, social workers, administrators, clergy, community leaders, attorneys, and sometimes professional ethicists. The committee meets to discuss and analyze the impact of the various potential decisions that may result. Typically, they will work until a consensus is achieved or until a majority agree. The U.S. federal government has established a website (www.ethicshare.org) to provide an online community that may support efforts to come up with the correct decision.

Many people believe that the Hippocratic Oath (Box 14-2 ■) provides a strong foundation for medical ethics. This is the oath that physicians must take upon their entry into the profession. The phrase "First, do no harm" is incorrectly attributed to this oath. Still, there is value to be gained in these words, honored by medical professionals for centuries.

BOX 14-2   **Hippocratic Oath**

Hippocratic Oath

I swear by Apollo the physician, and Asclepius, and Hygieia and Panacea and all the gods and goddesses as my witnesses, that, according to my ability and judgement, I will keep this Oath and this contract:

To hold him who taught me this art equally dear to me as my parents, to be a partner in life with him, and to fulfill his needs when required; to look upon his offspring as equals to my own siblings, and to teach them this art, if they shall wish to learn it, without fee or contract; and that by the set rules, lectures, and every other mode of instruction, I will impart a knowledge of the art to my own sons, and those of my teachers, and to students bound by this contract and having sworn this Oath to the law of medicine, but to no others.

I will use those dietary regimens which will benefit my patients according to my greatest ability and judgement, and I will do no harm or injustice to them.

I will not give a lethal drug to anyone if I am asked, nor will I advise such a plan; and similarly I will not give a woman a pessary to cause an abortion.

In purity and according to divine law will I carry out my life and my art.

I will not use the knife, even upon those suffering from stones, but I will leave this to those who are trained in this craft.

Into whatever homes I go, I will enter them for the benefit of the sick, avoiding any voluntary act of impropriety or corruption, including the seduction of women or men, whether they are free men or slaves.

Whatever I see or hear in the lives of my patients, whether in connection with my professional practice or not, which ought not to be spoken of outside, I will keep secret, as considering all such things to be private.

So long as I maintain this Oath faithfully and without corruption, may it be granted to me to partake of life fully and the practice of my art, gaining the respect of all men for all time. However, should I transgress this Oath and violate it, may the opposite be my fate.

Source: Michael North, National Library of Medicine, 2002.

Ethical Perspectives

Most people are taught throughout their childhood by their parents, their religion, or other authority about right and wrong behavior. Still, there are different perspectives on the ethical rightness and wrongness of some health care circumstances that create a challenge when making a decision. Life and death decisions are often the easy ones to make. However, health care processes and procedures can result in that gray area in between. Essentially, there are two overall perspectives of ethical decisions.

deontological
a perspective of ethical decision making that focuses on the obligation of one's oath or duty to care.

Deontological decisions are based on a duty or moral obligation stirred by oath or other circumstance. In health care, this perspective may lead a physician or other health care professional to perform a procedure because the technology, the skill, and the essential ability exists, and he or she feels it is their duty to do everything possible for the patient, regardless of the possible outcomes. For example, there is a surgical procedure that can be done for a particular patient. However, there is a 50 percent chance that the patient will come out of the procedure totally paralyzed. The physician feels that, in his duty to care for the patient, he must do everything possible to try to help the patient, regardless of what may happen afterward. A person with this view believes it is not the health care professional's business to consider what happens after the patient is discharged, it only matters that everything that can be done is done.

teleological
a perspective for ethical decision making based on the outcome of that decision.

Teleological decisions include considerations for the outcome of the action. This might be viewed as complying with the adage, "The end justifies the means." However, in health care, more often this ethical decision-making perspective views the consequences of the action as valuable as the ability to perform the procedure. For example, the procedure has a 70 percent chance of causing irreversible brain damage. Yes, the procedure can fix the aneurysm (which is what the procedure is designed to do); however, can the patient and the family live with the outcome? This perspective considers what will happen after the procedure, after the patient is discharged, as a significant part of the decision. The quality of life that will be available to the patient afterward is taken into regard.

Ethical Principles

Another challenge to making an ethical decision, especially in health care, is that emotion is virtually always involved in the situation. It might be simple for you, as the administrator, to determine that the patient and his or her family should make this decision, thereby taking this out of your hands. What would you do, however, if the patient and the physician disagree about the right thing to do? What if this decision involved a staff member's behavior, such as reporting a nurse for selling patient lists (violation of HIPAA) because he or she needs the money? There is no one else to make the decision for you.

To begin an objective process of making an ethical decision, you should take into account the four principles of ethical decision making:

- *Autonomy*: The state of being self-governing or essentially respecting an individual's right to make decisions for themselves. This goes further than a patient's constitutional right to refuse treatment. It encompasses each staff member's right to decide what is the right thing for him or her to do.
- *Non-maleficence*: The absence of harm or as it is attributed to the physician's oath to "do no harm." Maleficence is an action that is considered harmful or evil.
- *Beneficence*: Beneficence refers to the state of producing good acts. This, of course, is affected by one's personal definition of what is "good." However, there are general aspects of this principle that are common to most cultures and religions. In preparing to make an ethical decision, include the factors that focus on what will benefit the others involved in the situation.
- *Justice*: Society as a whole believes the principle of justice means that all people are treated fairly and equally. Some people believe this practice should be extended to identify a duty to help others in serious need and that the right to health care is a basic component of a just society.

Steps to Ethical Decision Making

Making decisions that are influenced by ethics is something that must be done quite often, especially when working in health care, so you may find worksheets and other guides to ethical decision making from many sources. Here are steps that most of these guides have in common:

1. *Specifically describe the question or issue.* Keep this description as short as possible. The point here is to carve out the real question from all of the rhetoric that surrounds it.
2. *Delineate the facts surrounding the question.* Itemize any social, economic, legal, cultural, and political influences and ramifications. In addition, identify any other external factors (e.g., an outside expert would need to be brought in; additional equipment would be required; the procedure is still considered experimental). If this relates to a patient's diagnosis and potential procedures, itemize the medical facts, including the prognosis and quality of life projections as well as patient and family preferences.
3. *Identify all individuals involved or affected by this decision and what your relationship to each may be.* This step is important in order for you to be able to consider the consequences of the decision (whatever they may be) as well as cull out whatever bias you may have to each. As you carefully reflect on your relationship to each person, ask yourself if this is someone: (a) to whom you made a promise or have some other type of loyalty; (b) you have harmed and feel you owe some type of reparation; (c) to whom you feel a debt of gratitude; (d) you feel deserves more consideration than others involved in this situation; (e) you feel is more needy than others; or (f) you believe needs more protection from harm. Note that, as the administrator, you must include the organization (facility) as an individual affected by this decision.
4. *Research guidance from all applicable resources.* Do not guess or assume that you remember; this is a time to confirm what the law requires or what this professional's contract guarantees. Use the Internet or consult with your professional advisors (i.e., attorneys, certified public accountants, union representatives) to assemble all the facts applicable to this situation.
5. *Ask for input.* Contact all of the individuals identified in number 3 and ask them what they want to happen and why. Do your best to trim away the emotion and gather as many straight facts as possible. Needless to say, there is a difference between someone whose feelings are hurt and someone who may be psychologically harmed. Make a bulleted list or some type of chart to help you weigh all of these opinions.
6. *Evaluate at least three decision scenarios.* List each possible decision and include the best and worst case outcomes for each. Match each option to the individuals involved and weigh the effect on each. Consider who may be harmed physically, psychologically, economically, and legally. Is the harm insurmountable? Which option will result in the most good or the least harm?
7. *Formulate the plan of action and implement it.* Once you have identified a decision that works as well as possible with all of the parameters, as best they can, ask yourself two more questions: Are you able to defend this decision to others? Are you confident in the reasonableness of this decision? If the answers are *yes*, go ahead and formulate the decision and put it into action.

CHAPTER REVIEW

SUMMARY

Legal and ethical decisions are required of everyone connected with the provision of health care services, and often, you as the administrator will be involved in making these decisions. At times, you will be the one who must make the decision. At other times, you may need to approve of a decision made by someone else. Therefore, you must become familiar with the laws that govern behaviors and actions in the health care industry; laws and regulations relating to patient care, your relationship with your staff members, and the way the facility is run, as a business. One thing known by most successful business professionals is that creating a culture of legal and ethical behavior begins in the administrative offices of every facility—large or small.

REVIEW QUESTIONS

MULTIPLE CHOICE

Choose the most accurate answer.

1. The legal doctrine that holds employers responsible for the actions of their employees is called
   a. EMTALA.
   b. Stark.
   c. respondeat superior.
   d. deontology.

2. Hospitals cannot turn away someone needing emergency care because of this patient's inability to pay as compelled by
   a. HIPAA.
   b. EMTALA.
   c. ADA.
   d. FMLA.

3. You must provide a safe workplace for your employees as required by
   a. FMLA.
   b. ADA.
   c. EMTALA.
   d. OSHA.

4. You cannot refuse to hire someone because of their race, sex, or age because this is prohibited by
   a. the EEO Act.
   b. OSHA.
   c. ADA.
   d. HIPAA.

5. Everyone in your organization is required to protect patient confidentiality as mandated by
   a. HIPAA.
   b. EMTALA.
   c. ADA.
   d. FMLA.

6. Dr. Smith becomes part owner of XYZ imaging center. From this point on, he refers all of his patients needing x-rays and MRIs to XYZ imaging only. Dr. Smith is breaking what law?
   a. False Claims Act
   b. Wage and Hour
   c. Stark
   d. Doctrine of Corporate Negligence

7. The ethical principle that states an individual should not do anything that might harm a patient or another staff member is known as
   a. beneficence.
   b. justice.
   c. autonomy.
   d. non-maleficence.

8. *"Everything that can be done should be done regardless of the outcome"* is a statement based on
   a. teleological decision making.
   b. deontological decision making.
   c. the ethical principle of beneficence.
   d. the ethical principle of autonomy.

9. When making an ethical decision, it is wise to begin by
   a. asking for input from everyone involved.
   b. speaking with an attorney.
   c. determining the social and economical ramifications.
   d. specifically describing the question.

10. As the decision maker, you should evaluate your relationship with everyone involved in this dilemma to identify if this is someone to whom you
    a. made a promise.
    b. feel a debt of gratitude.
    c. feel is more needy than others.
    d. all of the above.

FILL-IN-THE-BLANK

Fill in the blank with the accurate answer.

11. When a patient does not consent to treatment and a health care professional proceeds to treat despite this, that health care professional may be legally charged with _____.

12. The _____ law makes it illegal for a physician to refer a patient for treatment to another facility in which that physician has financial interest.

13. Hospitals that are participating providers for Medicare are forbidden by _____ to deny emergency services when the patient is unable to pay.

14. The Federal _____ prohibits the submission of any claim containing information that is untrue with the intention of obtaining reimbursement from Medicare or Medicaid.

15. The Comprehensive _____ Initiative seeks to strengthen the provision of primary care services by having public and private health care payers collaborate.

16. Ethical decisions that are _____ are based on a duty or moral obligation that is founded in an oath or other circumstance.

17. The state of producing good acts is known as _____.

18. A _____ is an action that is considered harmful or evil.

19. When individuals have the right to make decisions for themselves, this principle is known as _____.

20. The end justifies the means is an ethical perspective that is _____.

TRUE/FALSE

Determine if each of the following statements is true or false.

21. A health care professional can be charged with fraud if he or she performs a procedure on a patient without the patient's consent.

22. Any health care professionals failing to report a suspected case of child abuse as required by law may be charged with a crime.

23. Failure to do what is required by the standard of care can result in a professional being charged with malpractice.

24. If a physician enters "ABX" into a patient's chart and wants to change it to "ABC," he just needs to delete the error (or erase it, if it is on paper).

25. When working toward an ethically focused decision, you should confirm the applicable laws as well as the details of any contract involved.

26. If a staff member has a family emergency and needs some time off, OSHA mandates that you provide unpaid leave and ensure this individual has a job when he or she returns.

27. You are obligated to inform your supervisor if he or she directs you to do something that may cause risk to a patient or staff member. If you go ahead and do what you are told and someone is injured or harmed, you can be held personally liable.

28. An experimental surgical procedure is available to be done on a patient. However, there is a high chance that the patient may suffer severe brain damage as a result. The decision to go ahead with this procedure is a teleological one.

29. Not providing sharps disposal containers for your staff to throw away used syringes is an OSHA violation.

30. To protect a staff member, you altered a patient's chart so it would not show evidence of fraud. You can be charged with falsification of records.

WHEN YOU ARE THE ADMINISTRATOR . . .

Critical Thinking and Analysis

Case Study #1

Go to the Department of Health website for the state in which you live and download the list of diseases and conditions for which health care providers are required to report. Also research what the penalties are for failure to comply with this mandate. **Create a PowerPoint presentation that you might use to explain this mandate to your staff. Include specific consequences that** you as the administrator would assess if one of your employees failed to comply.

Case Study #2

One of your physicians wants the facility to go to court to gain permission to operate on an eighty-seven-year old patient because the patient's next of kin is refusing consent. The patient's son feels that the surgery would cause his father more suffering than ultimate benefit. **What will you, as the administrator, decide?**

(Continued)

Case Study #3

You have discovered that one of your physicians is violating the Stark law by sending patients to an imaging center in which she has an ownership percentage. She offers you a monthly consulting fee if you don't say anything and let her continue to refer patients. She tells you that the facility is good and the patients are not being harmed. **What will you do?**

 # INTERNET CONNECTIONS

County Indigent Health Care Program (CIHCP)

Department of State Health Services, State of Texas

This is an example of a state program to provide health services to those residents who are eligible for such care. Many levels of care are provided with a Basic Health Care Services program as well as additional Optional Health Care Services.

http://www.dshs.state.tx.us/cihcp/

Health Care Regulations

U.S. Department of Health & Human Services

This website lists all of the federal regulations divided by agency, such as Centers for Diseases Control and Prevention (CDC) or the Health Resources and Services Administration (HRSA).

http://www.hhs.gov/regulations/index.html

National Center for Ethics in Health Care

U.S. Department of Veterans Affairs

This group was founded in 1991 and consists of a multidisciplinary team that includes representatives from medicine, nursing, philosophy, law, policymaking, education, theology, social work, and health care administration. They work together to support clinical ethics, organizational ethics, and research ethics throughout the Veterans Health Administration.

http://www.ethics.va.gov/

CHAPTER 15

HEALTH CARE MARKETING, ADVERTISING, AND PUBLIC RELATIONS

LEARNING OBJECTIVES

Upon completion of this chapter, you should be able to:

- Define commonly used terms, abbreviations, and acronyms.
- Recognize the value of creating and implementing a marketing plan.
- Understand the purpose of marketing, advertising, and public relations.
- Prepare an effective message for your primary target market.
- Identify marketing strategies that will support the mission of the facility.
- Evaluate potential advertising vehicles appropriate for a health care facility.
- Analyze how to use public relations vehicles to interact with the community.
- Explain how to work with marketing and advertising agencies.

WHEN YOU ARE THE ADMINISTRATOR . . .

When you are the administrator overseeing a health care facility, you must take into account your responsibility to:

- Supervise the activities of all departments including clinical, human resources, finance (including accounts receivable and payable), operations, maintenance, housekeeping, marketing, and admissions/scheduling.
- Analyze data to identify trends of improvement and/or areas of importance to the patient populations, and ensure the message is clearly communicated via marketing, advertising, and public relations vehicles, as appropriate.

INTRODUCTION

Health care has changed a great deal over the decades. Eighty years ago, each town had its own physician who provided care for every resident from birth to death. There was no competition; there was no decision making about health care providers because there were no choices. Life expectancy in 1930 was 59.7 years of age and this rose, in 2010, to 78.7 years of age*. Evidently, the health care system is doing some things correctly, as the entire industry has expanded to provide more services, preventive care and guidance, and improved treatment options. With all this expansion and improvement came competition. More health care consumers (patients) have more choices of what service to have as well as from whom to get those services. Every business (remember, health care is a business) needs a certain number of customers (patients) to continue to exist; therefore, health care providers must extend a hand and promote themselves and the services they provide.

There are three basic components to self-promotion: marketing, advertising, and public relations. **Marketing**, when the term is used in this sense, refers to activities designed to build awareness, more specifically, **brand awareness**. **Advertising** is generally more direct, calling attention to something or someone, such as, "Buy this now!" **Public relations**, on the other hand, is the process of building goodwill and trust with the public.

A MARKETING PLAN

One of the elements to the formula for success is the creation of a **marketing plan** designed to let your patient population, both current and prospective, know who you are and what you do. A sign on the door stating "Doctor's Office" is no longer enough information.

The marketing plan should contain both short-term and long-term diagrams of how you will send out your message, using marketing, advertising, and public relations vehicles. A written plan will help to keep this very important initiative organized and prevent the waste of efforts and money. You want to be able to prevent knee-jerk reactions that will cost a great deal of money and provide little to no results benefitting the facility. The plan should establish the activities for two important stages: presence and reinforcement. Stage one establishes your facility's presence in the community and attaches the image of what kind of health care provider you are, and stage two will maintain that presence in between campaigns.

When you look at your entire community in relation to your potential patient population, you can generally figure it as 80-10-10. Ten percent of the community will never come to your facility because they don't go to the doctor—ever! Ten percent of the community will be on your doorstep the minute they have an appropriate need. Marketing, advertising, and public relations is all about conversing with the 80 percent in the middle to convince them that they can trust you to care for them when they are in need.

THE PURPOSE OF MARKETING, ADVERTISING, AND PUBLIC RELATIONS

It has been estimated that hospitals, medical centers, and clinics across the United States spent over $1.4 billion on marketing and advertising in 2011. In a single word, the reason why individual health care organizations spend thousands, possibly millions of dollars on marketing, advertising, and public relations activities is *communication*. They use television, radio, billboards, e-mail, postal mail, YouTube, Facebook, Twitter, Tumblr, and Foursquare, plus apps and more to carry messages addressing specific pieces of information of importance to a specific group of people—the patient population in general or a sub-set of the patient population. An organization must communicate with its customers (patients) and prospective customers (patients) to achieve understanding. This is the patient's understanding of what services the organization offers, and how those services match with the individual's wants and needs; in this case, as they relate to health care.

You might find it difficult to view health care services in the same manner with which you view laundry detergent and automobiles. Yet, the same basics of economics and consumerism—supply

---

Source: National Center for Health Statistics, *National Vital Statistics Reports.*

marketing
activities designed to build awareness, more specifically, brand awareness.

brand awareness
a marketing term used to describe activities that draw attention to both the name of the company or facility and the product or service itself.

advertising
direct methods for calling attention to something or someone.

public relations
the process of building good will and trust with the public.

marketing plan
a written document containing both short-term and long-term diagrams of how the facility's message will be dispersed, using marketing, advertising, and public relations vehicles.

and demand—now apply to the business of health care. This sensitivity to commercializing a physician or a hospital has been voiced as an ethical concern. Yet, as long as the truth is communicated in this effort, there is no breach of ethics. In any event, you should be considerate to the feelings of your team as well as your community. There are some aspects of health care professionals' advertising that may be legally questionable in some states. Therefore, it is a standing recommendation to consult a health care attorney to confirm that none of your efforts could be deemed illegal by your state's licensing board. The basic tenets are: always tell the complete truth, do not violate a patient's privacy, and do not make promises that cannot be kept or raise expectations that cannot be guaranteed. When communicating about procedures that include devices or components created by another organization, such as an artificial knee, discuss the success or skill of the medical personnel—the physician or the therapist—rather than the device over which you have no control. Pharmaceutical advertising has stricter legal parameters.

In the twenty-first century, there are many competitive aspects to the provision of health care. **Elective procedures**, including bariatric surgery, eye surgery (LASIK, or laser-assisted in situ keratomileusis), face-lift (rhytidectomy), and other cosmetic surgical procedures, are all typically prompted by the patient's desire to correct a concern, and all require a specialist. Medically speaking, any procedure that is nonemergency (not immediately medically necessary) is considered an elective procedure. This means the patient has the time to consider his or her options: have the procedure or not; determine who will perform the procedure and where the procedure will be performed. The average patient may ask his or her primary care physician for a recommendation; however, the final decision belongs to the patient. When your provider has credentials or accolades that support the patient by instilling more confidence about the outcome or reduce fear about having the procedure, you need to communicate this. The tried and true way to do this is with marketing, advertising, and public relations vehicles. How else can they know if you don't tell them? (Box 15-1 ▪).

Most patients stress out over choosing a health care provider. Typically, a person must determine in whom to place their trust, literally their lives, from a cold list of names and phone numbers—whether the list is generated by the third-party payer or the telephone directory. On what basis might an individual decide? Convenience, that is, which physician's office is closest to where the new patient lives or works is often a requisite. Or the recommendation of a co-worker or friend—typically based on the helpfulness of the provider or the length of time spent in the waiting room—may contribute to the decision-making process. Most states provide details about health care professionals on their websites, detailing degrees, certifications, training, and complaint history. Additionally, Hospital Compare and Nursing Home Compare are offered by CMS to assist with choosing a health care facility.

Reasons for choosing a health care facility can be happy ones, such as the delivery of a baby. Hospitals and birthing centers alike often reach out to woo expectant mothers. Some hospitals promote specialized, comfortable décor and elegant dinners for mom and dad after the baby is born, as well as room for the whole family to provide support for the occasion (Box 15-2 ▪).

Occasionally, health care communication between provider and patient must go through a third party—another provider who refers patients to a specialist or another facility. You want the opportunity to tell this provider what services you can offer to their patients. You will need to determine the most efficient and effective way to get this information across. (Remember, the anti-kickback law prohibits facilities from paying referral fees to physicians.) Your message to the referring provider would be similar to the message you communicate directly to patients: your organization's mission, your staff's skill and knowledge, accolades provided by accrediting bodies, and your assurance that you will give the best possible care to referred patients.

elective procedures
those procedures typically prompted by the patient's desire to correct a concern; a procedure that is not immediately medically necessary (nonemergency).

| BOX 15-1 | Examples of How Hospitals Use Their Websites to Communicate Accolades |

"Our bariatric surgery center has been recognized as one with a documented record of exceptional patient outcomes."

"Our cancer department is committed to delivering state-of-the-art care—from diagnosis through treatment—for patients with all stages of genitourinary malignancies, including prostate, bladder, kidney, and testicular cancers."

"Our physicians group has a long-standing commitment to provide the highest quality care to each patient every day."

BOX 15-2	Examples of How Marketing Can Communicate Treatment or Care Options

"We are the only midwife-based birthing center in this area that offers water births, natural births, and gentle birth choices. In addition, we pride ourselves on our knowledge of alternative birthing choices."

"Our family medicine group practice is dedicated to restoring the health of our patients of all ages, from newborns to adults. Come to us for your routine physicals and health screenings, sick (acute care) visits, immunization and flu shots . . . and more."

Each of these different communication paths has one ultimate goal: engagement. Engagement is the initial connection established between provider and patient. After your marketing, advertising, and public relations efforts result in an individual becoming a patient, a new and mutually beneficial relationship begins. At that point, the patient's own experiences, and that reality, will replace the messages you shared.

For all its detractors, the marketing, advertising and public relations communications of any health care organization work to establish that organization's reputation in the health care industry, even if the information only spreads as far as your local community. These promotional activities support not only efforts to attract new patients but also to attract the most highly qualified staff members as well.

RESEARCH AND THE MESSAGE

primary target market
your most likely customer; the largest group of people with the biggest and most frequent need or want for your product or service.

The first step to creating your marketing plan is to determine your audience. Regardless of the size of the budget, no organization has money to waste. To prevent this, you must have a clear identification of your **primary target market** so that you can create its profile. Once you have this profile, you must be certain that you spend all of your effort and money communicating with this target market. You will waste money talking to anyone else. For example, suppose your facility specializes in treating patients with cirrhosis (a chronic hepatic [liver] disease). Cirrhosis is twice as common among men over age fifty than any other population segment. It is easy to see that promoting your facility's services on Facebook, which is primarily used by a younger audience, will not reach as many potential 50+ male patients as might a promotion on ESPN, which is more male dominated and viewership skews older than Facebook.

The term *primary target market* refers to your most likely customer, in other words, the largest group of people with the biggest and most frequent need or want for your product or service. This is not a group of exclusion—you are not excluding sharing the message with anyone. This is the process of focus—you are honing in to share your message with those most likely to need your services. For example, 70 percent of those patients having a tonsillectomy in the United States are under the age of eighteen, and according to WebMD, is most common among children ages three to seven. Therefore, if you spend $100 to run a commercial on a classical music radio station whose listeners are known to be primarily age 50+, you are wasting $70 because only 30 percent of your audience has the potential to be one of your future patients or a parent of a future patient. However, when you know the facts and are clear about your primary target market profile, you can spend $100 for an ad in *Parents* magazine. This way, 100 percent of your purchase is likely to get the message to the right people—parents of young children.

Demographics and Psychographics

A target market profile consists of demographic and psychographic descriptors. These details will provide an accurate portrait of your most likely customer—the person with the most potential to become your patient.

Demographics involves a set of three basic classifications used to describe a person or group of persons. We look at the general population and divide it into segments determined by age, gender, and income. You want to start by narrowing your target market in each of these three areas. You might need to leave your description in a range, such as people aged twenty-five to thirty-four. Doing so is fine, but you need to try to keep the range as narrow as possible. And certainly, some categories may not apply. For example, your services may apply to both men and women equally, so the gender classification may be skipped. Be cautious; evaluate these situations carefully. For example, prostate exams are exclusively a male health care service. However, most men in their fifties (the age when regular prostate exams should begin) are married, and it is typically the wife who will convince her husband to get the exam. Therefore, you would be wise to expand your target market to include both men and women in this profile, so that you can take the opportunity to educate the wives about the need, as well.

Basic **psychographics** describes consumers using four elements: geographical location; job title or position; education level; and mind-set. Just as with the demographic identifiers, not all of these categories will necessarily apply; however, the same caution should be taken. Quite frequently, patients will choose a health care professional based on geographic location, selecting an office close to home or work. There are very few occasions where a patient will choose to go out of their way to establish a relationship with a provider. The second and third categories, job title and education level, will help you understand the best way to formulate your message. You never want to talk down to a prospective patient, but you don't want to talk over their heads, either. The fourth category, mind-set, refers to the consumers' frame of mind while experiencing your message. You must be certain to communicate with them when they are psychologically ready to absorb the information.

psychographics
four descriptors: geographical location; job title or position; education level; and mind-set used to identify specific groups of consumers.

Conducting Research

Depending upon your facility, determining the details of your primary target market profile could be easy or it may require some research to ensure accuracy. For example, an obstetrics office profile is quite easy: gender: female; age: eighteen to thirty-four (childbearing age); income (will impact whether infertility treatment is an affordable option); job situation (will directly relate to health insurance); and geographic location (the community surrounding the facility). The geographic scope should take into account any other obstetrical facilities in the area: the fewer competitive providers, the wider the geographical zone that will be viable for your patient population. Education level will give you insights into how to communicate about prenatal care or infertility treatments. And, of course, mind-set will generally correlate with age. The older the woman, the greater her motivation for receiving your services may be.

You can find this information in various ways. One of the first, and easiest, steps is to do a current patient survey. Of course, gender, age, employment, and geographical location can be pulled directly from the patient's original new-registration form. Your survey can ask what patients think of your services, what additional health concerns they might have, what led them to choose your facility, and other key questions whose answers can support your future marketing efforts. Patient surveys are particularly helpful to more generalized health care facilities, such as hospitals, clinics, and family practices (Box 15-3 ■).

Focus groups can also provide valuable understanding of your patient population. These are organized and run by companies who specialize in inviting members of the community who fit your profile and guiding discussions without influencing answers.

The bottom line is that before you can craft the right message, you have to understand with whom you are communicating, and you have to understand what they need to know.

Crafting the Message

All of your marketing, advertising, and public relations messages should relate to your primary target market profile and its relationship to your facility. Here are a few basic rules that will help ensure that your message will be more effective and successful:

1. **Wants, Needs, Benefits**: You should explain that you understand what they want or need from you, and explain the benefit to them for choosing your facility to address that want or need. Do not discuss the competition at all. You want their attention focused on what you can do for them. Help them relate to your facility and your providers; that connection will help them feel comfortable with you at the outset.
2. **The K.I.S.S. Principle**: Keep it short and sweet. Choose the most important benefit of your services and focus the message on that point. If you have several important benefits, consider creating a series of ads, with each concentrating on one key detail. If you try to communicate too much too quickly, your audience will end up coming away with nothing. Keep the visuals clear and clean. When visitors reach your website's home page, make it easy to figure out where to go next, without frustration or stress.

| BOX 15-3 | **Medicare Patient Experience Survey Questions** |

The survey asks patients to answer questions about five topics. The topics and questions are listed in the table below. Everyone taking the survey answers the same questions.

How often did the home health team give care in a professional way?

In the last two months of care. . .

- How often did home health providers from this agency seem informed and up to date about all the care or treatment you got at home? (Q9)
- How often did home health providers from this agency treat you as gently as possible? (Q16)
- How often did home health providers from this agency treat you with courtesy and respect? (Q19)
- Did you have any problems with the care you got through this agency? (Q24)

How well did the home health providers communicate with patients?

When you first started getting home health care from this agency. . .

- Did someone from the agency tell you what care and services you would get? (Q2)

In the last two months of care. . .

- How often did home health providers from this agency keep you informed about when they would arrive at your home? (Q15)
- How often did home health providers from this agency explain things in a way that was easy to understand? (Q17)
- How often did home health providers from this agency listen carefully to you? (Q18)
- When you contacted this agency's office, did you get the help or advice you needed? (Q22)

When you contacted this agency's office. . .

- How long did it take you to get the help or advice you needed? (Q23)

Did the home health providers discuss medicines, paid, and home safety with patients?

When you first started getting home health care from this agency. . .

- Did someone from the agency talk with you about how to set up your home so you can move around safely? (Q3)
- Did someone from the agency talk with you about all the prescription medicines you were taking? (Q4)
- Did someone from the agency ask to see all the prescription medicines you were taking? (Q5)

In the last two months of care. . .

- Did you and a home health provider from this agency talk about pain? (Q10)
- Did home health providers from this agency talk with you about the purpose for taking your new or changed prescription medicines? (Q12)
- Did home health providers from this agency talk with you about when to take these medicines? (Q13)
- Did home health providers from this agency talk with you about the important side effects of these medicines? (Q14)

How do patients rate the overall care from the home health agency?

- Using any number from 0 to 10, where 0 is the worst home health care possible and 10 is the best home health care possible, what number would you use to rate your care from this agency's home health providers? (Q20)

Would patients recommend the home health agency to friends and family?

- Would you recommend this agency to your family or friends if they needed home health care? (Q25)

Source: Centers for Medicare & Medicaid Services.

3. **Create an Identity That Is Yours Alone**: Your message and its design should not be "off the rack." Copying your competition will end up helping no one. Ads and other marketing vehicles draw more attention when they are distinctive and unique. After some time and repetition, your patient population should be able to see at a glance that the message is from you. Certainly, you need to ensure that this identity will strongly appeal to your primary target market. No matter what you or your Aunt Molly may think, your image and graphic identity must communicate to your target market in their language, express their wants and needs, and relate to what you can do for them.

4. **Be Consistent in Your Message**: You can create something beautiful and noticeable, something that sparks discussion and gets attention. However, ultimately, if the message provides nothing of substance to give the population a reason to make an appointment, it is just more noise. Don't lose sight of why you are doing all of this—to get patients to come to you for help. Any statements should be backed by facts that carry real meaning. When you make a statement, ask yourself what it will mean to your patient population. Do not expect them to work too hard to figure it out or read between the lines. They need to understand what you are stating right away, or they will go somewhere else. They are busy and cannot—will not—give you too much of their precious time trying to guess what you mean.

MARKETING

Marketing used to be the umbrella term under which advertising and public relations were placed. The marketing process, however, has become a valuable tool in its own right and involves the building of consciousness of consumer need intertwined with brand awareness. A marketing campaign can be used to establish a mind-set that "you have a problem," using an educational approach, followed by "we have a solution," suggesting your services as the best response to that need. Of course, health care problems must be handled delicately. Yet, educating patients on health issues, including preventive care and healthy habits, is part of the professional mandate. Many times patients cannot find answers alone, so establishing the partnership attitude is one that works well in today's physician-patient engagements.

Educational Approach

Health care providers taking an educational approach to marketing rather than a sales approach will find greater comfort in this nontraditional methodology for building a practice or patient population. This tactic fits squarely into the mind-set of health care providers as healers. As we all know, patient education is a key element of healing and caregiving.

Flyers and brochures on general good health, such as healthy eating, getting exercise, lifting heavy objects properly, and the like, stamped with the name and address of the health care facility or provider, support the patient by educating him or her about these important ongoing healthy habits, while at the same time reminding them about provider services. Share the knowledge about specific health concerns by having one of your physicians write an article, or series of articles, to be published in a local magazine, newspaper, or on Facebook or LinkedIn can also establish a relationship with potential patients. When a professional is open and available to help patients and prospective patients, this sparks a connection. Then, the next time that individual needs services you provide, there is a previously established connection and comfort level.

Building Brand Awareness

Brand awareness is a marketing term used to describe activities that draw attention to the name of the company or facility, as well as draw attention to the product or service itself, forging a connection between the two. This way, as soon as patients identify a need for a specific service, they will automatically know where to go.

You might have noticed this with specialists such as dentists and chiropractors. For example, when you get your teeth cleaned, does the dentist give you a new toothbrush? This gift will remind you to take good care of your teeth between cleanings—but look closely. The dentist's name and phone number is imprinted on the handle of that brush, so every time you use it, you are reminded of that dentist's services. When the time comes for your next appointment, the phone number is right there. This marketing opportunity builds good preventive care habits while simultaneously building brand awareness. Think of similar processes for each of your prospective patients.

Providers can build brand awareness in other ways. Health care facilities are investigated and ranked by many organizations. Those that rank high in quality and positive outcomes can publicize this fact and begin to establish themselves as the best, or one of the best, in a specific area of health care, such as heart surgery or oncology (cancer care). Many providers are known throughout the nation, or even throughout the world, for their continuing level of excellent care, such as the Mayo Clinic or MD Anderson Cancer Centers. The reputation of excellence directly connected to the name is a branding reaction. Marketing was used as a tool to inform the patient population of previous successful outcomes in patient care.

Creating a website is another way to empower patients and prospective patients so they can determine the best health care provider. Websites give you the opportunity to provide all of the information, related to each and every subset of your patient population's needs—bariatric surgery, obstetrics, cancer care, diabetes management, and so on. You can also provide all key components of the decision-making process, such as location/hours, third-party payers with whom you participate, and FAQ (frequently asked questions) pages.

Interacting with your patient population using social media vehicles (e.g., Facebook, Twitter) extends the reach of your message. Interaction between individuals and interaction between organizations and their consumers is commonplace in these arenas, and if your patient population is using these vehicles, you must use them, as well. It is your job to get your message to them, wherever they are, not the other way around. You are reaching out to them to encourage a comfort level, to provide support to their good health when they are healthy. Once established, when they are in need of services, they will turn to you. As long as you have a written and signed release, you might include some patient testimonials (if appropriate). This approach can provide support and comfort to potential patients similar to a friend or co-worker sharing his or her experience.

ADVERTISING

Advertising is the sales pitch, so to speak. From billboards to banner ads, television to online videos, radio broadcast to iTunes—wherever individuals are looking, reading, listening, or watching, there is usually a place for an advertisement. You can see for yourself—when you use your favorite search engine to get information on any health care procedure, service, or treatment, ads appear along with your search results.

As mentioned previously, advertising is more direct with its specific sell message. In order to address the wants and needs of the patient population, ads will provide a solution, along with describing the benefits offered by the provider. For example, one hospital ran a billboard campaign advertising a "thirty minutes or less" wait time in their emergency room (ER). You can see that this message addresses an issue that is the focus of countless complaints—lengthy wait times at the ER. (See Figure 15-1. ■)

Advertising comes in all shapes and sizes. Television and radio, known as the broadcast media, are often viewed as the entertainment, or show business, vehicles of advertising. An advertising agency, a production company, or the station itself can produce commercials, or "spots," as they are called in the industry. Essentially, you have ten seconds, fifteen seconds, or thirty seconds to get your message across. Accordingly, given these time constraints, it is critical to keep your message short and to the point. Some may incorrectly assume that television and radio advertising is not affordable for smaller health care facilities. This type of advertising may be less expensive than you imagine and can provide a powerful vehicle for your message. Radio attracts listeners by the station's format, such as country music, classical music, or talk radio. Each station chooses a particular audience to appeal to, and it focuses on that target group throughout the day. On the other hand, consumers watch television by specific program, with the exception of specialized stations such as sports or cooking channels, and television programming appeals to different types of people at various times of the day. Every TV and radio station conducts extensive research to determine their listening/viewing audience, and this listener/viewer profile can be compared to your target market profile to ensure you are spending your money in the most effective place.

Print media includes magazines and newspapers—in both paper and electronic formats. Print advertising is an excellent way to express your message, allowing you to go into a bit more detail because your audience can choose how much time to spend getting information from your

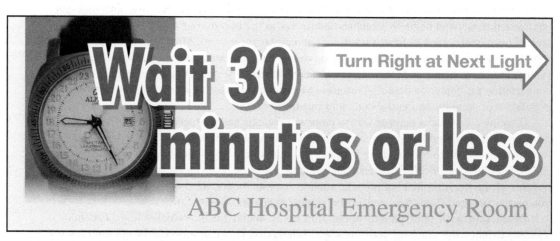

FIGURE 15-1 Billboard advertising for hospital ER.

ad. For example, readers can tear out your ad—or copy/paste it—for later reference. Another benefit of print ads is that you can make the response to this advertising tangible and quantitative by including a specific offer requiring the presentation of the ad, or a part thereof. The reader profile of the magazine or newspaper can be compared to your target market profile, so you ensure purchasing ad space in only those publications that match without wasting money.

Outdoor advertising (see Figure 15-1 as an example) includes the large signs alongside highways known as billboards. Billboards are an excellent way to get your message across, as well as direct patients to your door. Signage on bus stop shelters, inside the bus itself, signage in and on trains, and the kiosk signs along the walkways within shopping malls are all included in the category of outdoor advertising. You need to keep your message super short: the rule of thumb is no more than six words plus your logo. As you can see, the key to this type of advertising is large visuals that can be seen and identified with from a distance in a very short amount of time.

Online, the use of banner ads—those messages that appear with your search results on a browser, as well as next to blogs and other similar types of websites—has become an important advertising vehicle, allowing you to target a specific population and align your message accordingly. For example, you can design a banner ad (across the top of the screen or down one side) to promote your cancer care center and arrange for it to appear whenever someone enters certain key words—cancer, malignancy, breast surgery, prostate, and so on—into the search box.

Direct mail is a category of advertising that allows you to deliver a lengthier message. Direct mail pieces come in many sizes, ranging from postcards and brochures sent via the postal service to e-mail blasts that can carry a message and include a link to your website. The key to an effective and efficient direct-mail campaign is the mailing list. The mailing list needs to be current (no older than six months to a year). You can use your patient list; however, you must remember that this will not increase your patient base. This doesn't mean there is no value to sending information to your current patient population. You can remind them of services you offer, notify them of new services, and educate them on various health care issues.

To broaden your audience, you can purchase mailing lists from companies that specialize in these services. Again, you need assurance that the list is up to date (no more than one year since the last update). You can choose lists by gender, age range, geographic location (usually zip code), or other qualifiers, such as education level, job title, and more. Note that you cannot qualify by diagnosis because HIPAA makes such information illegal to collect. However, some companies do create lists from those who filled out a card stating they are interested in information about diabetes, hypertension, or other specific health issues. Perhaps you remember seeing one of these cards, possibly attached to a new product registration card or in a magazine.

In addition to solo mail (where you are the only one with a message on the single piece of mail), there are two other direct mail options: marriage mail and insertions/pre-prints. *Marriage mail* is the term used for the coupon packs you probably receive. It may be an envelope with several small sheets, each of which advertises a different company, or it may be an e-mail message with several companies combined, each with its own short message and link. You all are distributed together—married to each other, so to speak. Most companies will provide category exclusivity, so you will not be sharing with a direct competitor. Insertions, also known as pre-prints, are those flyers and brochures stuffed into your Sunday newspaper. Virtually all papers can dissect their distribution and limit your insertions to only those papers delivered within a specific zip code, so you can narrow your reach to only those that apply. The pre-print gives you more space to deliver your message, along with pictures and possibly a response card that can be mailed back to you requesting more information. These can be inserted into only those zones whose readership profile matches your target market profile.

Collateral materials is the term used to identify all printed materials used by your facility to deliver a message of any kind. This includes brochures, flyers, and other handouts. These materials are particularly important because you have the space to completely describe a type of procedure and provide all details necessary to get the patient to contact the provider regarding the service. Also, if you have a waiting area, or have a presence at a health fair or school function, these make great leave-behinds to deliver the message in a nonintrusive manner. Check with your pharmaceutical companies or medical device manufacturers. Many publish informational brochures that they will give you at little to no charge. Then, all you have to do is customize the brochure with your facility's information.

collateral materials
the term used to identify all printed materials used by your facility to deliver a message.

PUBLIC RELATIONS

Public relations is exactly what it sounds like, a means for relating to the public—your patient population. This methodology is the virtual opposite of advertising because it is subtle. Public relations activities encompass things such as sponsoring a charity run or bike ride or, better yet, having a team of employees participate. You might choose to take a position of knowledge and authority by offering a spokesperson to be interviewed on the local news about the importance of getting a flu shot or sharing prevention tips during an epidemic. This can also be viewed as marketing from within the community. You are not communicating *to* the community; you are demonstrating that you are *a part of* the community. (For an example, see Box 15-4 ■.) This type of public relations activity might involve inviting members of the community into your offices or facility to meet your staff in a social rather than a clinical environment, so they can ask questions and become better informed without the commitment of an official appointment.

Other community opportunities may be available to your facility to get the message of good health out to your patient population. You may volunteer your physician or head nurse (with their permission, of course) to talk to students at the local elementary, middle, or high school. Send a staff member to hand out brochures or other information (see section on collateral materials) at a community health fair—another way to maintain a visible presence in the area in a relatively noncommercial manner. See if staff members want to form a facility team to walk in the annual March of Dimes walkathon or work phones at the next cerebral palsy telethon and give them matching t-shirts with your facility logo to wear. When you match the charitable cause to your facility's mission, it is doing good on a higher level and will benefit your organization with brand awareness and a positive community relationship.

Public relations opportunities may even arise from a negative situation within the organization. When an organization has experienced a never event or some type of negative anomaly, it is best to get out your side of the story. It has been proven that this lessens liability, in many cases. For example, a nurse was preparing a newborn baby for discharge. As she was cutting off the hospital ID bracelet, she accidently cut off the baby's pinkie toe. Within hours, the hospital held a press conference and explained what happened, relayed that the baby had been taken into surgery immediately and the toe was successfully reattached with an excellent prognosis. In addition, they stated, the hospital was sincerely sorry and was going to provide the baby and both parents with lifelong free health care. They also mentioned that the nurse was put on paid leave pending an investigation. This event could have been cause for the community to turn against this hospital and ruin a reputation of excellent care that had been established over the years. By stepping in front of the negative press, this facility was able to get the community to reaffirm their faith in the organization and their staff and avert a lawsuit. They behaved honorably, and everyone came away respecting that. This is a true story and an example of excellent public relations.

WORKING WITH MARKETING PROFESSIONALS

Marketing and advertising agencies and public relations firms are very much like doctors. They are your partners, charged with helping you keep your facility's health in balance. They use their expertise to help sick companies get financially better and support healthy businesses in their quest to stay strong and get stronger. They have the professional expertise to ensure a valued message and placement of that message to accomplish your goals. While there are never guarantees, the money spent on marketing, advertising, and public relations should be viewed as an investment that will return more money in revenues, as any good investment should, even though this will appear on the "expenses" side of your facility's financial balance sheet.

| BOX 15-4 | **Giving the Community the Opportunity to Investigate** |

"On the first Saturday of each month, join us for an educational video and discussion about bariatric surgeries. Our physicians will be available to answer questions you and your family may have about the various alternatives—pros, cons, and previous outcomes."

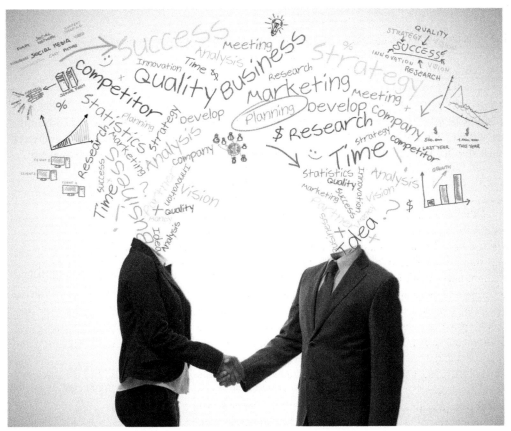

FIGURE 15-2 Working with marketing professionals can support your success with these efforts.

Photo credit: alphaspirit/Shutterstock.

Just as you would advise someone who is looking for a health care professional, you likewise want to be certain to check on the marketing agency's track record, ask about testimonials from other health care clients, and confirm they can understand your needs and guide you toward success. The agency should have access to primary and secondary research sources to support its philosophy for creating and presenting your message to your patient population. There are many intangibles to the creative aspects of marketing, advertising, and public relations; however, there is solid evidence, too. While it may appear on the surface to be all a matter of opinion, there is real method behind it all, psychological strategies and statistical evaluations that should be the foundation of every ad, commercial, and website. Hire a group with whom you feel chemistry (Figure 15-2 ■). They should care about results and be open to discussing and explaining their reasoning for every step in the plan. Do not be intimidated by an agency representative who tells you to just trust him or her. You should both agree on the goals for the campaign and the general direction it should take—before you enter into an agreement.

FUNDING THE INITIATIVE

You should already have a line item on your facility's budget to pay for marketing, advertising and public relations activities. In smaller groups and physician's offices, there may not be an existing program. Therefore, you may have to spearhead the initiative and find the funding. You can use a great deal of what you have learned in this chapter to support your proposal and help your board of directors understand how important these activities are. Start small and gradually increase your presence in the community.

CHAPTER REVIEW

SUMMARY

In twenty-first century health care, patients have more choices than ever before regarding health care services. Competition is greater, and health care providers must step forward to claim their patient population. Marketing, advertising, and public relations vehicles can provide a path of communication between provider and patient to build a strong, valuable relationship.

REVIEW QUESTIONS

MULTIPLE CHOICE

Choose the most accurate answer.

1. Life expectancies have _____ over the last eighty years.
   a. increased
   b. decreased
   c. remained the same
   d. not been measured

2. The three basic components of self-promotion include all EXCEPT
   a. marketing.
   b. advertising.
   c. brand awareness.
   d. public relations.

3. An elective procedure is one that is
   a. immediately medically necessary.
   b. not an emergency.
   c. not related to one's health.
   d. not a surgical procedure.

4. The marketing message for a successful procedure should always
   a. exaggerate the outcomes to give people hope.
   b. mention the patient's name—they will always be flattered.
   c. keep expectations high or people will be too afraid.
   d. tell the truth.

5. When marketing to a third-party, such as a primary care physician, you should
   a. offer to pay them a percentage for each patient referred.
   b. explain that you will take good care of their patients.
   c. offer to pay them a flat fee for each patient referred.
   d. never ask directly for a referral.

6. Educating patients on health issues can be accomplished using
   a. local television.
   b. Facebook.
   c. Twitter.
   d. all of the above.

7. The reputation of excellence directly connected to a facility's name is a(n)
   a. branding reaction.
   b. marketing ploy.
   c. educational approach.
   d. advertisement.

8. Social media vehicles include
   a. television.
   b. radio.
   c. Facebook.
   d. e-mail.

9. Having a spokesperson from your facility speak to the news media about an epidemic is an example of
   a. advertising.
   b. marketing.
   c. brand awareness.
   d. public relations.

10. You are permitted to use patient names and testimonials as long as you
    a. tell the truth about the procedure.
    b. get a signed release from the patient.
    c. include pictures.
    d. put it on your website only.

FILL-IN-THE-BLANK

Fill in the blank with the accurate answer.

11. With all the expansion and improvements in health care, comes _____.

12. Every health care business needs a certain number of _____ to continue to exist.

13. The reason why health care organizations spend money on marketing, advertising, and public relations is because they need to _____ with their patient population.

14. Communicating about your physician's credentials or accolades support a patient's _____ about the outcome of a procedure.

15. The various paths of communication have one ultimate goal: _____.

16. The marketing process includes the building of consciousness of consumer need intertwined with _____.

17. Educating patients on health issues including _____ and healthy habits is part of the professional mandate.

18. Brand awareness is a term used to describe activities that draw attention to the _____ of the company or facility.

19. Billboards, banner ads, online videos are all examples of _____.

20. As long as the _____ is communicated in marketing and advertising efforts, there is no breach of ethics.

TRUE/FALSE

Determine if each of the following statements is true or false.

21. The health care industry has gotten smaller and more condensed over the last century.

22. Public relations is the process of building good will and trust with the public.

23. When a procedure is elective, it means the patient has time to decide who will perform the treatment.

24. When communicating about a procedure that includes a device, such as an artificial hip, focus the message on the device rather than the physician.

25. The health care industry has expanded to provide more services, preventive care, and guidance, as well as treatment options.

26. A marketing campaign can be used to establish a mind-set that "you have a problem."

27. A dentist's name imprinted on a toothbrush is an example of public relations.

28. Your job is to get your message about your facility to your patient population wherever they are.

29. Advertising is subtle and does not have a direct sales message.

30. Once individuals become patients, their own experiences and that reality will replace the messages you shared.

WHEN YOU ARE THE ADMINISTRATOR . . .

Critical Thinking and Analysis

Case Study #1

Building Brand Awareness

Go to the website for a hospital or medical center in your area. **Analyze the way they present their facility and the services offered. Create a PowerPoint presentation on the marketing message presented by their website. Explain what the message is and what you believe the facility is trying to say to their patients and prospective patients. Identify the facility's**

patient population subsets and determine whether or not the facility is successful in delivering this communication to them.

Case Study #2

Advertising Health Care

Look through your local newspaper, local magazines, or look for any local outdoor advertising done by an area health care provider—whether hospital, clinic, doctor, dentist, or chiropractor. **Tear out the newspaper or magazine ad, or take a picture of a billboard. Write an analysis of this advertising. Is the message clear? Can you identify the patient population subset?**

(Continued)

Case Study #3

Public Relations

You are the administrator of a new urgent care clinic in a medium-sized community that is mostly rural. The residents are skeptical because they view you and your staff as outsiders. **Create a public relations plan that will help the residents of the area accept your facility as a valued member of the community. List several events or circumstances that could help earn their trust.**

 INTERNET CONNECTIONS

2013 Healthcare Marketing Trends Report

This report is created annually to identify consumer trends on health care engagement.

There are good explanations of the key points to providing health care and what the patient populations want and need.

franklinstreet.com/franklinstreet_2013_trendsreport.pdf

Ragan's Health Care Communication News

This publication features several articles on health care and the marketing of services, including this article on health care trends.

http://www.healthcarecommunication.com/Main/Articles/4_health_care_trends_for_2013_10319.aspx#

Health Care Marketing

This single webpage offers several articles about various aspects of health care marketing, advertising, and public relations. Find several discussion opportunities, including these articles:

- Why Your Hospital Needs a Strong Brand Right Now
- Taboo Topics: Health Care and Marketing to Men
- Marketing Cardiac Services in Health Care

http://gojunto.com/

CASE STUDIES

These are actual case summaries from the websites of the Office of the Inspector General and the Department of Justice. These agencies investigate various aspects of health care organizations. Use this appendix for further critical thinking, analysis, and evaluation of some of the concepts shared in this textbook.

Case 1.

Former Owner of Wilkesboro Clinical Laboratory Pleads Guilty to Criminal Health Care Fraud and Tax Charges and Agrees to Pay $300,000 to Settle Civil Fraud Allegations

FOR IMMEDIATE RELEASE   April 25, 2013

United States Attorney Anne M. Tompkins
Western District of North Carolina

CHARLOTTE, N.C. – The former owner of Wilkesboro Clinical Laboratory ("WCL") pleaded guilty today in U.S. District Court for his involvement in a health care fraud scheme in which he and his company billed Medicare for services which were not rendered, announced Anne M. Tompkins, U.S. Attorney for the Western District of North Carolina. Louis Francis Curte, 49, also admitted he filed false tax returns from 2007 to 2010.

In a separate civil settlement with the U.S. Attorney's Office, Curte also agreed to pay $300,000 to resolve civil fraud allegations that he and his company violated the Physician Self-Referral Act or "Stark Law."

U.S. Attorney Tompkins is joined in making today's announcement by Derrick Jackson, Special Agent in Charge, Department of Health and Human Services, Office of the Inspector General (HHS-OIG), Office of Investigations, Atlanta Region; Jeannine A. Hammett, Special Agent in Charge of the Internal Revenue Service, Criminal Investigation Division (IRS-CI); and John A. Strong, Special Agent in Charge of the Federal Bureau of Investigation (FBI), Charlotte Division.

Curte appeared before U.S. Magistrate Judge David C. Keesler today and pleaded guilty to four counts of health care fraud and one count of filing a false tax return. According to court documents and today's plea hearing, Curte was the owner and operator of Wilkesboro Clinical Laboratory ("WCL"), which was enrolled with the Medicare program and provided microbiology and other laboratory services. Court records show that from at least 2007 to in or about 2009, Curte defrauded Medicare by submitting false and fraudulent claims for microbiology services which were never rendered.

Court documents indicate that Curte and WCL used another company ("Company #1") for certain types of microbiology testing that could not be performed by WCL in house. Court records show that WCL generally submitted specimens to Company #1 to test for the presence of infection-causing bacteria. If an infection was present in a specimen, Company #1 then typically performed one or two additional tests to identify the type of pathogen present ("identification test") and the type of antibiotic to which the pathogen was susceptible ("susceptibility test").

Pursuant to the scheme to defraud, Curte routinely billed Medicare for identification and susceptibility tests, when, in fact, no such tests were performed and even when the initial testing indicated that no pathogen was actually present in the specimen. According to the plea agreement, the intended loss to Medicare by the defendant was between $10,000 and $30,000.

At today's hearing, Curte also pleaded guilty to filing false tax returns for the years 2007 through 2010. According to filed documents and court proceedings, Curte filed false tax returns which substantially understated his gross income, and therefore, the tax owed to the United States. Court records indicate that Curte maintained false books in an attempt to mask a prohibited business relationship with a physician, identified in court documents as Dr. T.M. According to the plea agreement, the amount of tax loss was more than $30,000 but less than $50,000.

At sentencing, Curte faces a maximum term of 10 years in prison and a $250,000 fine for the health care fraud charges and a maximum term of three years in prison and a $250,000 fine for the tax fraud charge. In his plea agreement, Curte agreed to pay full restitution to Medicare and to IRS for any losses. The final restitution amount will be determined by the Court at Curte's sentencing hearing, which has not been scheduled yet. Curte has been released on bond pending sentencing.

Curte's prohibited relationship with Dr. T. M. forms the basis for Curte's civil settlement agreement. According to the civil settlement agreement, from January 1, 2006 through April 30, 2009, Curte and WCL violated the Stark Law by knowingly having a prohibited financial relationship with Dr. T.M.

Dr. T.M. owned and operated a billing company, now defunct, which submitted all of WCL's reimbursement claims to Medicare. Dr. T.M.'s billing company was paid on a "per claim" basis for the reimbursement claims submitted to Medicare on behalf of WCL. As an owner of the billing company, Dr. T.M. benefited directly from WCL's payments to his billing company. Investigators also found that Dr. T.M. referred blood and tissue specimens to WCL for pathology testing.

The Stark Law forbids a medical provider from billing Medicare and Medicaid for certain services referred by physicians who have a financial relationship with the medical provider. A prohibited financial relationship includes an agreement between the medical provider and a physician to compensate the physician based on the volume of the physician's referrals or the revenue realized through those referrals.

Under the terms of the settlement agreement, Curte is required to reimburse the government for the amount he wrongfully received from Medicare in violation of the Stark Law and to pay penalties back to the program, for a total of $300,000.

The investigation into Curte was handled by HHS-OIG and IRS, with the assistance of the FBI. The criminal prosecution was handled by Assistant U.S. Attorney Kelli Ferry. Assistant U.S. Attorney Don Caldwell handled the civil settlement.

The investigation and charges are the work of the Western District's joint Health Care Fraud Task Force. The Task Force is multi-agency team of experienced federal and state investigators, working in conjunction with criminal and civil Assistant United States Attorneys, dedicated to identifying and prosecuting those who defraud the health care system, and reducing the potential for health care fraud in the future. The Task Force focuses on the coordination of cases, information sharing, identification of trends in health care fraud throughout the region, staffing of all whistleblower complaints, and the creation of investigative teams so that individual agencies may focus their unique areas of expertise on investigations. The Task Force builds upon existing partnerships between the agencies and its work reflects a heightened effort to reduce fraud and recover taxpayer dollars.

Source:
The United States Attorney's Office.

Case 2.

City Dentist Charged with Health Care Fraud

OKLAHOMA CITY, OKLAHOMA – ROBIN R. LOCKWOOD, 44, a dentist from Oklahoma City, has been charged with committing health care fraud, announced Sanford C. Coats, United States Attorney for the Western District of Oklahoma.

Lockwood is a dentist licensed to practice in the State of Oklahoma and was employed under contract by Ocean Dental at offices located at 1610 Southwest 74th Avenue, Oklahoma City. Ocean Dental's dentists provided dental care to Medicaid-eligible children. The Medicaid Program is a cooperative program that provides federal and state funds to pay for health care benefits for individuals with insufficient incomes to meet the costs of necessary medical expenses. In Oklahoma, Medicaid is administered as "SoonerCare" by the Oklahoma Health Care Authority ("OHC"), a state governmental agency. Ocean Dental submitted claims to the OHCA for reimbursement of dentists' services based on patient treatment notes created by the dentists. Ocean Dental paid Lockwood a percentage of the funds that OHCA reimbursed to Ocean Dental for services she personally rendered.

The information alleges that from July 12, 2007 through December 31, 2010, Lockwood engaged in a scheme to defraud Medicaid by submitting claims for dental services that she did not provide. Specifically, it is alleged that Lockwood recorded

in the patient's treatment notes that she had placed dental restorations on certain teeth when, in fact, she had not treated the teeth at all. It is also alleged that on other teeth, Lockwood recorded that she had placed dental restorations on more surfaces of the tooth than she had, in fact, restored or recorded that she had placed a dental restoration on the tooth when, in fact, she had placed on the tooth a type of treatment that is nonreimbursable by Medicaid. Relying upon Lockwood's treatment notes, Ocean Dental submitted claims for reimbursement to Medicaid and paid Lockwood a percentage of those reimbursements. It is alleged that Lockwood used the proceeds of the fraud for her own personal benefit.

If convicted, Lockwood faces up to 10 years in prison and a $250,000 fine.

These charges are the result of an investigation conducted by the Federal Bureau of Investigation and the Department of Health and Human Services—Office of Inspector General, and is being prosecuted by Assistant U.S. Attorney Amanda Maxfield Green.

The public is reminded that an Information is merely a formal charge that a defendant has committed a violation of the federal criminal laws, and that the defendant is presumed innocent unless, and until, proven guilty. Reference is made to the Information and other public filings for further information.

Source:
Department of Justice.

Case 3.

Harmon Memorial Hospital and Hollis Physician Pay $1.5 Million to Settle Health Care Fraud Case

OKLAHOMA CITY, OKLAHOMA – Sanford C. Coats, United States Attorney for the Western District of Oklahoma, and Scott E. Pruitt, Oklahoma Attorney General, jointly announce that the Harmon County Healthcare Authority (Harmon Memorial Hospital) and Dr. Akram R. Abraham, of Hollis, Oklahoma, have agreed to pay $1,550,000 to settle claims of health care fraud of the Medicare and Medicaid programs.

The settlement concludes a lawsuit styled United States of America and State of Oklahoma ex rel. Randy L. Curry v. Harmon County Healthcare Authority, Akram R. Abraham, M.D., P.C., and Akram R. Abraham, M.D., Case No CIV-09-1321-D, filed in Oklahoma City federal court. This suit was brought under the qui tam or whistleblower, provisions of the federal False Claims Act (FCA) and the Oklahoma Medicaid False Claims Act (OMFCA). These Acts allow private citizens with knowledge of fraud to bring civil actions for health care fraud of the federal and state health care programs on behalf of the United States and State of Oklahoma and share in any recovery.

Randy L. Curry is from Harmon County and served as the hospital Administrator of Harmon County Healthcare Authority (HCHA) from 2008 to 2009. HCHA operates the Harmon Memorial Hospital in Hollis, Oklahoma. Dr. Akram R. Abraham, M.D., is a medical doctor licensed to practice in the

State of Oklahoma who has a medical practice and resides in Hollis, Oklahoma.

The United States and State of Oklahoma alleged that from July 1, 2001, through May 30, 2008, both HCHA and Dr. Abraham violated the FCA and the OMFCA by submitting claims, or causing claims to be submitted, to the Medicare and Medicaid programs that violated the federal "Stark" regulations and Anti-Kickback Statute. Specifically, the government alleged that there was a prohibited contractual relationship between HCHA and Dr. Abraham resulting in excessive remuneration which was not commercially reasonable in the absence of health care referrals and that HCHA and Dr. Abraham made false certifications that the Medicare and Medicaid claims they submitted were in compliance with federal and state regulations. The alleged improper remuneration included, but was not limited to, free rent of office space, free billing and staff personnel, reimbursement of uncollected accounts receivable, duplicative per encounter payments for emergency room services, and improper payment of locum tenens physician services. HCHA and Dr. Abraham have each denied liability.

In the settlement, HCHA agreed to pay $550,000 and Dr. Abraham agreed to pay $1,000,000 to resolve the claims. In addition, both HCHA and Dr. Abraham have entered into five-year corporate integrity agreements with the United States Department of Health and Human Services Office of the Inspector General which requires additional regulatory compliance reporting and monitoring. Under the qui tam provisions of the FCA and OMFCA, Randy Curry will receive a share of the settlement proceeds.

Since January 2009, the Department of Justice has recovered over $11.1 billion under the False Claims Act. Of this amount, more than $7.4 billion was recovered in health care fraud matters. Last year, more than 630 qui tam matters were filed with the Department of Justice—more than in any other year in the history of the FCA and an increase of more than 47 percent since 2009. More than two-thirds of these qui tam cases alleged false claims to government health care programs.

The OMFCA went into effect on November 1, 2007, and its focus is solely on fraud perpetrated against the Oklahoma Medicaid Program. Since its passage, over 351 qui tam cases have been filed on behalf of the State of Oklahoma. The State has received over $63.8 million in civil recoveries resulting from cases alleging fraud on the Oklahoma Medicaid system. The Oklahoma Attorney General's MFCU is the only Oklahoma law enforcement agency dedicated to the investigation and prosecution of Medicaid fraud.

This case was investigated by the U.S. Department of Health and Human Services Office of Inspector General Office of Investigations and the Office of Audit Services, and the Oklahoma Medicaid Fraud Control Unit. The case was prosecuted by Executive Assistant U.S. Attorney Bob Troester and Assistant Attorneys General Niki Batt and Lory Dewey.

Source:
Department of Justice.

Case 4.

Ambulance Company Agrees to Pay $5.4 Million to Settle Claims of Fraudulent Medicare Billing

BIRMINGHAM – A medical transport corporation operating in several states, including Alabama and Kentucky, will pay $5.4 million to settle claims that the company improperly billed Medicare, announced U.S. Attorney Joyce White Vance for the Northern District of Alabama, U.S. Attorney David J. Hale for the Western District of Kentucky, and Derrick L. Jackson, special agent in charge of the U.S. Department of Health and Human Services Office of Inspector General for the Atlanta Region.

The payment of $5,426,000 by **Rural/Metro Corporation, Rural/Metro of Central Alabama, Inc., and Mercury Ambulance Service**, doing business as Rural/Metro Ambulance, settles a lawsuit that claimed the ambulance company violated the False Claims Act by submitting false claims for payment on ambulance services that were never provided or were medically unnecessary.

"The resolution of this lawsuit means millions of taxpayer dollars that were used to reimburse false claims by Rural Metro's ambulance service have been recovered," Vance said. "A whistleblower who worked for the ambulance company in Alabama brought these claims to light. We encourage anyone with information about potential wrongdoing to come forward and help us stop fraud and abuse in our health care services," she said.

"Our office led an extensive investigation of conduct occurring in Kentucky, and we are pleased with the outcome announced today," Hale said. "Coordinating our efforts with federal and state law enforcement partners, in Kentucky and Alabama, we avoided duplication of efforts and contributed significantly to today's recovery of taxpayer dollars."

"This is a substantial recovery for the taxpayer," Jackson said. "Today's action sends a message to greedy ambulance companies that improperly bill the Medicare and Medicaid systems. The Office of Inspector General will continue to ensure that federal health care programs pay for services that are proper and necessary."

According to the settlement agreement, the government claimed that Rural/Metro ambulance services in Alabama and Tennessee sought Medicare reimbursement from January 2008 through December 2010 for nonemergency transportation for Medicare beneficiaries to receive dialysis services. The government also claimed that from January 2008 through August 2011, a Rural/Metro company in Kentucky, Mercury Ambulance, also sought reimbursement for nonemergency transportation for Medicare beneficiaries to receive dialysis services.

The lawsuit that originally asserted the False Claims Act violations against Rural/Metro was filed against the company in 2009 in U.S. District Court for the Northern District of Alabama. It was filed as a whistleblower action by a former employee of Rural/Metro of Central Alabama. The United States intervened in the lawsuit in March 2011.

Rural/Metro Corporation, through its subsidiaries and affiliates, is engaged in the business of providing medical transportation services to individuals, including ambulance transportation services to Medicare and Medicaid beneficiaries, in approximately 20 states.

In conjunction with several federal and state law enforcement agencies, the U.S. Attorney's Office for the Western District of Kentucky investigated conduct occurring in that state and worked with the U.S. Attorney's Office in Alabama to include the Kentucky-based claims in the Alabama lawsuit. Under the whistleblowing statute, the offices will share the reimbursed funds with the whistleblower and his attorneys, who will receive $1,030,940 plus fees and costs.

Medicare's regulations cover the reimbursement of certain ambulance services only if those services are furnished to a beneficiary whose medical condition dictates that other means of transportation are not advised. This generally means that ambulance transportation is appropriate if the beneficiary is bed-confined or if the beneficiary's medical condition, regardless of bed confinement, is such that transportation by ambulance is medically required.

The United States' complaint alleged that the defendants created and submitted fraudulent records and claims for payment by governmental health care providers. According to the complaint, Rural/Metro falsely represented that transported patients were either bed-confined or that transportation by ambulance was, otherwise, medically required. Many of those patients, however, were neither bed-confined nor needed to be moved on stretchers, and did not require ambulance transportation or qualify for ambulance transport under the applicable Medicare requirements.

The allegations in the complaint do not relate to the quality of the care provided by the defendants during the transportation.

The lawsuit was filed under the qui tam provisions of the False Claims Act, which permit private parties to sue on behalf of the United States when they believe that defendants submitted false claims for government funds. The law provides that the whistleblowers are entitled to receive a share of any funds recovered through the lawsuit. The False Claims Act permits the government to recover three times its damages plus civil penalties.

This settlement is neither an admission of liability by the defendants, nor is it a concession by the United States that its claims are not well founded.

This resolution is part of the government's emphasis on combating health care fraud and another step for the Health Care Fraud Prevention and Enforcement Action Team (HEAT) initiative, which was announced by Attorney General Eric Holder and Department of Health and Human Services Secretary Kathleen Sebelius in May 2009. The partnership between the two departments has focused efforts to reduce and prevent Medicare and Medicaid financial fraud through enhanced cooperation.

The U.S. Attorney's Office for the Northern District of Alabama prosecuted the case. The U.S. Attorney's Office for the Western District of Kentucky joined the Northern District of Alabama Office, along with the Health and Human Services' Office of Inspector General, the FBI, the Medicaid Fraud and Abuse Control Division of the Kentucky Attorney General's

Office and the Office of the Inspector General of the U.S. Railroad Retirement Board in investigating the case.

Source:

Department of Justice.

Case 5.

Miami-Area Resident Pleads Guilty to Participating in $63 Million Medicare Fraud Scheme

WASHINGTON – A Miami-area resident pleaded guilty today in U.S. District Court in Miami for her role in a health care fraud scheme that resulted in the submission of more than $63 million in fraudulent claims to Medicare and Medicaid, announced the Department of Justice, the FBI and the Department of Health and Human Services (HHS).

Sarah Da Silva Keller, 27, pleaded guilty before U.S. District Judge Marcia G. Cooke in Miami to one count of conspiracy to commit health care fraud. Keller admitted to participating in a fraud scheme that was orchestrated by the owner and operators of Health Care Solutions Network (HCSN), which operated purported partial hospitalization programs (PHPs), a form of intensive mental health treatment for severe mental illness.

According to an indictment unsealed on May 2, 2012, HCSN paid kickbacks to owners and operators of assisted living facilities in exchange for referring Medicare beneficiaries to HCSN for PHP treatment that was unnecessary and, in many instances, not provided. According to court documents, Keller admitted that she falsified records at the direction of others so that HCSN could bill Medicare for patients who did not receive the services from HCSN. Keller knew that the falsification of these records was part of a plan for HCSN to commit health care fraud.

At sentencing, scheduled for Oct. 17, 2012, Keller faces a maximum of 10 years in prison and a $250,000 fine for each count.

Nine other charged defendants, including the owner and operators of HCSN, await trial before U.S. District Judge Cecilia M. Altonaga. Defendants are presumed innocent until proven guilty at trial.

Today's guilty plea was announced by Assistant Attorney General Lanny A. Breuer of the Justice Department's Criminal Division; U.S. Attorney Wifredo A. Ferrer of the Southern District of Florida; Xanthi C. Mangum, Acting Special Agent-in-Charge of the FBI's Miami Field Office; and Special Agent-in-Charge Christopher B. Dennis of the HHS Office of Inspector General (HHS-OIG), Office of Investigations Miami office.

The case is being prosecuted by Trial Attorneys Steven Kim, William Parente and Allan Medina of the Criminal Division's Fraud Section. The case was investigated by the FBI, HHS-OIG and Medicaid Fraud Control Unit and was brought as part of the Medicare Fraud Strike Force, supervised by the Criminal Division's Fraud Section and the U.S. Attorney's Office for the Southern District of Florida.

Since their inception in March 2007, Medicare Fraud Strike Force operations in nine locations have charged more than 1,330 defendants who collectively have falsely billed the Medicare program for more than $4 billion. In addition, HHS's Centers for Medicare and Medicaid Services, working in conjunction with the HHS-OIG, are taking steps to increase accountability and decrease the presence of fraudulent providers.

Source:

Department of Justice.

Case 6.

Houston Man Headed to Federal Prison for Health Care Fraud

HOUSTON – Kelvin Washington, 49, of Houston, has been handed a 24-month federal sentence following his convictions of health care fraud, conspiracy and violations of the anti-kickback statute, United States Attorney Kenneth Magidson announced today. Washington was convicted after six days of trial and three and a half hours of deliberation on Dec. 8, 2011.

Today, U.S. District Court Judge Nancy Atlas, who presided over the trial, sentenced Washington to 24 months for each of the six convictions of health care fraud, conspiracy conviction and three counts of violating the anti-kickback statute, all to be served concurrently. The court additionally ordered three years supervised release, of which the first 12 months of to be served as home confinement. He was ordered to pay approximately $480,000 in restitution to Medicare and Medicaid.

The evidence in the weeklong trial showed that from 2003 to 2007, Washington received illegal payments for the referral of dialysis patients to a Houston ambulance transport service. In addition, he conspired with others to have unsuspecting doctors sign transport prescriptions for dialysis patients never admitted to a Sugar Land nursing home where he worked.

Testimony at trial showed Washington was paid for the referral of dialysis patients to an ambulance service that was under contract with the nursing home where he worked. The evidence also showed he would present prescriptions to doctors who worked at the nursing home. The doctors testified at trial that they would not have signed the prescriptions if they had known the various patients were never admitted to the nursing home.

The jury also heard evidence that the ambulance service paid the Washington in checks totaling $22,200, with many tied to specific patients. Washington did not report all the income he made to the Internal Revenue Service (IRS) from the ambulance service. At trial, an undercover video and audio tape showed one of the managers of the ambulance company bribing a patient to ride with the ambulance company. The ambulance company would later bill Medicare for this patient, a paid informant whose own doctors would not sign a prescription for him. The bill to Medicare was based upon a false script from Washington. In a search warrant executed on a co-conspirator's home, "The List" was discovered which detailed payments made not only to Washington but also to patients who rode with the ambulance service. A computer file from that home also showed detailed records tracking payments for patients, the check numbers for those payments and the fact that payments were made to the defendant.

The false scripts alone resulted in $1.2 million billed to Medicare and Medicaid and approximately $480,000 paid.

Washington was permitted to remain on bond pending transfer to a U.S. Bureau of Prisons facility to be determined in the near future.

The charges are the result of the investigative efforts of Health and Human Services—Office of Inspector General, Office of Investigations; Texas Attorney General's Medicaid Fraud Unit, FBI and the United States Attorney's Office. Special Assistant United States Attorney Suzanne Bradley and Assistant United States Attorney Al Balboni prosecuted the case.

Source:

Department of Justice.

Case 7.

Detroit-Area Clinic Owner Pleads Guilty to $16 Million Psychotherapy Fraud Scheme

WASHINGTON – Detroit-area resident Louisa Thompson pleaded guilty today for her role in a $16 million fraud scheme, announced the Department of Justice, the FBI and the Department of Health and Human Services (HHS).

Thompson, 63, pleaded guilty today before U.S. District Judge Nancy D. Edmunds in the Eastern District of Michigan to one count of conspiracy to commit health care fraud. At sentencing, scheduled for Oct. 18, 2012, Thompson faces a maximum penalty of 10 years in prison and a $250,000 fine.

According to the plea documents, in approximately January 2006, Thompson began billing Medicare for psychotherapy services through two companies, TGW Medical, Inc. and Caldwell Thompson Manor, Inc. The services billed by Thompson at TGW and Caldwell Thompson were never performed or were performed by unlicensed staff who were not authorized to perform services reimbursed by Medicare. The unlicensed staff members also fabricated therapy notes for patients that were never seen and billed Medicare using document templates created by Thompson.

According to court documents, Thompson also received payments from the owner of P&C Adult Day Care, Inc., a psychotherapy clinic. Those payments to Thompson were, in part, for the use of Thompson's provider number by P&C. Thompson also admitted signing therapy documents for P&C patients she never saw or treated. P&C, like TGW and Caldwell Thompson, billed for psychotherapy services that were either not performed or performed by unlicensed staff. Caldwell Thompson and P&C shared Medicare beneficiaries and/or beneficiary information.

Thompson admitted to submitting or causing to be submitted approximately $15.9 million in fraudulent psychotherapy claims on behalf of TGW, Caldwell Thompson and P&C. Medicare paid approximately $4.9 million of those claims.

The guilty plea was announced by Assistant Attorney General Lanny A. Breuer of the Justice Department's Criminal Division; U.S. Attorney for the Eastern District of Michigan Barbara L. McQuade; Acting Special Agent in Charge of the

FBI's Detroit Field Office Edward J. Hanko; and Special Agent in Charge Lamont Pugh III of the HHS Office of Inspector General's (HHS-OIG), Chicago Regional Office.

The case is being prosecuted by Trial Attorney Gejaa T. Gobena of the Criminal Division's Fraud Section and Assistant U.S. Attorney for the Eastern District of Michigan Philip A. Ross. The case was investigated by the FBI and HHS-OIG, and was brought as part of the Medicare Fraud Strike Force, supervised by the Criminal Division's Fraud Section and the U.S. Attorney's Office for the Eastern District of Michigan.

Since its inception in March 2007, Medicare Fraud Strike Force operations in nine locations have charged more than 1,330 individuals and organizations that collectively have billed the Medicare program for more than $4 billion. In addition, HHS's Centers for Medicare and Medicaid Services, working in conjunction with the HHS-OIG, are taking steps to increase accountability and decrease the presence of fraudulent providers.

Source:
Department of Justice.

Case 8.

Brooklyn Doctor Convicted for Role in Medicare and Private Insurance Fraud Scheme

WASHINGTON – A Brooklyn board-certified colorectal surgeon, who owned and operated a New York medical clinic, was convicted for his role in a fraud scheme that billed Medicare and numerous private insurance companies for surgeries and other complex medical procedures that were never performed, the Department of Justice, FBI and Department of Health and Human Services (HHS) announced today.

On Wednesday, June 13, 2012, after a two-week trial in federal court in Brooklyn, a jury found Boris Sachakov, M.D., 43, guilty of one count of health care fraud and five counts of health care false statements.

The trial evidence showed that from January 2008 to January 2010, Sachakov, who owned and operated a clinic called Colon and Rectal Care of New York, P.C., defrauded Medicare and private insurance companies by billing for surgeries and medical services that he never provided. According to trial testimony, several private insurance companies began investigating Sachakov after receiving complaints from patients that Sachakov had submitted claims for surgeries, including hemorrhoidectomies, that he never performed.

At trial, 11 of Dr. Sachakov's patients testified that they had not received the surgeries and other medical services for which Sachakov had billed their insurance companies. The evidence presented at trial showed that the medical records Dr. Sachakov created and maintained on these patients, including letters to the patient's referring doctors, did not support the extensive billings he submitted. After Dr. Sachakov was confronted by two insurance companies about complaints of billings for surgeries that did not happen, the evidence at trial showed that Dr. Sachakov sent letters to his patients, asking them to falsely certify in writing that they had received the phony surgeries.

The indictment alleged that Sachakov submitted and caused the submission of over $22.6 million in false and fraudulent claims to Medicare and private insurance companies, and received more than $9 million on those claims.

At sentencing, scheduled for Sept. 24, 2012, Sachakov faces a maximum penalty of 35 years in prison and an $18 million fine.

The charges were announced by Assistant Attorney General Lanny A. Breuer of the Justice Department's Criminal Division; Assistant Director-in-Charge Janice K. Fedarcyk of the FBI's New York field office; and Special Agent-in-Charge Thomas O'Donnell of the HHS Office of Inspector General (HHS-OIG).

The case is being prosecuted by Trial Attorney Sarah M. Hall and Assistant Chief William Pericak of the Criminal Division's Fraud Section. The case was investigated by the FBI, HHS, the New York State Office of Medicaid Inspector General and the New York State Department of Financial Services, Criminal Investigative Division.

The case was brought as part of the Medicare Fraud Strike Force, supervised by the Criminal Division's Fraud Section. The Medicare Fraud Strike Force operations are part of the Health Care Fraud Prevention & Enforcement Action Team (HEAT), a joint initiative announced in May 2009 between the Department of Justice and HHS to focus their efforts to prevent and deter fraud and enforce current antifraud laws around the country.

Since their inception in March 2007, strike force operations in nine districts have charged 1,330 defendants who collectively have falsely billed the Medicare program for more than $4 billion. In addition, the HHS Centers for Medicare and Medicaid Services, working in conjunction with the HHS-OIG, are taking steps to increase accountability and decrease the presence of fraudulent providers.

Source:
Department of Justice.

Case 9.

Texas County Memorial Hospital (TCMH), Texas, agreed to pay $20,000 to resolve its liability for Civil Monetary Penalties under the patient dumping statute. The OIG alleged that TCMH failed to provide an adequate medical screening examination for a minor. Specifically, the minor presented to TCMH's emergency department (ED) and was accompanied by a family member. TCMH's registration clerk informed the family member that the minor should be treated by her family physician rather than be admitted to TCMH's ED. The minor left TCMH without receiving a medical screen.

Source:
Office of the Inspector General.

Case 10.

Northside Hospital (Northside), Florida, agreed to pay $38,000 to resolve its liability for Civil Monetary Penalties under the patient dumping statute. The OIG alleged that Northside failed to provide an appropriate medical screening examination and stabilizing treatment to a patient with a history of mitral valve replacement. Specifically, the patient presented to Northside's emergency department (ED) by ambulance with flu symptoms and a high fever. A triage nurse instructed the patient to go home and to follow his primary care physician's orders. Two days later the patient presented again to Northside's ED and was admitted to their intensive care unit. On August 8, 2009, the patient died due to influenza A (H1N1).

Source:

Office of the Inspector General.

Case 11.

Fort Lauderdale Hospital, Inc. (FLH), Florida, agreed to pay $45,000 to resolve its liability for Civil Monetary Penalties under the patient dumping statute. The OIG alleged that FLH failed to provide an appropriate medical screening examination and stabilizing treatment to an autistic patient that presented to FLH's emergency department after physically attacking his mother. A clinical psychologist asked for the patient's insurance information. FLH did not accept the patient's insurance, and the patient's mother was instructed to take the patient to another facility. The patient was seen at another facility and admitted for six days due to a diagnosis of depression.

Source:

Office of the Inspector General.

Case 12.

Randolph, N.J., Otolaryngologist, Sentenced to Two Years in Prison for Health Care Fraud Court-Ordered Forfeiture and Restitution Total More than $1.4 Million

NEWARK, N.J. – A North Caldwell, N.J., doctor was sentenced today to 24 months in prison for his role in defrauding Blue Cross Blue Shield of more than $725,000 by submitting false claims for services he never performed, U.S. Attorney Paul J. Fishman announced.

Dr. Michael P. Stein, 63, previously pleaded guilty before U.S. District Judge Esther Salas to an Information charging him with one count of defrauding Blue Cross Blue Shield by filing false claims for services that were not rendered and office visits that did not occur. Judge Salas also imposed the sentence today in Newark federal court.

According to documents filed in this case and statements made in court:

Between August 2004 and September 2010 Stein was the owner and operator of Randolph Otolaryngology, P.C., a medical treatment facility. Stein treated a patient with the initials J.F. for nasal problems and billed Blue Cross Blue Shield for the services he purportedly performed.

Stein admitted he filed fraudulent claims with Blue Cross Blue Shield for medical procedures that were not performed

during office visits. Stein submitted claims for approximately 900 nasal endoscopies he purportedly conducted on the patient, when only a few were actually performed. Stein also admitted he filed fraudulent claims for office visits and medical procedures that purportedly occurred while he was away on vacation. Between Sept. 6, 2010, and Sept. 27, 2010, Stein billed Blue Cross Blue Shield for 11 nasal endoscopies and 10 office outpatient visits for purported services rendered to J.F. In truth, J.F. ceased seeing Stein around Sept. 3, 2010, and Stein was in Germany from Sept. 11, 2010 through Sept. 27, 2010. Stein received $725,156.45 from Blue Cross Blue Shield as a result of his submission of the false claims, and, under the plea agreement, agreed to pay restitution and forfeiture in the same amount.

In addition to the prison term, Judge Salas sentenced Stein to three years of supervised release and ordered him to forfeit $725,156.45 and pay restitution of $725,156.45. He has also surrendered his medical license.

U.S. Attorney Fishman credited special agents and investigators of the FBI, under the direction of Special Agent in Charge Michael B. Ward; Health and Human Services/OIG under the direction of Special Agent in Charge Thomas O'Donnell; and the Railroad Retirement Board/OIG under the direction of Special Agent in Charge Michael Angelucci with the investigation leading to today's sentence.

The government is represented by Assistant U.S. Attorney Jacob T. Elberg, deputy chief of the U.S. Attorney's Office Health Care and Government Fraud Unit, and Assistant U.S. Attorney Jacques S. Pierre of the Health Care and Government Fraud Unit.

Source:

Department of Justice.

Case 13.

Tennessee State Medicaid Fraud Control Unit: 2012 Onsite Review

SUMMARY:

WHY WE DID THIS STUDY

OIG is responsible for overseeing the activities of all Medicaid Fraud Control Units (MFCU or Unit). As part of this oversight, OIG conducts periodic reviews of all Units and prepares public reports based on these reviews. The reviews describe the Units' caseloads; assess performance in accordance with the 12 MFCU performance standards; identify any opportunities for improvement; and identify any instances of noncompliance with laws, regulations, and policy transmittals.

HOW WE DID THIS STUDY

We based our review on an analysis of data from seven sources: (1) a review of policies, procedures and documentation of the Unit's operations, staffing, and caseload; (2) a review of financial documentation; (3) structured interviews with key stakeholders; (4) a survey of Unit staff; (5) structured interviews with the Unit director and supervisors; (6) an onsite review of case files; and (7) an onsite review of Unit operations.

WHAT WE FOUND

For federal fiscal years 2009 through 2011, the Tennessee Unit obtained 96 criminal convictions and 22 civil settlements, and reported recoveries of over $181 million. We identified one instance of noncompliance with applicable laws, regulations, and policy transmittals: the Unit investigated a case that was not eligible for federal funding under federal regulations. With the exception of this instance, our review of compliance issues found no evidence of significant noncompliance with applicable laws, regulations, or policy transmittals. We identified two instances in which the Unit did not fully meet Performance Standards. The Unit referred all convicted health care providers to OIG for program exclusion, but did not refer nonprovider convictions. Although the Unit had a training plan, it did not establish training hour requirements for each professional discipline. Additionally, despite Unit efforts to increase referrals, the State Medicaid Agency and managed care organizations sent a small number of fraud referrals to the Unit. Finally, Unit staff and stakeholders reported that involvement on various task forces was key to the Unit's productivity.

WHAT WE RECOMMEND

On the basis of these findings, we recommend that the Tennessee Unit: (1) repay grant funds spent on the case that, under federal regulations, was not eligible for federal funding; (2) refer all convictions to OIG, including nonprovider convictions, within 30 days; and (3) establish training hour requirements for professional disciplines. The Unit stated that it felt the case in question was within its purview. We disagree with the Unit's opinion because the case in question was not one of the three eligible case types specified by Medicaid statute and federal regulations: investigation of allegations of fraud in the administration of the Medicaid program, in the provision of Medicaid services, or in the activities of Medicaid providers. The Unit should work with OIG to determine ineligible costs.

Source:

Office of the Inspector General.

Case 14.

United States Settled with Temple University and Dr. Joseph Kubacki over Improper Billing

PHILADELPHIA – Dr. Joseph Kubacki and Temple University - Of the Commonwealth System of Higher Education ("Temple") have agreed to pay the United States a combined $1,088,574.93, resolving Temple's voluntary disclosure that it improperly billed the United States for medical services provided by residents but that Temple billed as though they had been performed by attending physicians.

The False Claims Act makes it illegal for any person or entity to present a false or fraudulent claim to the United States for payment and/or to retain overpayments that were improperly

received. Federal programs only reimburse hospitals for services which attending physicians performed or which attending physicians were present for the critical portions. Those physicians certify that they were present when the critical portion of the services were performed as part of the charting and billing process.

Dr. Kubacki, formerly the Chairman of Temple's Ophthalmology Department, was convicted by a jury on August 22, 2011 of 73 counts of health care fraud, 73 counts of false statements in health care matters, and four counts of wire fraud. The evidence at his trial showed that he had billed the United States for performing services that were performed by residents when he was not even physically present in the hospital. The settlement with Temple pertains both to this fraud and to other fraud discovered in Temple's plastic surgery department, where attending physicians were present in the hospital at the time services were performed but were not actually present for the critical portions of the services for which they submitted claims.

Although Temple trained its physicians in charting and billing requirements, this training did not prevent the fraud from occurring.

"Combating Medicare fraud and overbilling is an increasingly critical issue," said Memeger. "Every year we lose tens of billions of dollars to Medicare and Medicaid fraud. Those billions represent health care dollars that could be spent on medicine, elder care or emergency room visits. This is unacceptable, and we are committed to working with health care providers like Temple and with the Department of Health and Human Services to eradicate it."

Temple brought this case to the government's attention by voluntarily disclosing the improper billing. Memeger complimented Temple on its approach to these issues, stating "When health care providers come forward, forthrightly acknowledge improper conduct, and take steps to prevent that conduct from recurring in the future, everyone benefits. Temple's decision to disclose the misconduct, to reveal the results of their internal investigation, and to cooperate with our investigation demonstrated that they were serious about providing patients with appropriate medical care and about compliance with the law. Temple also improved its compliance program, promptly terminated its relationship with the physicians implicated in this fraud, and agreed to voluntarily repay both the federal and private payors who had been defrauded. These are critical factors in our decision whether to pursue health care providers in litigation or whether to reach an amicable resolution."

In light of Temple's voluntary disclosure and self-audit, and upon the evaluation of Temple's compliance structure by the Office of the Inspector General of the Department of Health and Human Services, Temple will continue to implement its corporate compliance program without the need for a Corporate Integrity Agreement overseen by the Office of the Inspector General.

This resolution is part of the Eastern District of Pennsylvania's Special Focus Team Health Care Initiative. The case was investigated civilly by the Department of Health and Human Services Office of the Inspector General and Assistant

United States Attorneys Paul Kaufman and Susan Dein Bricklin. Dr. Kubacki was prosecuted criminally by Assistant United States Attorneys Anthony Kyriakakis and Matthew Hogan.

Source:

Department of Justice.

Case 15.

FOR IMMEDIATE RELEASE   Thursday, April 25, 2013

Supervisor of $63 Million Health Care Fraud Scheme Convicted

A federal jury today convicted a Miami-area supervisor of a mental health care company, Health Care Solutions Network (HCSN), for helping to orchestrate a fraud scheme that crossed state lines and that resulted in the submission of more than $63 million in fraudulent claims to Medicare and Florida Medicaid.

The announcement was made by Acting Assistant Attorney General Mythili Raman of the Justice Department's Criminal Division; U.S. Attorney Wifredo A. Ferrer of the Southern District of Florida; Michael B. Steinbach, Special Agent in Charge of the FBI's Miami Field Office; and Special Agent in Charge Christopher B. Dennis of the U.S. Department of Health and Human Services Office of Inspector General (HHS-OIG), Office of Investigation's Miami office.

After a five-day trial, a jury in the Southern District of Florida found Wondera Eason, 51, guilty of conspiracy to commit health care fraud. Sentencing is scheduled for July 8, 2013.

Eason was employed as the Director of Medical Records at HCSN's Partial Hospitalization Program (PHP). A PHP is a form of intensive treatment for severe mental illness. In Florida, HCSN operated community mental health centers at two locations. After stealing millions from Medicare and Medicaid in Florida, HCSN's owner, Armando Gonzalez, exported the scheme to North Carolina, opening a third HCSN location in Hendersonville.

Evidence at trial showed that at all three locations, Eason, a certified medical records technician, oversaw the alteration, fabrication, and forgery of thousands of documents, which purported to support the fraudulent claims HCSN submitted to Medicare and Florida Medicaid. Many of these medical records were created weeks or months after the patients were admitted to HCSN facilities in Florida for purported PHP treatment and were utilized to support false and fraudulent billing to government sponsored health care benefit programs, including Medicare and Florida Medicaid. Eason directed therapists to

fabricate documents, and she also forged the signature of therapists and others on documents that she was in charge of maintaining. Eason interacted with Medicare and Medicaid auditors, providing them with false and fraudulent documents, while certifying the documents were accurate.

The "therapy" at HCSN oftentimes consisted of nothing more than patients watching Disney movies, playing bingo, and having barbeques. Eason directed therapists to remove any references to these recreational activities in the medical records.

According to evidence at trial, Eason was aware that HCSN in Florida paid illegal kickbacks to owners and operators of Miami-Dade County Assisted Living Facilities (ALF) in exchange for patient referral information to be used to submit false and fraudulent claims to Medicare and Medicaid. Eason also knew that many of the ALF referral patients were ineligible for PHP services because many patients suffered from mental retardation, dementia, and Alzheimer's disease.

From 2004 through 2011, HCSN billed Medicare and the Florida Medicaid program approximately $63 million for purported mental health services.

Fifteen defendants have been charged for their alleged roles in the HCSN health care fraud scheme, and 12 defendants have pleaded guilty. On Monday, Feb. 25, 2013, Gonzalez was sentenced to serve 168 months in prison for his role in the scheme. Alleged co-conspirators Alina Feas and Lisset Palmero are scheduled for trial on June 3, 2013. Defendants are presumed innocent until proven guilty at trial.

This case is being investigated by the FBI and HHS-OIG and was brought as part of the Medicare Fraud Strike Force, supervised by the Criminal Division's Fraud Section and the U.S. Attorney's Office for the Southern District of Florida. This case was prosecuted by Trial Attorneys Allan J. Medina and Steven Kim, former Special Trial Attorney William Parente and Deputy Chief Benjamin D. Singer of the Criminal Division's Fraud Section.

Since its inception in March 2007, the Medicare Fraud Strike Force, now operating in nine cities across the country, has charged more than 1,480 defendants who have collectively billed the Medicare program for more than $4.8 billion. In addition, HHS's Centers for Medicare and Medicaid Services, working in conjunction with HHS-OIG, is taking steps to increase accountability and decrease the presence of fraudulent providers.

To learn more about the Health Care Fraud Prevention and Enforcement Action Team (HEAT), go to: www.stopmedicare-fraud.gov.

Source:

Department of Justice.

APPENDIX B

WEBSITES FOR ADDITIONAL INFORMATION

Use this appendix to support learning for all chapters.

Agency for Healthcare Research and Quality	http://www.ahrq.gov/
American College of Health Care Administrators	http://www.achca.org
American College of Healthcare Executives	http://www.ache.or
American College of Medical Practice Executives	http://www.mgma.com/acmpe
American College of Physician Executives	http://www.acpe.org
American Dental Association	http://www.ada.org
American Health Lawyers Association	http://www.healthlawyers.org
American Hospital Association	http://www.aha.org
American Medical Association	http://www.ama-assn.org/
Centers for Disease Control and Prevention	http://www.cdc.gov
Centers for Medicare and Medicaid Services	http://www.cms.gov
Code of Federal Regulations	http://www.gpoaccess.gov/cfr/retrieve.html
Department of Health & Human Services	http://www.dhhs.gov
Federal Bureau of Investigation	http://www.fbi.gov
Federal Register	http://gpoaccess.gov/fr/index.html
Find Law	http://www.findlaw.com
Florida Agency for Health Care Administration	http://www.fdhc.state.fl.us
Health.gov (health information)	http://www.health.gov
Healthcare.gov	http://www.healthcare.gov
Healthcare Finance News	http://www.healthcarefinancenews.com
Healthcare Financial Management Association (HFMA)	http://www.hfma.org
Healthcare IT News	http://www.healthcareitnews.com
Health Leaders Magazine	http://www.healthleadersmedia.com
Health Resources and Services Administration	http://www.hrsa.gov
Internal Revenue Service	http://www.irs.gov
Joint Commission	http://www.jointcommission.org
Journal of Medical Case Reports	http://www.jmedicalcasereports.com/
Kaiser Health News	http://www.kaiserhealthnews.org
Library of Congress THOMAS	http://thomas.loc.gov
Medical Cases for Health Care Providers	http://npic.orst.edu/mcapro/index.html
Medical Group Management Association	http://www.mgma.com
MedlinePlus (NIH encyclopedia)	http://www.nlm.nih.gov/medlineplus
National Association of Health Services Executives	http://www.nahse.org
National Center for Health Workforce Analysis	http://bhpr.hrsa.gov/healthworkforce/index.html
National Guideline Clearinghouse (AHRQ)	http://www.guideline.gov/
National Institutes of Health (NIH)	http://www.nih.gov

Occupational Safety and Health Administration	http://www.osha.gov
Office of the Inspector General	http://www.oig.hhs.gov
Quick Health Data Online (DHHS)	http://www.healthstatus2020.com/owh
Substance Abuse and Mental Health Administration	http://www.samhsa.gov
U.S. Census Bureau	http://www.census.gov
U.S. Department of Justice	http://www.doj.gov

COMPLIANCE PLAN GUIDANCE FOR INDIVIDUAL AND SMALL GROUP PHYSICIAN PRACTICES

Use this appendix to support learning about compliance plans. For **Compliance Plan Guidance for Hospitals**, see the Federal Register at https://oig.hhs.gov/authorities/docs/cpghosp.pdf

Federal Register / Vol. 65, No. 194 / Thursday, October 5, 2000 /

DEPARTMENT OF HEALTH AND HUMAN SERVICES

Office of Inspector General

OIG Compliance Program for Individual and Small Group Physician Practices

AGENCY: Office of Inspector General (OIG), HHS.

ACTION: Notice.

SUMMARY: This **Federal Register** notice sets forth the recently issued Compliance Program Guidance for Individual and Small Group Physician Practices developed by the Office of Inspector General (OIG). The OIG has previously developed and published voluntary compliance program guidance focused on several other areas and aspects of the health care industry. We believe that the development and issuance of this voluntary compliance program guidance for individual and small group physician practices will serve as a positive step towards assisting providers in preventing the submission of erroneous claims or engaging in unlawful conduct involving the Federal health care programs.

FOR FURTHER INFORMATION CONTACT: Kimberly Brandt, Office of Counsel to the Inspector General, (202) 619-2078.

SUPPLEMENTARY INFORMATION

Background

The creation of compliance program guidances is a major initiative of the OIG in its effort to engage the private health care community in preventing the submission of erroneous claims and in combating fraudulent conduct. In the past several years, the OIG has developed and issued compliance program guidances directed at a variety of segments in the health care industry. The development of these types of compliance program guidances is based on our belief that a health care provider can use internal controls to more efficiently monitor adherence to applicable statutes, regulations and program requirements.

Copies of these compliance program guidances can be found on the OIG web site at http://www.hhs.gov/oig.

Developing the Compliance Program Guidance for Individual and Small Group Physician Practices

On September 8, 1999, the OIG published a solicitation notice seeking information and recommendations for developing formal guidance for individual and small group physician practices (64 FR 48846). In response to that solicitation notice, the OIG received 83 comments from various outside sources. We carefully considered those comments, as well as previous OIG publications, such as other compliance program guidance and Special Fraud Alerts, in developing a guidance for individual and small group physician practices. In addition, we have consulted with the Health Care Financing Administration and the Department of Justice. In an effort to ensure that all parties had a reasonable opportunity to provide input into a final product, draft guidance for individual and small group physician practices was published in the **Federal Register** on June 12, 2000 (65 FR 36818) for further comments and recommendations.

Components of an Effective Compliance Program

This compliance program guidance for individual and small group physician practices contains seven components that provide a solid basis upon which a physician practice can create a voluntary compliance program:

- Conducting internal monitoring and auditing;
- Implementing compliance and practice standards;
- Designating a compliance officer or contact;
- Conducting appropriate training and education;
- Responding appropriately to detected offenses and developing corrective action;
- Developing open lines of communication; and
- Enforcing disciplinary standards through well-publicized guidelines.

Similar components have been contained in previous guidances issued by the OIG. However, unlike other guidances issued by OIG, this guidance for physicians does not suggest that physician practices implement all seven components of a full scale compliance program. Instead, the guidance emphasizes a step-by-step approach to follow in developing and implementing a voluntary compliance program. This change is in recognition of the financial by physician practices. The guidance should not be viewed as mandatory or as an all-inclusive discussion of the advisable components of a compliance program. Rather, the document is intended to present guidance to assist physician practices that voluntarily choose to develop a compliance program.

Office of Inspector General's Compliance Program Guidance for Individual and Small Group Physician Practices

I. INTRODUCTION

This compliance program guidance is intended to assist individual and small group physician practices ("physician practices") in developing a voluntary compliance program that promotes adherence to statutes and regulations applicable to the Federal health care programs ("Federal health care program requirements"). The goal of voluntary compliance programs is to provide a tool to strengthen the efforts of health care providers to prevent and reduce improper conduct. These programs can also benefit physician practices by helping to streamline business operations.

Many physicians have expressed an interest in better protecting their practices from the potential for erroneous or fraudulent conduct through the implementation of voluntary compliance programs. The Office of Inspector General (OIG) believes that the great majority of physicians are honest and share our goal of protecting the integrity of Medicare and other Federal health care programs. To that end, all health care providers have a duty to ensure that the claims submitted to Federal health care programs are true and accurate. The development of voluntary compliance programs and the active application of compliance principles in physician practices will go a long way toward achieving this goal.

Through this document, the OIG provides its views on the fundamental components of physician practice compliance programs, as well as the principles that a physician practice might consider when developing and implementing a voluntary compliance program. While this document presents basic procedural and structural guidance for designing a voluntary compliance program, it is not in and of itself a compliance program. Indeed, as recognized by the OIG and the health care industry, there is no "one size fits all" compliance program, especially for physician practices. Rather, it is a set of guidelines that physician practices can consider if they choose to develop and implement a compliance program.

As with the OIG's previous guidance, these guidelines are not mandatory. Nor do they represent an all-inclusive document containing all components of a compliance program. Other OIG outreach efforts, as well as other Federal agency efforts to promote compliance, can also be used in developing a compliance program. However, as explained later, if a physician practice adopts a voluntary and active compliance program, it may well lead to benefits for the physician practice.

A. *Scope of the Voluntary Compliance Program Guidance*
This guidance focuses on voluntary compliance measures related to claims submitted to the Federal health care programs. Issues related to private payor claims may also be covered by a compliance plan if the physician practice so desires.

The guidance is also limited in scope by focusing on the development of voluntary compliance programs for individual and small group physician practices. The difference between a small practice and a large practice cannot be determined by stating a particular number of physicians. Instead, our intent in narrowing the guidance to the small practices subset was to provide guidance to those physician practices whose financial or staffing resources would not allow them to implement a full scale, institutionally structured compliance program as set forth in the Third-Party Medical Billing Guidance or other previously released OIG guidance. A compliance program can be an important tool for physician practices of all sizes and does not have to be costly, resource-intensive or time-intensive.

B. *Benefits of a Voluntary Compliance Program*
The OIG acknowledges that patient care is, and should be, the first priority of a physician practice. However, a practice's focus on patient care can be enhanced by the adoption of a voluntary compliance program. For example, the increased accuracy of documentation that may result from a compliance program will actually assist in enhancing patient care. The OIG believes that physician practices can realize numerous other benefits by implementing a compliance program. A well-designed compliance program can:
- Speed and optimize proper payment of claims;
- Minimize billing mistakes;
- Reduce the chances that an audit will be conducted by HCFA or the OIG; and
- Avoid conflicts with the self-referral and anti-kickback statutes.

The incorporation of compliance measures into a physician practice should not be at the expense of patient care, but instead should augment the ability of the physician practice to provide quality patient care.

Voluntary compliance programs also provide benefits by not only helping to prevent erroneous or fraudulent claims, but also by showing that the physician practice is making additional good faith efforts to submit claims appropriately. Physicians should view compliance programs as analogous to practicing preventive medicine for their practice. Practices that embrace the active application of compliance principles in their practice culture and put efforts towards compliance on a continued basis can help to prevent problems from occurring in the future.

A compliance program also sends an important message to a physician practice's employees that while the practice recognizes that mistakes will occur, employees have an affirmative, ethical duty to come forward and report erroneous or fraudulent conduct, so that it may be corrected.

C. *Application of Voluntary Compliance Program Guidance*
The applicability of these recommendations will depend on the circumstances and resources of the particular physician practice.

Each physician practice can undertake reasonable steps to implement compliance measures, depending on the size and resources of that practice. Physician practices can rely, at least in part, upon standard protocols and current practice procedures to develop an appropriate compliance program for that practice. In fact, many physician practices already have established the framework of a compliance program without referring to it as such.

D. The Difference Between "Erroneous" and "Fraudulent" Claims To Federal Health Programs

There appear to be significant misunderstandings within the physician community regarding the critical differences between what the Government views as innocent "erroneous" claims on the one hand and "fraudulent" (intentionally or recklessly false) health care claims on the other. Some physicians feel that Federal law enforcement agencies have maligned medical professionals, in part, by a perceived focus on innocent billing errors. These physicians are under the impression that innocent billing errors can subject them to civil penalties, or even jail. These impressions are mistaken.

To address these concerns, the OIG would like to emphasize the following points. First, the OIG does not disparage physicians, other medical professionals or medical enterprises. In our view, the great majority of physicians are working ethically to render high quality medical care and to submit proper claims.

Second, under the law, physicians are not subject to criminal, civil or administrative penalties for innocent errors, or even negligence. The Government's primary enforcement tool, the civil False Claims Act, covers only offenses that are committed with actual knowledge of the falsity of the claim, reckless disregard, or deliberate ignorance of the falsity of the claim. The False Claims Act does not encompass mistakes, errors, or negligence. The Civil Monetary Penalties Law, an administrative remedy, similar in scope and effect to the False Claims Act, has exactly the same standard of proof. The OIG is very mindful of the difference between innocent errors ("erroneous claims") on one hand, and reckless or intentional conduct ("fraudulent claims") on the other. For criminal penalties, the standard is even higher—criminal intent to defraud must be proved beyond a reasonable doubt.

Third, even ethical physicians (and their staffs) make billing mistakes and errors through inadvertence or negligence. When physicians discover that their billing errors, honest mistakes, or negligence result in erroneous claims, the physician practice should return the funds erroneously claimed, but without penalties. In other words, absent a violation of a civil, criminal or administrative law, erroneous claims result only in the return of funds claimed in error.

Fourth, innocent billing errors are a significant drain on the Federal health care programs. All parties (physicians, providers, carriers, fiscal intermediaries, Government agencies, and beneficiaries) need to work cooperatively to reduce the overall error rate.

Finally, it is reasonable for physicians (and other providers) to ask: what duty do they owe the Federal health care programs? The answer is that all health care providers have a duty to reasonably ensure that the claims submitted to Medicare and other Federal health care programs are true and accurate. The OIG continues to engage the provider community in an extensive, good faith effort to work cooperatively on voluntary compliance to minimize errors and to prevent potential penalties for improper billings before they occur. We encourage all physicians and other providers to join in this effort.

II. DEVELOPING A VOLUNTARY COMPLIANCE PROGRAM

A. The Seven Basic Components of a Voluntary Compliance Program

The OIG believes that a basic framework for any voluntary compliance program begins with a review of the seven basic components of an effective compliance program. A review of these components provides physician practices with an overview of the scope of a fully developed and implemented compliance program. The following list of components, as set forth in previous OIG compliance program guidances, can form the basis of a voluntary compliance program for a physician practice:

- Conducting internal monitoring and auditing through the performance of periodic audits;
- Implementing compliance and practice standards through the development of written standards and procedures;
- Designating a compliance officer or contact(s) to monitor compliance efforts and enforce practice standards;
- Conducting appropriate training and education on practice standards and procedures;
- Responding appropriately to detected violations through the investigation of allegations and the disclosure of incidents to appropriate Government entities;
- Developing open lines of communication, such as (1) discussions at staff meetings regarding how to avoid erroneous or fraudulent conduct and (2) community bulletin boards, to keep practice employees updated regarding compliance activities; and
- Enforcing disciplinary standards through well-publicized guidelines.

These seven components provide a solid basis upon which a physician practice can create a compliance program. The OIG acknowledges that full implementation of all components may not be feasible for all physician practices. Some physician practices may never fully implement all of the components. However, as a first step, physician practices can begin by adopting only those components which, based on a practice's specific history with billing problems and other compliance issues, are most likely to provide an identifiable benefit.

The extent of implementation will depend on the size and resources of the practice. Smaller physician practices may incorporate each of the components in a manner that best suits the practice. By contrast, larger physician practices often have the means to incorporate the components in a more systematic manner. For example, larger physician practices can use both this guidance and the Third-Party Medical Billing Compliance Program Guidance, which provides a more detailed compliance program structure, to create a compliance program unique to the practice.

The OIG recognizes that physician practices need to find the best way to achieve compliance for their given circumstances. Specifically, the OIG encourages physician practices to participate in other provider's compliance programs, such as the compliance programs of the hospitals or other settings in which the physicians practice. Physician Practice Management companies also may serve as a source of compliance program guidance. A physician practice's participation in such compliance programs could be a way, at least partly, to augment the practice's own compliance efforts.

The opportunities for collaborative compliance efforts could include participating in training and education programs or using another entity's policies and procedures as a template from which the physician practice creates its own version. The OIG encourages this type of collaborative effort, where the content is appropriate to the setting involved (i.e., the training is relevant to physician practices as well as the sponsoring provider), because it provides a means to promote the desired objective without imposing excessive burdens on the practice or requiring physicians to undertake duplicative action. However, to prevent possible anti-kickback or self-referral issues, the OIG recommends that physicians consider limiting their participation in a sponsoring provider's compliance program to the areas of training and education or policies and procedures.

The key to avoiding possible conflicts is to ensure that the entity providing compliance services to a physician practice (its referral source) is not perceived as nor is it operating the practice compliance program at no charge. For example, if the sponsoring entity conducted claims review for the physician practice as part of a compliance program or provided compliance oversight without charging the practice fair market value for those services, the anti-kickback and Stark self-referral laws would be implicated. The payment of fair market value by referral sources for compliance services will generally address these concerns.

B. *Steps for Implementing a Voluntary Compliance Program*
As previously discussed, implementing a voluntary compliance program can be a multi-tiered process. Initial development of the compliance program can be focused on practice risk areas that have been problematic for the practice such as coding and billing. Within this area, the practice should examine its claims denial history or claims that have resulted in repeated overpayments, and identify and correct the most frequent sources of those denials or overpayments. A review of claim denials will help the practice scrutinize a significant risk area and improve its cash flow by submitting correct claims that will be paid the first time they are submitted. As this example illustrates, a compliance program for a physician practice often makes sound business sense.

The following is a suggested order of the steps a practice could take to begin the development of a compliance program. The steps outlined below articulate all seven components of a compliance program and there are numerous suggestions for implementation within each component. Physician practices should keep in mind, as stated earlier, that it is up to the practice to determine the manner in which and the extent to which the practice chooses to implement these voluntary measures.

Step One: Auditing and Monitoring
An ongoing evaluation process is important to a successful compliance program. This ongoing evaluation includes not only whether the physician practice's standards and procedures are in fact current and accurate, but also whether the compliance program is working, *i.e.*, whether individuals are properly carrying out their responsibilities and claims are submitted appropriately. Therefore, an audit is an excellent way for a physician practice to ascertain what, if any, problem areas exist and focus on the risk areas that are associated with those problems. There are two types of reviews that can be performed as part of this evaluation: (1) A standards and procedures review; and (2) a claims submission audit.

1. Standards and Procedures
    It is recommended that an individual(s) in the physician practice be charged with the responsibility of periodically reviewing the practice's standards and procedures to determine if they are current and complete. If the standards and procedures are found to be ineffective or outdated, they should be updated to reflect changes in Government regulations or compendiums generally relied upon by physicians and insurers (*i.e.*, changes in Current Procedural Terminology (CPT) and ICD–9–CM codes).

2. Claims Submission Audit
    In addition to the standards and procedures themselves, it is advisable that bills and medical records be reviewed for compliance with applicable coding, billing and documentation requirements. The individuals from the physician practice involved in these self-audits would ideally include the person in charge of billing (if the practice has such a person) and a medically trained person (*e.g.*, registered nurse or preferably a physician (physicians can rotate in this position)). Each physician practice needs to decide for itself whether to review claims retrospectively or concurrently with the claims submission. In the Third-Party Medical Billing Compliance Program Guidance, the OIG recommended that a baseline, or "snapshot," be used to enable a practice to judge over time its progress in reducing or eliminating potential areas of vulnerability. This practice, known as "benchmarking," allows a practice to chart its compliance efforts by showing a reduction or increase in the number of claims paid and denied.

The practice's self-audits can be used to determine whether:

- Bills are accurately coded and accurately reflect the services provided (as documented in the medical records);
- Documentation is being completed correctly;
- Services or items provided are reasonable and necessary; and
- Any incentives for unnecessary services exist.

A baseline audit examines the claim development and submission process, from patient intake through claim submission and payment, and identifies elements within this process that may contribute to non-compliance or that may need to be the focus for improving execution. This audit will establish a consistent methodology for selecting and examining records, and this methodology will then serve as a basis for future audits.

There are many ways to conduct a baseline audit. The OIG recommends that claims/services that were submitted and paid during the initial three months after implementation of the education and training program be examined, so as to give the physician practice a benchmark against which to measure future compliance effectiveness.

Following the baseline audit, a general recommendation is that periodic audits be conducted at least once each year to ensure that the compliance program is being followed. Optimally, a randomly selected number of medical records could be reviewed to ensure that the coding was performed accurately. Although there is no set formula to how many medical records should be reviewed, a basic guide is five or more medical records per Federal payor (*i.e.*, Medicare, Medicaid), or five to ten medical records per physician. The OIG realizes that physician practices receive reimbursement from a number of different payors, and we would encourage a physician practice's auditing/ monitoring process to consist of a review of claims from all Federal payors from which the practice receives reimbursement. Of course, the larger the sample size, the larger the comfort level the physician practice will have about the results. However, the OIG is aware that this may be burdensome for some physician practices, so, at a minimum, we would encourage the physician practice to conduct a review of claims that have been reimbursed by Federal health care programs.

If problems are identified, the physician practice will need to determine whether a focused review should be conducted on a more frequent basis. When audit results reveal areas needing additional information or education of employees and physicians, the physician practice will need to analyze whether these areas should be incorporated into the training and educational system.

There are many ways to identify the claims/services from which to draw the random sample of claims to be audited. One methodology is to choose a random sample of claims/services from either all of the claims/services a physician has received reimbursement for or all claims/ services from a particular payor. Another method is to identify risk areas or potential billing vulnerabilities. The codes associated with these risk areas may become the universe of claims/services from which to select the sample. The OIG recommends that the physician practice evaluate claims/services selected to determine if the codes billed and reimbursed were accurately ordered, performed, and reasonable and necessary for the treatment of the patient.

One of the most important components of a successful compliance audit protocol is an appropriate response when the physician practice identifies a problem. This action should be taken as soon as possible after the date the problem is identified. The specific action a physician practice takes should depend on the circumstances of the situation. In some cases, the response can be as straight forward as generating a repayment with appropriate explanation to Medicare or the appropriate payor from which the overpayment was received. In others, the physician practice may want to consult with a coding/billing expert to determine the next best course of action. There is no boilerplate solution to how to handle problems that are identified.

It is a good business practice to create a system to address how physician practices will respond to and report potential problems. In addition, preserving information relating to identification of the problem is as important as preserving information that tracks the physician practice's reaction to, and solution for, the issue.

Step Two: Establish Practice Standards and Procedures
After the internal audit identifies the practice's risk areas, the next step is to develop a method for dealing with those risk areas through the practice's standards and procedures. Written standards and procedures are a central component of any compliance program. Those standards and procedures help to reduce the prospect of erroneous claims and fraudulent activity by identifying risk areas for the practice and establishing tighter internal controls to counter those risks, while also helping to identify any aberrant billing practices. Many physician practices already have something similar to this called "practice standards" that include practice policy statements regarding patient care, personnel matters and practice standards and procedures on complying with Federal and State law.

The OIG believes that written standards and procedures can be helpful to all physician practices, regardless of size and capability. If a lack of resources to develop such standards and procedures is genuinely an issue, the OIG recommends that a physician practice focus first on those risk areas most likely to arise in its particular practice. Additionally, if the physician practice works with a physician practice management company (PPMC), independent practice association (IPA), physician-hospital organization, management services organization (MSO) or third-party billing company, the practice can incorporate the compliance standards and procedures of those entities, if appropriate, into its own standards and procedures. Many physician practices have found that the adoption of a third party's compliance standards and procedures, as appropriate, has many benefits and the result is a consistent set of standards and procedures for a community of physicians as well as having just one entity that can then monitor and refine the process as needed. This sharing of compliance responsibilities assists physician practices in rural areas that do not have the staff to perform these functions, but do belong to a group that does have the resources. Physician practices using another entity's compliance materials will need to tailor those materials to the physician practice where they will be applied.

Physician practices that do not have standards or procedures in place can develop them by: (1) Developing a written standards and procedures manual; and (2) updating clinical forms periodically to make sure they facilitate and encourage clear and complete documentation of patient care. A practice's standards could also identify the clinical protocol(s), pathway(s), and other treatment guidelines followed by the practice.

Creating a resource manual from publicly available information may be a cost-effective approach for developing additional standards and procedures. For example, the practice can develop a "binder" that contains the practice's written standards and procedures, relevant HCFA directives and carrier bulletins, and summaries of informative OIG documents (*e.g.*, Special Fraud Alerts, Advisory Opinions, inspection and audit reports). If the practice chooses to adopt this idea, the binder should be updated as appropriate and located in a readily accessible location.

If updates to the standards and procedures are necessary, those updates should be communicated to employees to keep them informed regarding the practice's operations. New employees can be made aware of the standards and procedures when hired and can be trained on their contents as part of their orientation to the practice. The OIG recommends that the communication of updates and training of new employees occur as soon as possible after either the issuance of a new update or the hiring of a new employee.

1. Specific Risk Areas

The OIG recognizes that many physician practices may not have in place standards and procedures to prevent erroneous or fraudulent conduct in their practices. In order to develop standards and procedures, the physician practice may consider what types of fraud and abuse related topics need to be addressed based on its specific needs. One of the most important things in making that determination is a listing of risk areas where the practice may be vulnerable.

To assist physician practices in performing this initial assessment, the OIG has developed a list of four potential risk areas affecting physician practices. These risk areas include: (a) Coding and billing; (b) reasonable and necessary services; (c) documentation; and (d) improper inducements, kickbacks and self-referrals. This list of risk areas is not exhaustive, or all-encompassing. Rather, it should be viewed as a starting point for an internal review of potential

vulnerabilities within the physician practice. The objective of such an assessment is to ensure that key personnel in the physician practice are aware of these major risk areas and that steps are taken to minimize, to the extent possible, the types of problems identified. While there are many ways to accomplish this objective, clear written standards and procedures that are communicated to all employees are important to ensure the effectiveness of a compliance program. Specifically, the following are discussions of risk areas for physician practices:

a. *Coding and Billing.* A major part of any physician practice's compliance program is the identification of risk areas associated with coding and billing. The following risk areas associated with billing have been among the most frequent subjects of investigations and audits by the OIG:

• Billing for items or services not rendered or not provided as claimed;
• Submitting claims for equipment, medical supplies and services that are not reasonable and necessary;
• Double billing resulting in duplicate payment;
• Billing for non-covered services as if covered;
• Knowing misuse of provider identification numbers, which results in improper billing;
• Unbundling (billing for each component of the service instead of billing or using an all-inclusive code);
• Failure to properly use coding modifiers;
• Clustering; and
• Upcoding the level of service provided.

The physician practice written standards and procedures concerning proper coding reflect the current reimbursement principles set forth in applicable statutes, regulations and Federal, State or private payor health care program requirements and should be developed in tandem with coding and billing standards used in the physician practice. Furthermore, written standards and procedures should ensure that coding and billing are based on medical record documentation. Particular attention should be paid to issues of appropriate diagnosis codes and individual Medicare Part B claims (including documentation guidelines for evaluation and management services). A physician practice can also institute a policy that the coder and/or physician review all rejected claims pertaining to diagnosis and procedure codes. This step can facilitate a reduction in similar errors.

b. *Reasonable and Necessary Services.* A practice's compliance program may provide guidance that claims are to be submitted only for services that the physician practice finds to be reasonable and necessary in the particular case. The OIG recognizes that physicians should be able to order any tests, including screening tests, they believe are appropriate for the treatment of their patients. However, a physician practice should be aware that Medicare will only pay for services that meet the Medicare definition of reasonable and necessary.

Medicare (and many insurance plans) may deny payment for a service that is not reasonable and necessary according to the Medicare reimbursement rules. Thus, when a physician provides services to a Medicare beneficiary, he or she should only bill those services that meet the Medicare standard of being reasonable and necessary for the diagnosis and treatment of a patient. A physician practice can bill in order to receive a denial for services, but only if the denial is needed for reimbursement from the secondary payor. Upon request, the physician practice should be able to provide documentation, such as a patient's medical records and physician's orders, to support the appropriateness of a service that the physician has provided.

c. *Documentation.* Timely, accurate and complete documentation is important to clinical patient care. This same documentation serves as a second function when a bill is submitted for payment, namely, as verification that the bill is accurate as submitted. Therefore, one of the most important physician practice compliance issues is the appropriate documentation of diagnosis and treatment. Physician documentation is necessary to determine the appropriate medical treatment for the patient and is the basis for coding and billing determinations. Thorough and accurate documentation also helps to ensure accurate recording and timely transmission of information.

i. Medical Record Documentation. In addition to facilitating high quality patient care, a properly documented medical record verifies and documents precisely what services were actually provided. The medical record may be used to validate: (a) The site of the service; (b) the appropriateness of the services provided; (c) the accuracy of the billing; and (d) the identity of the caregiver (service provider). Examples of internal documentation guidelines a practice might use to ensure accurate medical record documentation include the following:

- The medical record is complete and legible;
- The documentation of each patient encounter includes the reason for the encounter; any relevant history; physical examination findings; prior diagnostic test results; assessment, clinical impression, or diagnosis; plan of care; and date and legible identity of the observer;
- If not documented, the rationale for ordering diagnostic and other ancillary services can be easily inferred by an independent reviewer or third party who has appropriate medical training;
- CPT and ICD–9–CM codes used for claims submission are supported by documentation and the medical record; and
- Appropriate health risk factors are identified. The patient's progress, his or her response to, and any changes in, treatment, and any revision in diagnosis is documented.

The CPT and ICD–9–CM codes reported on the health insurance claims form should be supported by documentation in the medical record and the medical chart should contain all necessary information. Additionally, HCFA and the local carriers should be able to determine the person who provided the services. These issues can be the root of investigations of inappropriate or erroneous conduct, and have been identified by HCFA and the OIG as a leading cause of improper payments.

One method for improving quality in documentation is for a physician practice to compare the practice's claim denial rate to the rates of other practices in the same specialty to the extent that the practice can obtain that information from the carrier. Physician coding and diagnosis distribution can be compared for each physician within the same specialty to identify variances.

ii. HCFA 1500 Form. Another documentation area for physician practices to monitor closely is the proper completion of the HCFA 1500 form. The following practices will help ensure that the form has been properly completed:

- Link the diagnosis code with the reason for the visit or service;
- Use modifiers appropriately;
- Provide Medicare with all information about a beneficiary's other insurance coverage under the Medicare Secondary Payor (MSP) policy, if the practice is aware of a beneficiary's additional coverage.

d. *Improper Inducements, Kickbacks and Self-Referrals.* A physician practice would be well advised to have standards and procedures that encourage compliance with the anti-kickback statute and the physician self-referral law. Remuneration for referrals is illegal because it can distort medical decision-making, cause overutilization of services or supplies, increase costs to Federal health care programs, and result in unfair competition by shutting out competitors who are unwilling to pay for referrals. Remuneration for referrals can also affect the quality of patient care by encouraging physicians to order services or supplies based on profit rather than the patients' best medical interests.

In particular, arrangements with hospitals, hospices, nursing facilities, home health agencies, durable medical equipment suppliers, pharmaceutical manufacturers and vendors are areas of potential concern. In general the anti-kickback statute prohibits knowingly and willfully giving or receiving anything of value to induce referrals of Federal health care program business. It is generally recommended that all business arrangements wherein physician practices refer business to, or order services or items from, an outside entity should be on a fair market value basis. Whenever a physician practice intends to enter into a business arrangement that involves making referrals, the arrangement should be reviewed by legal counsel familiar with the anti-kickback statute and physician self-referral statute.

In addition to developing standards and procedures to address arrangements with other health care providers and suppliers, physician practices should also consider implementing measures to avoid offering inappropriate inducements to patients. Examples of such inducements include routinely waiving coinsurance or deductible amounts without a good faith determination that the patient is in financial need or failing to make reasonable efforts to collect the cost-sharing amount.

Possible risk factors relating to this risk area that could be addressed in the practice's standards and procedures include:

- Financial arrangements with outside entities to whom the practice may refer Federal health care program business;
- Joint ventures with entities supplying goods or services to the physician practice or its patients;
- Consulting contracts or medical directorships;
- Office and equipment leases with entities to which the physician refers; and
- Soliciting, accepting or offering any gift or gratuity of more than nominal value to or from those who may benefit from a physician practice's referral of Federal health care program business.

In order to keep current with this area of the law, a physician practice may obtain copies, available on the OIG web site or in hard copy from the OIG, of all relevant OIG Special Fraud Alerts and Advisory Opinions that address the application of the anti-kickback and physician self-referral laws to ensure that the standards and procedures reflect current positions and opinions.

2. Retention of Records

In light of the documentation requirements faced by physician practices, it would be to the practice's benefit if its standards and procedures contained a section on the retention of compliance, business and medical records. These records primarily include documents relating to patient care and the practice's business activities. A physician practice's designated compliance contact could keep an updated binder or record of these documents, including information relating to compliance activities. The primary compliance documents that a practice would want to retain are those that relate to educational activities, internal investigations and internal audit results. We suggest that particular attention should be paid to documenting investigations of potential violations uncovered by the compliance program and the resulting remedial action. Although there is no requirement that the practice retain its compliance records, having all the relevant documentation relating to the practice's compliance efforts or handling of a particular problem can benefit the practice should it ever be questioned regarding those activities.

Physician practices that implement a compliance program might also want to provide for the development and implementation of a records retention system. This system would establish standards and procedures regarding the creation, distribution, retention, and destruction of documents. If the practice decides to design a record system, privacy concerns and Federal or State regulatory requirements should be taken into consideration.

While conducting its compliance activities, as well as its daily operations, a physician practice would be well advised, to the extent it is possible, to document its efforts to comply with applicable Federal health care program requirements. For example, if a physician practice requests advice from a Government agency (including a Medicare carrier) charged with administering a Federal health care program, it is to the benefit of the practice to document and retain a record of the request and any written or oral response (or nonresponse). This step is extremely important if the practice intends to rely on that response to guide it in future decisions, actions, or claim reimbursement requests or appeals.

In short, it is in the best interest of all physician practices, regardless of size, to have procedures to create and retain appropriate documentation. The following record retention guidelines are suggested:

- The length of time that a practice's records are to be retained can be specified in the physician practice's standards and procedures (Federal and State statutes should be consulted for specific time frames, if applicable);
- Medical records (if in the possession of the physician practice) need to be secured against loss, destruction, unauthorized access, unauthorized reproduction, corruption, or damage; and
- Standards and procedures can stipulate the disposition of medical records in the event the practice is sold or closed.

Step Three. Designation of a Compliance Officer/Contact(s)
After the audits have been completed and the risk areas identified, ideally one member of the physician practice staff needs to accept the responsibility of developing a corrective action plan, if necessary, and oversee the practice's adherence to that plan. This person can either be in charge of all compliance activities for the practice or play a limited role merely to resolve the current issue. In a formalized institutional compliance program there is a compliance officer who is responsible for overseeing the implementation and day-to-day operations of the compliance program. However, the resource constraints of physician practices make it so that it is often impossible to designate one person to be in charge of compliance functions.

It is acceptable for a physician practice to designate more than one employee with compliance monitoring responsibility. In lieu of having a designated compliance officer, the physician practice could instead describe in its standards and procedures the compliance functions for which designated employees, known as "compliance contacts," would be responsible. For example, one employee could be responsible for preparing written standards and procedures, while another could be responsible for conducting or arranging for periodic audits and ensuring that billing questions are answered. Therefore, the compliance-related responsibilities of the designated person or persons may be only a portion of his or her duties.

Another possibility is that one individual could serve as compliance officer for more than one entity. In situations where staffing limitations mandate that the practice cannot afford to designate a person(s) to oversee compliance activities, the practice could outsource all or part of the functions of a compliance officer to a third party, such as a consultant, PPMC, MSO, IPA or third-party billing company. However, if this role is outsourced, it is beneficial for the compliance officer to have sufficient interaction with the physician practice to be able to effectively understand the inner workings of the practice. For example, consultants that are not in close geographic proximity to a practice may not be effective compliance officers for the practice.

One suggestion for how to maintain continual interaction is for the practice to designate someone to serve as a liaison with the outsourced compliance officer. This would help ensure a strong tie between the compliance officer and the practice's daily operations. Outsourced compliance officers, who spend most of their time offsite, have certain limitations that a physician practice should consider before making such a critical decision. These limitations can include lack of understanding as to the inner workings of the practice, accessibility and possible conflicts of interest when one compliance officer is serving several practices.

If the physician practice decides to designate a particular person(s) to oversee all compliance activities, not just those in conjunction with the audit-related issue, the following is a list of suggested duties that the practice may want to assign to that person(s):

- Overseeing and monitoring the implementation of the compliance program;
- Establishing methods, such as periodic audits, to improve the practice's efficiency and quality of services, and to reduce the practice's vulnerability to fraud and abuse;
- Periodically revising the compliance program in light of changes in the needs of the practice or changes in the law and in the standards and procedures of Government and private payor health plans;
- Developing, coordinating and participating in a training program that focuses on the components of the compliance program, and seeks to ensure that training materials are appropriate;
- Ensuring that the HHS–OIG's List of Excluded Individuals and Entities, and the General Services Administration's (GSA's) List of Parties Debarred from Federal Programs have been checked with respect to all employees, medical staff and independent contractors; and
- Investigating any report or allegation concerning possible unethical or improper business practices, and monitoring subsequent corrective action and/or compliance.

Each physician practice needs to assess its own practice situation and determine what best suits that practice in terms of compliance oversight.

Step Four. Conducting Appropriate Training and Education
Education is an important part of any compliance program and is the logical next step after problems have been identified and the practice has designated a person to oversee educational training. Ideally, education programs will be tailored to the physician practice's needs, specialty and size and will include both compliance and specific training.

There are three basic steps for setting up educational objectives:
- Determining who needs training (both in coding and billing and in compliance);
- Determining the type of training that best suits the practice's needs (*e.g.*, seminars, in-service training, self-study or other programs); and
- Determining when and how often education is needed and how much each person should receive.

Training may be accomplished through a variety of means, including in-person training sessions (*i.e.*, either on site or at outside seminars), distribution of newsletters, or even a readily accessible office bulletin board. Regardless of the training modality used, a physician practice should ensure that the necessary education is communicated effectively and that the practice's employees come away from the training with a better understanding of the issues covered.

1. Compliance Training
   Under the direction of the designated compliance officer/contact, both initial and recurrent training

in compliance is advisable, both with respect to the compliance program itself and applicable statutes and regulations. Suggestions for items to include in compliance training are: The operation and importance of the compliance program; the consequences of violating the standards and procedures set forth in the program; and the role of each employee in the operation of the compliance program.

There are two goals a practice should strive for when conducting compliance training: (1) All employees will receive training on how to perform their jobs in compliance with the standards of the practice and any applicable regulations; and (2) each employee will understand that compliance is a condition of continued employment. Compliance training focuses on explaining why the practice is developing and establishing a compliance program. The training should emphasize that following the standards and procedures will not get a practice employee in trouble, but violating the standards and procedures may subject the employee to disciplinary measures. It is advisable that new employees be trained on the compliance program as soon as possible after their start date and employees should receive refresher training on an annual basis or as appropriate.

2. Coding and Billing Training
   Coding and billing training on the Federal health care program requirements may be necessary for certain members of the physician practice staff depending on their respective responsibilities. The OIG understands that most physician practices do not employ a professional coder and that the physician is often primarily responsible for all coding and billing. However, it is in the practice's best interest to ensure that individuals who are directly involved with billing, coding or other aspects of the Federal health care programs receive extensive education specific to that individual's responsibilities. Some examples of items that could be covered in coding and billing training include:
   - Coding requirements;
   - Claim development and submission processes;
   - Signing a form for a physician without the physician's authorization;
   - Proper documentation of services rendered;
   - Proper billing standards and procedures and submission of accurate bills for services or items rendered to Federal health care program beneficiaries; and
   - The legal sanctions for submitting deliberately false or reckless billings.

3. Format of the Training Program
   Training may be conducted either in-house or by an outside source.

   Training at outside seminars, instead of internal programs and in-service sessions, may be an effective way to achieve the practice's training goals. In fact, many community colleges offer certificate or associate degree programs in billing and coding,

and professional associations provide various kinds of continuing education and certification programs. Many carriers also offer billing training.

The physician practice may work with its third-party billing company, if one is used, to ensure that documentation is of a level that is adequate for the billing company to submit accurate claims on behalf of the physician practice. If it is not, these problem areas should also be covered in the training. In addition to the billing training, it is advisable for physician practices to maintain updated ICD–9, HCPCS and CPT manuals (in addition to the carrier bulletins construing those sources) and make them available to all employees involved in the billing process. Physician practices can also provide a source of continuous updates on current billing standards and procedures by making publications or Government documents that describe current billing policies available to its employees.

Physician practices do not have to provide separate education and training programs for the compliance and coding and billing training. All in-service training and continuing education can integrate compliance issues, as well as other core values adopted by the practice, such as quality improvement and improved patient service, into their curriculum.

4. Continuing Education on Compliance Issues
   There is no set formula for determining how often training sessions should occur. The OIG recommends that there be at least an annual training program for all individuals involved in the coding and billing aspects of the practice. Ideally, new billing and coding employees will be trained as soon as possible after assuming their duties and will work under an experienced employee until their training has been completed.

Step Five. Responding to Detected Offenses and Developing Corrective Action Initiatives
When a practice determines it has detected a possible violation, the next step is to develop a corrective action plan and determine how to respond to the problem. Violations of a physician practice's compliance program, significant failures to comply with applicable Federal or State law, and other types of misconduct threaten a practice's status as a reliable, honest, and trustworthy provider of health care. Consequently, upon receipt of reports or reasonable indications of suspected noncompliance, it is important that the compliance contact or other practice employee look into the allegations to determine whether a significant violation of applicable law or the requirements of the compliance program has indeed occurred, and, if so, take decisive steps to correct the problem. As appropriate, such steps may involve a corrective action plan, the return of any overpayments, a report to the Government, and/or a referral to law enforcement authorities.

One suggestion is that the practice, in developing its compliance program, develop its own set of monitors and warning indicators. These might include: Significant changes in the number and/or types of claim rejections and/or reductions; correspondence from the carriers and insurers challenging the medical necessity or validity of claims; illogical patterns or unusual changes in the pattern of CPT–4, HCPCS or ICD–9 code utilization; and high volumes of unusual charge or payment adjustment transactions. If any of these warning indicators become apparent, then it is recommended that the practice follow up on the issues. Subsequently, as appropriate, the compliance procedures of the practice may need to be changed to prevent the problem from recurring.

For potential criminal violations, a physician practice would be well advised in its compliance program procedures to include steps for prompt referral or disclosure to an appropriate Government authority or law enforcement agency. In regard to overpayment issues, it is advised that the physician practice take appropriate corrective action, including prompt identification and repayment of any overpayment to the affected payor.

It is also recommended that the compliance program provide for a full internal assessment of all reports of detected violations. If the physician practice ignores reports of possible fraudulent activity, it is undermining the very purpose it hoped to achieve by implementing a compliance program.

It is advised that the compliance program standards and procedures include provisions to ensure that a violation is not compounded once discovered. In instances involving individual misconduct, the standards and procedures might also advise as to whether the individuals involved in the violation either be retrained, disciplined, or, if appropriate, terminated. The physician practice may also prevent the compounding of the violation by conducting a review of all confirmed violations, and, if appropriate, self-reporting the violations to the applicable authority.

The physician practice may consider the fact that if a violation occurred and was not detected, its compliance program may require modification. Physician practices that detect violations could analyze the situation to determine whether a flaw in their compliance program failed to anticipate the detected problem, or whether the compliance program's procedures failed to prevent the violation. In any event, it is prudent, even absent the detection of any violations, for physician practices to periodically review and modify their compliance programs.

Step Six. Developing Open Lines of Communication
In order to prevent problems from occurring and to have a frank discussion of why the problem happened in the first place, physician practices need to have open lines of communication. Especially in a smaller practice, an open line of communication is an integral part of implementing a compliance program. Guidance previously issued by the OIG has encouraged the use of several forms of communication between the compliance officer/ committee and provider personnel, many of which focus on formal processes and are more costly to implement (*e.g.,* hotlines

and e-mail). However, the OIG recognizes that the nature of some physician practices is not as conducive to implementing these types of measures. The nature of a small physician practice dictates that such communication and information exchanges need to be conducted through a less formalized process than that which has been envisioned by prior OIG guidance.

In the small physician practice setting, the communication element may be met by implementing a clear "open door" policy between the physicians and compliance personnel and practice employees. This policy can be implemented in conjunction with less formal communication techniques, such as conspicuous notices posted in common areas and/or the development and placement of a compliance bulletin board where everyone in the practice can receive up-to-date compliance information.

A compliance program's system for meaningful and open communication can include the following:
- The requirement that employees report conduct that a reasonable person would, in good faith, believe to be erroneous or fraudulent;
- The creation of a user-friendly process (such as an anonymous drop box for larger practices) for effectively reporting erroneous or fraudulent conduct;
- Provisions in the standards and procedures that state that a failure to report erroneous or fraudulent conduct is a violation of the compliance program;
- The development of a simple and readily accessible procedure to process reports of erroneous or fraudulent conduct;
- If a billing company is used, communication to and from the billing company's compliance officer/contact and other responsible staff to coordinate billing and compliance activities of the practice and the billing company, respectively. Communication can include, as appropriate, lists of reported or identified concerns, initiation and the results of internal assessments, training needs, regulatory changes, and other operational and compliance matters;
- The utilization of a process that maintains the anonymity of the persons involved in the reported possible erroneous or fraudulent conduct and the person reporting the concern; and
- Provisions in the standards and procedures that there will be no retribution for reporting conduct that a reasonable person acting in good faith would have believed to be erroneous or fraudulent.

The OIG recognizes that protecting anonymity may not be feasible for small physician practices. However, the OIG believes all practice employees, when seeking answers to questions or reporting potential instances of erroneous or fraudulent conduct, should know to whom to turn for assistance in these matters and should be able to do so without fear of retribution. While the physician practice may strive to maintain the anonymity of an employee's identity, it also needs to make clear that there may be a point at which the individual's identity may become known or may have to be revealed in certain instances.

Step Seven. Enforcing Disciplinary Standards Through Well-Publicized Guidelines

Finally, the last step that a physician practice may wish to take is to incorporate measures into its practice to ensure that practice employees understand the consequences if they behave in a non-compliant manner. An effective physician practice compliance program includes procedures for enforcing and disciplining individuals who violate the practice's compliance or other practice standards. Enforcement and disciplinary provisions are necessary to add credibility and integrity to a compliance program.

The OIG recommends that a physician practice's enforcement and disciplinary mechanisms ensure that violations of the practice's compliance policies will result in consistent and appropriate sanctions, including the possibility of termination, against the offending individual. At the same time, it is advisable that the practice's enforcement and disciplinary procedures be flexible enough to account for mitigating or aggravating circumstances. The procedures might also stipulate that individuals who fail to detect or report violations of the compliance program may also be subject to discipline. Disciplinary actions could include: Warnings (oral); reprimands (written); probation; demotion; temporary suspension; termination; restitution of damages; and referral for criminal prosecution. Inclusion of disciplinary guidelines in in-house training and procedure manuals is sufficient to meet the "well publicized" standard of this element.

It is suggested that any communication resulting in the finding of non-compliant conduct be documented in the compliance files by including the date of incident, name of the reporting party, name of the person responsible for taking action, and the follow-up action taken. Another suggestion is for physician practices to conduct checks to make sure all current and potential practice employees are not listed on the OIG or GSA lists of individuals excluded from participation in Federal health care or Government procurement programs.

C. Assessing A Voluntary Compliance Program

A practice's commitment to compliance can best be assessed by the active application of compliance principles in the day-to-day operations of the practice. Compliance programs are not just written standards and procedures that sit on a shelf in the main office of a practice, but are an everyday part of the practice operations. It is by integrating the compliance program into the practice culture that the practice can best achieve maximum benefit from its compliance program.

III. CONCLUSION

Just as immunizations are given to patients to prevent them from becoming ill, physician practices may view the implementation of a voluntary compliance program as comparable to a form of preventive medicine for the practice. This voluntary compliance program guidance is intended to assist physician practices in developing and implementing internal controls and procedures that promote adherence to Federal health care program requirements.

As stated earlier, physician compliance programs do not need to be time or resource intensive and can be developed in a manner that best reflects the nature of each individual practice. Many of the recommendations set forth in this document are ones that many physician practices already have in place and are simply good business practices that can be adhered to with a reasonable amount of effort. By implementing an effective compliance program, appropriate for its size and resources, and making compliance principles an active part of the practice culture, a physician practice can help prevent and reduce erroneous or fraudulent conduct in its practice. These efforts can also streamline and improve the business operations within the practice and therefore inoculate itself against future problems.

Dated: September 27, 2000.

June Gibbs Brown,
Inspector General.

APPENDIX A: ADDITIONAL RISK AREAS

Appendix A describes additional risk areas that a physician practice may wish to address during the development of its compliance program. If any of the following risk areas are applicable to the practice, the practice may want to consider addressing the risk areas by incorporating them into the practice's written standards and procedures manual and addressing them in its training program.

I. REASONABLE AND NECESSARY SERVICES

A. Local Medical Review Policy

An area of concern for physicians relating to determinations of reasonable and necessary services is the variation in local medical review policies (LMRPs) among carriers. Physicians are supposed to bill the Federal health care programs only for items and services that are reasonable and necessary. However, in order to determine whether an item or service is reasonable and necessary under Medicare guidelines, the physician must apply the appropriate LMRP.

With the exception of claims that are properly coded and submitted to Medicare solely for the purpose of obtaining a written denial, physician practices are to bill the Federal health programs only for items and services that are covered. In order to determine if an item or service is covered for Medicare, a physician practice must be knowledgeable of the LMRPs applicable to its practice's jurisdiction. The practice may contact its carrier to request a copy of the pertinent LMRPs, and once the practice receives the copies, they can be incorporated into the practice's written standards and procedures manual. When the LMRP indicates that an item or service may not be covered by Medicare, the physician practice is responsible to convey this information to the patient so that the patient can make an informed decision concerning the health care services he/she may want to receive. Physician practices convey this information through Advance Beneficiary Notices (ABNs).

B. *Advance Beneficiary Notices*

Physicians are required to provide ABNs before they provide services that they know or believe Medicare does not consider reasonable and necessary. (The one exception to this requirement is for services that are performed pursuant to EMTALA requirements as described in section II.A.) A properly executed ABN acknowledges that coverage is uncertain or yet to be determined, and stipulates that the patient promises to pay the bill if Medicare does not. Patients who are not notified before they receive such services are not responsible for payment. The ABN must be sufficient to put the patient on notice of the reasons why the physician believes that the payment may be denied. The objective is to give the patient sufficient information to allow an informed choice as to whether to pay for the service.

Accordingly, each ABN should:

i.   Be in writing;
ii. Identify the specific service that may be denied (procedure name and CPT/HCPC code is recommended);
iii. State the specific reason why the physician believes that service may be denied; and
iv. Be signed by the patient acknowledging that the required information was provided and that the patient assumes responsibility to pay for the service.

The Medicare Carrier's Manual provides that an ABN will not be acceptable if: (1) The patient is asked to sign a blank ABN form; or (2) the ABN is used routinely without regard to a particularized need. The routine use of ABNs is generally prohibited because the ABN must state the specific reason the physician anticipates that the specific service will not be covered.

A common risk area associated with ABNs is in regard to diagnostic tests or services. There are three steps that a physician practice can take to help ensure it is in compliance with the regulations concerning ABNs for diagnostic tests or services:

1. Determine which tests are not covered under national coverage rules;
2. Determine which tests are not covered under local coverage rules such as LMRPs (contact the practice's carrier to see if a listing has been assembled); and
3. Determine which tests are only covered for certain diagnoses. The OIG is aware that the use of ABNs is an area where physician practices experience numerous difficulties. Practices can help to reduce problems in this area by educating their physicians and office staff on the correct use of ABNs, obtaining guidance from the carrier regarding their interpretation of whether an ABN is necessary where the service is not covered, developing a standard form for all diagnostic tests (most carriers have a developed model), and developing a process for handling patients who refuse to sign ABNs.

C. *Physician Liability for Certifications in the Provision of Medical Equipment and Supplies and Home Health Services*

In January 1999, the OIG issued a Special Fraud Alert on this topic, which is available on the OIG web site at www.hhs.gov/oig/frdalrt/index.htm. The following is a summary of the Special Fraud Alert.

The OIG issued the Special Fraud Alert to reiterate to physicians the legal and programmatic significance of physician certifications made in connection with the ordering of certain items and services for Medicare patients. In light of information obtained through OIG provider audits, the OIG deemed it necessary to remind physicians that they may be subject to criminal, civil and administrative penalties for signing a certification when they know that the information is false or for signing a certification with reckless disregard as to the truth of the information. (*See Appendix B* and *Appendix C* for more detailed information on the applicable statutes.)

Medicare has conditioned payment for many items and services on a certification signed by a physician attesting that the physician has reviewed the patient's condition and has determined that an item or service is reasonable and necessary. Because Medicare primarily relies on the professional judgment of the treating physician to determine the reasonable and necessary nature of a given service or supply, it is important that physicians provide complete and accurate information on any certifications they sign. Physician certification is obtained through a variety of forms, including prescriptions, orders, and Certificates of Medical Necessity (CMNs). Two areas where physician certification as to whether an item or service is reasonable and necessary is essential and which are vulnerable to abuse are: (1) Home health services; and (2) durable medical equipment.

By signing a CMN, the physician represents that:

1. He or she is the patient's treating physician and that the information regarding the physician's address and unique physician identification number (UPIN) is correct;
2. the entire CMN, including the sections filled out by the supplier, was completed *prior* to the physician's signature; and
3. the information in section B relating to whether the item or service is reasonable and necessary is true, accurate, and complete to the best of the physician's knowledge.

Activities such as signing blank CMNs, signing a CMN without seeing the patient to verify the item or service is reasonable and necessary, and signing a CMN for a service that the physician knows is not reasonable and necessary are activities that can lead to criminal, civil and administrative penalties.

Ultimately, it is advised that physicians carefully review any form of certification (order, prescription or CMN) before signing it to verify that the information contained in the certification is both complete and accurate.

D. Billing for Non-covered Services as if Covered

In some instances, we are aware that physician practices submit claims for services in order to receive a denial from the carrier, thereby enabling the patient to submit the denied claim for payment to a secondary payer.

A common question relating to this risk area is: If the medical services provided are not covered under Medicare, but the secondary or supplemental insurer requires a Medicare rejection in order to cover the services, then would the original submission of the claim to Medicare be considered fraudulent? Under the applicable regulations, the OIG would not consider such submissions to be fraudulent. For example, the denial may be necessary to establish patient liability protections as stated in section 1879 of the Social Security Act (the Act) (codified at 42 U.S.C. 1395pp). As stated, Medicare denials may also be required so that the patient can seek payment from a secondary insurer. In instances where a claim is being submitted to Medicare for this purpose, the physician should indicate on the claim submission that the claim is being submitted for the purpose of receiving a denial, in order to bill a secondary insurance carrier. This step should assist carriers and prevent inadvertent payments to which the physician is not entitled.

In some instances, however, the carrier pays the claim even though the service is non-covered, and even though the physician did not intend for payment to be made. When this occurs, the physician has a responsibility to refund the amount paid and indicate that the service is not covered.

II. PHYSICIAN RELATIONSHIPS WITH HOSPITALS

A. The Physician Role in EMTALA

The Emergency Medical Treatment and Active Labor Act (EMTALA), 42 U.S.C. 1395dd, is an area that has been receiving increasing scrutiny. The statute is intended to ensure that all patients who come to the emergency department of a hospital receive care, regardless of their insurance or ability to pay. Both hospitals and physicians need to work together to ensure compliance with the provisions of this law.

The statute imposes three fundamental requirements upon hospitals that participate in the Medicare program with regard to patients requesting emergency care. First, the hospital must conduct an appropriate medical screening examination to determine if an emergency medical condition exists. Second, if the hospital determines that an emergency medical condition exists, it must either provide the treatment necessary to stabilize the emergency medical condition or comply with the statute's requirements to effect a proper transfer of a patient whose condition has not been stabilized. A hospital is considered to have met this second requirement if an individual refuses the hospital's offer of additional examination or treatment, or refuses to consent to a transfer, after having been informed of the risks and benefits.

If an individual's emergency medical condition has not been stabilized, the statute's third requirement is activated.

A hospital may not transfer an individual with an unstable emergency medical condition unless: (1) The individual or his or her representative makes a written request for transfer to another medical facility after being informed of the risk of transfer and the transferring hospital's obligation under the statute to provide additional examination or treatment; (2) a physician has signed a certification summarizing the medical risks and benefits of a transfer and certifying that, based upon the information available at the time of transfer, the medical benefits reasonably expected from the transfer outweigh the increased risks; or (3) if a physician is not physically present when the transfer decision is made, a qualified medical person signs the certification after the physician, in consultation with the qualified medical person, has made the determination that the benefits of transfer outweigh the increased risks. The physician must later countersign the certification.

Physician and/or hospital misconduct may result in violations of the statute. One area of particular concern is physician on-call responsibilities. Physician practices whose members serve as on-call emergency room physicians with hospitals are advised to familiarize themselves with the hospital's policies regarding on-call physicians. This can be done by reviewing the medical staff bylaws or policies and procedures of the hospital that must define the responsibility of on-call physicians to respond to, examine, and treat patients with emergency medical conditions. Physicians should also be aware of the requirement that, when medically indicated, on-call physicians must generally come to the hospital to examine the patient. The exception to this requirement is that a patient may be sent to see the on-call physician at a hospital-owned contiguous or on-campus facility to conduct or complete the medical screening examination as long as:

1. All persons with the same medical condition are moved to this location;
2. there is a bona fide medical reason to move the patient; and
3. qualified medical personnel accompany the patient.

B. Teaching Physicians

Special regulations apply to teaching physicians' billings. Regulations provide that services provided by teaching physicians in teaching settings are generally payable under the physician fee schedule only if the services are personally furnished by a physician who is not a resident or the services are furnished by a resident in the presence of a teaching physician.

Unless a service falls under a specified exception, such as the Primary Care Exception, the teaching physician must be present during the key portion of any service or procedure for which payment is sought. Physicians should ensure the following with respect to services provided in the teaching physician setting

- Only services actually provided are billed;
- Every physician who provides or supervises the provision of services to a patient is responsible for the correct documentation of the services that were rendered;

- Every physician is responsible for assuring that in cases where the physician provides evaluation and management (E&M) services, a patient's medical record includes appropriate documentation of the applicable key components of the E&M services provided or supervised by the physician (*e.g.,* patient history, physician examination, and medical decision making), as well as documentation to adequately reflect the procedure or portion of the services provided by the physician; and

- Unless specifically excepted by regulation, every physician must document his or her presence during the key portion of any service or procedure for which payment is sought.

C. *Gainsharing Arrangements and Civil Monetary Penalties for Hospital Payments to Physicians to Reduce or Limit Services to Beneficiaries*

In July 1999, the OIG issued a Special Fraud Alert on this topic, which is available on the OIG web site at *www.hhs. gov/oig/frdalrt/index.htm*. The following is a summary of the Special Fraud Alert.

The term "gainsharing" typically refers to an arrangement in which a hospital gives a physician a percentage share of any reduction in the hospital's costs for patient care attributable in part to the physician's efforts. The civil monetary penalty (CMP) that applies to gainsharing arrangements is set forth in 42 U.S.C. 1320a–7a(b)(1). This section prohibits any hospital or critical access hospital from knowingly making a payment directly or indirectly to a physician as an inducement to reduce or limit services to Medicare or Medicaid beneficiaries under a physician's care.

It is the OIG's position that the Civil Monetary Penalties Law clearly prohibits any gainsharing arrangements that involve payments by, or on behalf of, a hospital to physicians with clinical care responsibilities to induce a reduction or limitation of services to Medicare or Medicaid beneficiaries. However, hospitals and physicians are not prohibited from working together to reduce unnecessary hospital costs through other arrangements. For example, hospitals and physicians may enter into personal services contracts where hospitals pay physicians based on a fixed fee at fair market value for services rendered to reduce costs rather than a fee based on a share of cost savings.

D. *Physician Incentive Arrangements*

The OIG has identified potentially illegal practices involving the offering of incentives by entities in an effort to recruit and retain physicians. The OIG is concerned that the intent behind offering incentives to physicians may not be to recruit physicians, but instead the offer is intended as a kickback to obtain and increase patient referrals from physicians. These recruitment incentive arrangements are implicated by the Anti-Kickback Statute because they can constitute remuneration offered to induce, or in return for, the referral of business paid for by Medicare or Medicaid.

Some examples of questionable incentive arrangements are:
- Provision of free or significantly discounted billing, nursing, or other staff services;
- Payment of the cost of a physician's travel and expenses for conferences;
- Payment for a physician's services that require few, if any, substantive duties by the physician; and
- Guarantees that if the physician's income fails to reach a predetermined level, the entity will supplement the remainder up to a certain amount.

III. PHYSICIAN BILLING PRACTICES

A. *Third-Party Billing Services*

Physicians should remember that they remain responsible to the Medicare program for bills sent in the physician's name or containing the physician's signature, even if the physician had no actual knowledge of a billing impropriety. The attestation on the HCFA 1500 form, *i.e.,* the physician's signature line, states that the physician's services were billed properly. In other words, it is no defense for the physician if the physician's billing service improperly bills Medicare.

One of the most common risk areas involving billing services deals with physician practices contracting with billing services on a percentage basis. Although percentage based billing arrangements are not illegal *per se,* the Office of Inspector General has a longstanding concern that such arrangements may increase the risk of intentional upcoding and similar abusive billing practices.

A physician may contract with a billing service on a percentage basis. However, the billing service cannot directly receive the payment of Medicare funds into a bank account that it solely controls. Under 42 U.S.C. 1395u(b)(6), Medicare payments can only be made to either the beneficiary or a party (such as a physician) that furnished the services and accepted assignment of the beneficiary's claim. A billing service that contracts on a percentage basis does not qualify as a party that furnished services to a beneficiary, thus a billing service cannot directly receive payment of Medicare funds. According to the *Medicare Carriers Manual* Section 3060(A), a payment is considered to be made directly to the billing service if the service can convert the payment to its own use and control without the payment first passing through the control of the physician. For example, the billing service should not bill the claims under its own name or tax identification number. The billing service should bill claims under the physician's name and tax identification number. Nor should a billing service receive the payment of Medicare funds directly into a bank account over which the billing service maintains sole control. The Medicare payments should instead be deposited into a bank account over which the provider has signature control.

Physician practices should review the third-party medical billing guidance for additional information on third-party billing companies and the compliance risk areas associated with billing companies.

B. *Billing Practices by Non-Participating Physicians*

Even though nonparticipating physicians do not accept payment directly from the Medicare program, there are a number of laws that apply to the billing of Medicare beneficiaries by non-participating physicians.

Limiting Charges

42 U.S.C. 1395w–4(g) prohibits a nonparticipating physician from knowingly and willfully billing or collecting on a repeated basis an actual charge for a service that is in excess of the Medicare limiting charge. For example, a nonparticipating physician may not bill a Medicare beneficiary $50 for an office visit when the Medicare limiting charge for the visit is $25. Additionally, there are numerous provisions that prohibit nonparticipating physicians from knowingly and willfully charging patients in excess of the statutory charge limitations for certain specified procedures, such as cataract surgery, mammography screening and coronary artery bypass surgery. Failure to comply with these sections can result in a fine of up to $10,000 per violation or exclusion from participation in Federal health care programs for up to 5 years.

Refund of Excess Charges

42 U.S.C. 1395w–4(g) mandates that if a nonparticipating physician collects an actual charge for a service that is in excess of the limiting charge, the physician must refund the amount collected above the limiting charge to the individual within 30 days notice of the violation. For example, if a physician collected $50 from a Medicare beneficiary for an office visit, but the limiting charge for the visit was $25, the physician must refund $25 to the beneficiary, which is the difference between the amount collected ($50) and the limiting charge ($25). Failure to comply with this requirement may result in a fine of up to $10,000 per violation or exclusion from participation in Federal health care programs for up to 5 years.

Specifically, 42 U.S.C. 1395u(l)(A)(iii) mandates that a nonparticipating physician must refund payments received from a Medicare beneficiary if it is later determined by a Peer Review Organization or a Medicare carrier that the services were not reasonable and necessary. Failure to comply with this requirement may result in a fine of up to $10,000 per violation or exclusion from participation in Federal health care programs for up to 5 years.

C. *Professional Courtesy*

The term "professional courtesy" is used to describe a number of analytically different practices. The traditional definition is the practice by a physician of waiving all or a part of the fee for services provided to the physician's office staff, other physicians, and/or their families. In recent times, "professional courtesy" has also come to mean the waiver of coinsurance obligations or other out-of-pocket expenses for physicians or their families (*i.e.*, "insurance only" billing), and similar payment arrangements by hospitals or other institutions for services provided to their medical staffs or employees. While only the first of these practices is truly "professional courtesy," in the interests of clarity and completeness, we will address all three.

In general, whether a professional courtesy arrangement runs afoul of the fraud and abuse laws is determined by two factors: (i) How the recipients of the professional courtesy are selected; and (ii) how the professional courtesy is extended. If recipients are selected in a manner that directly or indirectly takes into account their ability to affect past or future referrals, the anti-kickback statute—which prohibits giving anything of value to generate Federal health care program business—may be implicated. If the professional courtesy is extended through a waiver of copayment obligations (*i.e.*, "insurance only" billing), other statutes may be implicated, including the prohibition of inducements to beneficiaries, section 1128A(a)(5) of the Act (codified at 42 U.S.C. 1320a–7a(a)(5)). Claims submitted as a result of either practice may also implicate the civil False Claims Act.

The following are general observations about professional courtesy arrangements for physician practices to consider:

- A physician's regular and consistent practice of extending professional courtesy by waiving the entire fee for services rendered to a group of persons (including employees, physicians, and/or their family members) may not implicate any of the OIG's fraud and abuse authorities so long as membership in the group receiving the courtesy is determined in a manner that does not take into account directly or indirectly any group member's ability to refer to, or otherwise generate Federal health care program business for, the physician.

- A physician's regular and consistent practice of extending professional courtesy by waiving otherwise applicable copayments for services rendered to a group of persons (including employees, physicians, and/or their family members), would not implicate the anti-kickback statute so long as membership in the group is determined in a manner that does not take into account directly or indirectly any group member's ability to refer to, or otherwise generate Federal health care program business for, the physician.

- Any waiver of copayment practice, including that described in the preceding bullet, does implicate section 1128A(a)(5) of the Act if the patient for whom the copayment is waived is a Federal health care program beneficiary who is not financially needy.

The legality of particular professional courtesy arrangements will turn on the specific facts presented, and, with respect to the anti-kickback statute, on the specific intent of the parties. A physician practice may wish to consult with an attorney if it is uncertain about its professional courtesy arrangements.

IV. OTHER RISK AREAS

A. Rental of Space in Physician Offices by Persons or Entities to Which Physicians Refer

In February 2000, the OIG issued a Special Fraud Alert on this topic, which is available on the OIG web site at *www. hhs.gov/oig/frdalrt/index.htm*. The following is a summary of the Special Fraud Alert.

Among various relationships between physicians and labs, hospitals, home health agencies, etc., the OIG has identified potentially illegal practices involving the rental of space in a physician's office by suppliers that provide items or services to patients who are referred or sent to the supplier by the physician-landlord. An example of a suspect arrangement is the rental of physician office space by a durable medical equipment (DME) supplier in a position to benefit from referrals of the physician's patients. The OIG is concerned that in such arrangements the rental payments may be disguised kickbacks to the physician-landlord to induce referrals.

Space Rental Safe Harbor to the Anti-Kickback Statute

To avoid potentially violating the anti-kickback statute, the OIG recommends that rental agreements comply with all of the following criteria for the space rental safe harbor:

- The agreement is set out in writing and signed by the parties.
- The agreement covers all of the space rented by the parties for the term of the agreement and specifies the space covered by the agreement.
- If the agreement is intended to provide the lessee with access to the space for periodic intervals of time rather than on a full-time basis for the term of the rental agreement, the rental agreement specifies exactly the schedule of such intervals, the precise length of each interval, and the exact rent for each interval.
- The term of the rental agreement is for not less than one year.
- The aggregate rental charge is set in advance, is consistent with fair market value, and is not determined in a manner that takes into account the volume or value of any referrals or business otherwise generated between the parties for which payment may be made in whole or in part under Medicare or a State health care program.
- The aggregate space rented does not exceed that which is reasonably necessary to accomplish the commercially reasonable business purpose of the rental.

B. Unlawful Advertising

42 U.S.C. 1320b–10 makes it unlawful for any person to advertise using the names, abbreviations, symbols, or emblems of the Social Security Administration, Health Care Financing Administration, Department of Health and Human Services, Medicare, Medicaid or any combination or variation of such words, abbreviations, symbols or emblems in a manner that such person knows or should know would convey the false impression that the advertised item is endorsed by the named entities. For instance, a physician may not place an ad in the newspaper that reads "Dr. X is a cardiologist approved by both the Medicare and Medicaid programs." A violation of this section may result in a penalty of up to $5,000 ($25,000 in the case of a broadcast or telecast) for each violation.

APPENDIX B: CRIMINAL STATUTES

This Appendix contains a description of criminal statutes related to fraud and abuse in the context of health care. The Appendix is not intended to be a compilation of all Federal statutes related to health care fraud and abuse. It is merely a summary of some of the more frequently cited Federal statutes.

I. HEALTH CARE FRAUD (18 U.S.C. 1347)

Description of Unlawful Conduct

It is a crime to knowingly and willfully execute (or attempt to execute) a scheme to defraud any health care benefit program, or to obtain money or property from a health care benefit program through false representations. Note that this law applies not only to Federal health care programs, but to most other types of health care benefit programs as well.

Penalty for Unlawful Conduct

The penalty may include the imposition of fines, imprisonment of up to 10 years, or both. If the violation results in serious bodily injury, the prison term may be increased to a maximum of 20 years. If the violation results in death, the prison term may be expanded to include any number of years, or life imprisonment.

Examples

1. Dr. X, a chiropractor, intentionally billed Medicare for physical therapy and chiropractic treatments that he never actually rendered for the purpose of fraudulently obtaining Medicare payments.
2. Dr. X, a psychiatrist, billed Medicare, Medicaid, TRICARE, and private insurers for psychiatric services that were provided by his nurses rather than himself.

II. THEFT OR EMBEZZLEMENT IN CONNECTION WITH HEALTH CARE (18 U.S.C. 669)

Description of Unlawful Conduct

It is a crime to knowingly and willfully embezzle, steal or intentionally misapply any of the assets of a health care benefit program. Note that this law applies not only to Federal health care programs, but to most other types of health care benefit programs as well.

Penalty for Unlawful Conduct

The penalty may include the imposition of a fine, imprisonment of up to 10 years, or both. If the value of the asset is $100 or less, the penalty is a fine, imprisonment of up to a year, or both.

Example

An office manager for Dr. X knowingly embezzles money from the bank account for Dr. X's practice. The bank account includes reimbursement received from the Medicare program;

thus, intentional embezzlement of funds from this account is a violation of the law.

III. FALSE STATEMENTS RELATING TO HEALTH CARE MATTERS (18 U.S.C. 1035)

Description of Unlawful Conduct

It is a crime to knowingly and willfully falsify or conceal a material fact, or make any materially false statement or use any materially false writing or document in connection with the delivery of or payment for health care benefits, items or services. Note that this law applies not only to Federal health care programs, but to most other types of health care benefit programs as well.

Penalty for Unlawful Conduct

The penalty may include the imposition of a fine, imprisonment of up to 5 years, or both.

Example

Dr. X certified on a claim form that he performed laser surgery on a Medicare beneficiary when he knew that the surgery was not actually performed on the patient.

IV. OBSTRUCTION OF CRIMINAL INVESTIGATIONS OF HEALTH CARE OFFENSES (18 U.S.C. 1518)

Description of Unlawful Conduct

It is a crime to willfully prevent, obstruct, mislead, delay or attempt to prevent, obstruct, mislead, or delay the communication of records relating to a Federal health care offense to a criminal investigator. Note that this law applies not only to Federal health care programs, but to most other types of health care benefit programs as well.

Penalty for Unlawful Conduct

The penalty may include the imposition of a fine, imprisonment of up to 5 years, or both.

Examples

1. Dr. X instructs his employees to tell OIG investigators that Dr. X personally performs all treatments when, in fact, medical technicians do the majority of the treatment and Dr. X is rarely present in the office.
2. Dr. X was under investigation by the FBI for reported fraudulent billings. Dr. X altered patient records in an attempt to cover up the improprieties.

V. MAIL AND WIRE FRAUD (18 U.S.C. 1341 AND 1343)

Description of Unlawful Conduct

It is a crime to use the mail, private courier, or wire service to conduct a scheme to defraud another of money or property. The term "wire services" includes the use of a telephone, fax machine or computer. Each use of a mail or wire service to further fraudulent activities is considered a separate crime. For instance, each fraudulent claim that is submitted electronically to a carrier would be considered a separate violation of the law.

Penalty for Unlawful Conduct

The penalty may include the imposition of a fine, imprisonment of up to 5 years, or both.

Examples

1. Dr. X knowingly and repeatedly submits electronic claims to the Medicare carrier for office visits that he did not actually provide to Medicare beneficiaries with the intent to obtain payments from Medicare for services he never performed.
2. Dr. X, a neurologist, knowingly submitted claims for tests that were not reasonable and necessary and intentionally upcoded office visits and electromyograms to Medicare.

VI. CRIMINAL PENALTIES FOR ACTS INVOLVING FEDERAL HEALTH CARE PROGRAMS (42 U.S.C. 1320A–7B)

Description of Unlawful Conduct

False Statement and Representations
It is a crime to knowingly and willfully:

1. make, or cause to be made, false statements or representations in applying for benefits or payments under all Federal health care programs;
2. make, or cause to be made, any false statement or representation for use in determining rights to such benefit or payment;
3. conceal any event affecting an individual's initial or continued right to receive a benefit or payment with the intent to fraudulently receive the benefit or payment either in an amount or quantity greater than that which is due or authorized;
4. convert a benefit or payment to a use other than for the use and benefit of the person for whom it was intended;
5. present, or cause to be presented, a claim for a physician's service when the service was not furnished by a licensed physician;
6. for a fee, counsel an individual to dispose of assets in order to become eligible for medical assistance under a State health program, if disposing of the assets results in the imposition of an ineligibility period for the individual.

Anti-Kickback Statute

It is a crime to knowingly and willfully solicit, receive, offer, or pay remuneration of any kind (*e.g.,* money, goods, services):

- for the referral of an individual to another for the purpose of supplying items or services that are covered by a Federal health care program; or
- for purchasing, leasing, ordering, or arranging for any good, facility, service, or item that is covered by a Federal health care program.

There are a number of limited exceptions to the law, also known as "safe harbors," which provide immunity from criminal prosecution and which are described in greater detail in the statute and related regulations (found at 42 CFR 1001.952 and www.hhs.gov/oig/ak). Current safe harbors include:

- investment interests;
- space rental;
- equipment rental;

- personal services and management contracts;
- sale of practice;
- referral services;
- warranties;
- discounts;
- employment relationships;
- waiver of Part A co-insurance and deductible amounts;
- group purchasing organizations;
- increased coverage or reduced cost sharing under a risk-basis or prepaid plan; and
- charge reduction agreements with health plans.

Penalty for Unlawful Conduct

The penalty may include the imposition of a fine of up to $25,000, imprisonment of up to 5 years, or both. In addition, the provider can be excluded from participation in Federal health care programs. The regulations defining the aggravating and mitigating circumstances that must be reviewed by the OIG in making an exclusion determination are set forth in 42 CFR part 1001.

Examples

1. Dr. X accepted payments to sign Certificates of Medical Necessity for durable medical equipment for patients she never examined.
2. Home Health Agency disguises referral fees as salaries by paying referring physician Dr. X for services Dr. X never rendered to the Medicare beneficiaries or by paying Dr. X a sum in excess of fair market value for the services he rendered to the Medicare beneficiaries.

APPENDIX C: CIVIL AND ADMINISTRATIVE STATUTES

This Appendix contains a description of civil and administrative statutes related to fraud and abuse in the context of health care. The Appendix is not intended to be a compilation of all federal statutes related to health care fraud and abuse. It is merely a summary of some of the more frequently cited Federal statutes.

I. THE FALSE CLAIMS ACT (31 U.S.C. 3729– 3733)

Description of Unlawful Conduct

This is the law most often used to bring a case against a health care provider for the submission of false claims to a Federal health care program. The False Claims Act prohibits knowingly presenting (or causing to be presented) to the Federal Government a false or fraudulent claim for payment or approval. Additionally, it prohibits knowingly making or using (or causing to be made or used) a false record or statement to get a false or fraudulent claim paid or approved by the Federal Government or its agents, like a carrier, other claims processor, or State Medicaid program.

Definitions

False Claim—A "false claim" is a claim for payment for services or supplies that were not provided specifically as presented or for which the provider is otherwise not entitled to payment. Examples of false claims for services or supplies that were not provided specifically as presented include, but are not limited to:

- a claim for a service or supply that was never provided.
- a claim indicating the service was provided for some diagnosis code other than the true diagnosis code in order to obtain reimbursement for the service (which would not be covered if the true diagnosis code were submitted).
- a claim indicating a higher level of service than was actually provided.
- a claim for a service that the provider knows is not reasonable and necessary.
- a claim for services provided by an unlicensed individual.

Knowingly—To "knowingly" present a false or fraudulent claim means that the provider: (1) Has actual knowledge that the information on the claim is false; (2) acts in deliberate ignorance of the truth or falsity of the information on the claim; or (3) acts in reckless disregard of the truth or falsity of the information on the claim. It is important to note the provider does not have to deliberately intend to defraud the Federal Government in order to be found liable under this Act. The provider need only "knowingly" present a false or fraudulent claim in the manner described above.

Deliberate Ignorance—To act in "deliberate ignorance" means that the provider has deliberately chosen to ignore the truth or falsity of the information on a claim submitted for payment, even though the provider knows, or has notice, that information may be false. An example of a provider who submits a false claim with deliberate ignorance would be a physician who ignores provider update bulletins and thus does not inform his/her staff of changes in the Medicare billing guidelines or update his/her billing system in accordance with changes to the Medicare billing practices. When claims for non-reimbursable services are submitted as a result, the False Claims Act has been violated.

Reckless Disregard—To act in "reckless disregard" means that the provider pays no regard to whether the information on a claim submitted for payment is true or false. An example of a provider who submits a false claim with reckless disregard would be a physician who assigns the billing function to an untrained office person without inquiring whether the employee has the requisite knowledge and training to accurately file such claims.

Penalty for Unlawful Conduct

The penalty for violating the False Claims Act is a minimum of $5,500 up to a maximum of $11,000 for *each* false claim submitted. In addition to the penalty, a provider could be found liable for damages of up to three times the amount unlawfully claimed.

Examples

- A physician submitted claims to Medicare and Medicaid representing that he had personally performed certain services when, in reality, the services were performed by a nonphysician and they were not reimbursable under the Federal health care programs.
- Dr. X intentionally upcoded office visits and angioplasty consultations that were submitted for payment to Medicare.
- Dr. X, a podiatrist, knowingly submitted claims to the Medicare and Medicaid programs for non-routine surgical

procedures when he actually performed routine, non-covered services such as the cutting and trimming of toenails and the removal of corns and calluses.

II. CIVIL MONETARY PENALTIES LAW (42 U.S.C. 1320A–7A)

Description of Unlawful Conduct

The Civil Monetary Penalties Law (CMPL) is a comprehensive statute that covers an array of fraudulent and abusive activities and is very similar to the False Claims Act. For instance, the CMPL prohibits a health care provider from presenting, or causing to be presented, claims for services that the provider "knows or should know" were:

* not provided as indicated by the coding on the claim;
* not medically necessary;
* furnished by a person who is not licensed as a physician (or who was not properly supervised by a licensed physician);
* furnished by a licensed physician who obtained his or her license through misrepresentation of a material fact (such as cheating on a licensing exam);
* furnished by a physician who was not certified in the medical specialty that he or she claimed to be certified in; or
* furnished by a physician who was excluded from participation in the Federal health care program to which the claim was submitted.

Additionally, the CMPL contains various other prohibitions, including:

* offering remuneration to a Medicare or Medicaid beneficiary that the person knows or should know is likely to influence the beneficiary to obtain items or services billed to Medicare or Medicaid from a particular provider;
* employing or contracting with an individual or entity that the person knows or should know is excluded from participation in a Federal health care program.

The term "should know" means that a provider: (1) Acted in deliberate ignorance of the truth or falsity of the information; or (2) acted in reckless disregard of the truth or falsity of the information. The Federal Government does not have to show that a provider specifically intended to defraud a Federal health care program in order to prove a provider violated the statute.

Penalty for Unlawful Conduct

Violation of the CMPL may result in a penalty of up to $10,000 per item or service and up to three times the amount unlawfully claimed. In addition, the provider may be excluded from participation in Federal health care programs. The regulations defining the aggravating and mitigating circumstances that must be reviewed by the OIG in making an exclusion determination are set forth in 42 CFR part 1001.

Examples

1. Dr. X paid Medicare and Medicaid beneficiaries $20 each time they visited him to receive services and have tests performed that were not preventive care services and tests.
2. Dr. X hired Physician Assistant P to provide services to Medicare and Medicaid beneficiaries without conducting a background check on P. Had Dr. X performed a background check by reviewing the HHS– OIG List of Excluded Individuals/Entities, Dr. X would have discovered that he should not hire P because P is excluded from participation in Federal health care programs for a period of 5 years.
3. Dr. X and his oximetry company billed Medicare for pulse oximetry that they knew they did not perform and services that had been intentionally upcoded.

III. LIMITATIONS ON CERTAIN PHYSICIAN REFERRALS ("STARK LAWS") (42 U.S.C. 1395NN)

Description of Unlawful Conduct

Physicians (and immediate family members) who have an ownership, investment or compensation relationship with an entity providing "designated health services" are prohibited from referring patients for these services where payment may be made by a Federal health care program unless a statutory or regulatory exception applies. An entity providing a designated health service is prohibited from billing for the provision of a service that was provided based on a prohibited referral. Designated health services include: clinical laboratory services; physical therapy services; occupational therapy services; radiology services, including magnetic resonance imaging, axial tomography scans, and ultrasound services; radiation therapy services and supplies; durable medical equipment and supplies; parenteral and enteral nutrients, equipment and supplies; prosthetics, orthotics, prosthetic devices and supplies; home health services; outpatient prescription drugs; and inpatient and outpatient hospital services.

New regulations clarifying the exceptions to the Stark Laws are expected to be issued by HCFA shortly. Current exceptions articulated within the Stark Laws include the following, provided all conditions of each exception as set forth in the statute and regulations are satisfied.

Exceptions for Ownership or Compensation Arrangements

* physician's services;
* in-office ancillary services; and
* prepaid plans.

Exceptions for Ownership or Investment in Publicly Traded Securities and Mutual Funds

* ownership of investment securities which may be purchased on terms generally available to the public;
* ownership of shares in a regulated investment company as defined by Federal law, if such company had, at the end of the company's most recent fiscal year, or on average, during the previous 3 fiscal years, total assets exceeding $75,000,000;
* hospital in Puerto Rico;
* rural provider; and
* hospital ownership (whole hospital exception).

Exceptions Relating to Other Compensation Arrangements

- rental of office space and rental of equipment;
- bona fide employment relationship;
- personal service arrangement;
- remuneration unrelated to the provision of designated health services;
- physician recruitment;
- isolated transactions;
- certain group practice arrangements with a hospital (pre-1989); and
- payments by a physician for items and services.

Penalty for Unlawful Conduct

Violations of the statute subject the billing entity to denial of payment for the designated health services, refund of amounts collected from improperly submitted claims, and a civil monetary penalty of up to $15,000 for each improper claim submitted. Physicians who violate the statute may also be subject to additional fines per prohibited referral. In addition, providers that enter into an arrangement that they know or should know circumvents the referral restriction law may be subject to a civil monetary penalty of up to $100,000 per arrangement.

Examples

1. Dr. A worked in a medical clinic located in a major city. She also owned a free standing laboratory located in a major city. Dr. A referred all orders for laboratory tests on her patients to the laboratory she owned.
2. Dr. X agreed to serve as the Medical Director of Home Health Agency, HHA, for which he was paid a sum substantially above the fair market value for his services. In return, Dr. X routinely referred his Medicare and Medicaid patients to HHA for home health services.
3. Dr. Y received a monthly stipend of $500 from a local hospital to assist him in meeting practice expenses. Dr. Y performed no specific service for the stipend and had no obligation to repay the hospital. Dr. Y referred patients to the hospital for in-patient surgery.

IV. EXCLUSION OF CERTAIN INDIVIDUALS AND ENTITIES FROM PARTICIPATION IN MEDICARE AND OTHER FEDERAL HEALTH CARE PROGRAMS (42 U.S.C. 1320A–7)

Mandatory Exclusion

Individuals or entities convicted of the following conduct must be excluded from participation in Medicare and Medicaid for a minimum of 5 years:

1. a criminal offense related to the delivery of an item or service under Medicare or Medicaid;
2. a conviction under Federal or State law of a criminal offense relating to the neglect or abuse of a patient;
3. a conviction under Federal or State law of a felony relating to fraud, theft, embezzlement, breach of fiduciary responsibility or other financial misconduct against a health care program financed by any Federal, State, or local government agency;

4. a conviction under Federal or State law of a felony relating to the unlawful manufacture, distribution, prescription, or dispensing of a controlled substance.

If there is one prior conviction, the exclusion will be for 10 years. If there are two prior convictions, the exclusion will be permanent.

Permissive Exclusion

Individuals or entities convicted of the following offenses, may be excluded from participation in Federal health care programs for a minimum of 3 years:

1. a criminal offense related to the delivery of an item or service under Medicare or Medicaid;
2. a misdemeanor related to fraud, theft, embezzlement, breach of fiduciary responsibility or other financial misconduct against a health care program financed by any Federal, State, or local government agency;
3. interference with, or obstruction of, any investigation into certain criminal offenses;
4. a misdemeanor related to the unlawful manufacture, distribution, prescription or dispensing of a controlled substance;
5. exclusion or suspension under a Federal or State health care program;
6. submission of claims for excessive charges, unnecessary services or services that were of a quality that fails to meet professionally recognized standards of health care;
7. violating the Civil Monetary Penalties Law or the statute entitled "Criminal Penalties for Acts Involving Federal Health Care Programs;"
8. ownership or control of an entity by a sanctioned individual or immediate family member (spouse, natural or adoptive parent, child, sibling, stepparent, stepchild, stepbrother or stepsister, in-laws, grandparent and grandchild);
9. failure to disclose information required by law;
10. failure to supply claims payment information; and
11. defaulting on health education loan or scholarship obligations.

The above list of offenses is not all inclusive. Additional grounds for permissive exclusion are detailed in the statute.

Examples

1. Nurse R was excluded based on a conviction involving obtaining dangerous drugs by forgery. She also altered prescriptions that were given for her own health problems before she presented them to the pharmacist to be filled.
2. Practice T was excluded due to its affiliation with its excluded owner. The practice owner, excluded from participation in the Federal health care programs for soliciting and receiving illegal kickbacks, was still participating in the day-to-day operations of the practice after his exclusion was effective.

APPENDIX D: OIG–HHS CONTACT INFORMATION

I. OIG HOTLINE NUMBER

One method for providers to report potential fraud, waste, and abuse problems is to contact the OIG Hotline number. All HHS and contractor employees have a responsibility to assist in combating fraud, waste and abuse in all departmental programs. As such, providers are encouraged to report matters involving fraud, waste and mismanagement in any departmental program to the OIG. The OIG maintains a hotline that offers a confidential means for reporting these matters.

Contacting the OIG Hotline

By Phone: 1–800–HHS–TIPS (1–800–447– 8477) By E-Mail: *HTips@os.dhhs.gov* By Mail: Office of Inspector General, Department of Health and Human Services, Attn: HOTLINE, 330 Independence Ave., SW., Washington, DC 20201

When contacting the Hotline, please provide the following information to the best of your ability:

- Type of Complaint:

Medicare Part A Medicare Part B Indian Health Service TRICARE Other (please specify)

- HHS Department or program being affected by your allegation of fraud, waste, abuse/mismanagement: Health Care Financing Administration (HCFA) Indian Health Service Other (please specify)

Please provide the following information. (However, if you would like your referral to be submitted anonymously, please indicate such in your correspondence or phone call.)

Your Name, Your Street Address, Your City/County, Your State, Your Zip Code, Your email Address

- Subject/Person/Business/Department that allegation is against. Name of Subject Title of Subject Subject's Street Address Subject's City/County Subject's State Subject's Zip Code

Please provide a brief summary of your allegation and the relevant facts.

II. PROVIDER SELF-DISCLOSURE PROTOCOL

The recommended method for a provider to contact the OIG regarding potential fraud or abuse issues that may exist in the provider's own organization is through the use of the Provider Self-Disclosure Protocol. This program encourages providers to voluntarily disclose irregularities in their dealings with Federal health care programs. While voluntary disclosure under the protocol does not guarantee a provider protection from civil, criminal, or administrative actions, the fact that a provider voluntarily disclosed possible wrongdoing is a mitigating factor in OIG's recommendations to prosecuting agencies. Although other agencies may not have formal policies offering immunity or mitigation for self-disclosure, they typically view self-disclosure favorably for the self-disclosing entity. Self-reporting offers providers the opportunity to minimize the potential cost and disruption of a full-scale audit and investigation, to negotiate a fair monetary settlement, and to avoid an OIG permissive exclusion preventing the provider from doing business with Federal health care programs. In addition, if the provider is obligated to enter into an Integrity Agreement (IA) as part of the resolution of a voluntary disclosure, there are three benefits the provider might receive as a result of self-reporting:

- If the provider has an effective compliance program and agrees to maintain its compliance program as part of the False Claims Act settlement, the OIG may not even require an IA;
- In cases where the provider's own audits detected the disclosed problem, the OIG may consider alternatives to the IA's auditing provisions. The provider may be able to perform some or all of its billing audits through internal auditing methods rather than be required to retain an independent review organization to perform the billing review; and
- Self-disclosing can help to demonstrate a provider's trustworthiness to the OIG and may result in the OIG determining that it can sufficiently safeguard the Federal health care programs through an IA without the exclusion remedy for a material breach, which is typically included in an IA.

Specific instructions on how a physician practice can submit a voluntary disclosure under the Provider Self-Disclosure Protocol can be found on the OIG's Internet site at www.hhs. gov/oig or in the **Federal Register** at 63 FR 58399 (1998). A physician practice may, however, wish to consult with an attorney prior to submitting a disclosure to the OIG.

The Provider Self-Disclosure Protocol can also be a useful tool for baseline audits. The protocol details the OIG's views on the appropriate elements of an effective investigative and audit plan for providers. Physician practices can use the self-disclosure protocol as a model for conducting audits and self-assessments.

In relying on the protocol for audit design and sample selection, a physician practice should pay close attention to the sections on self-assessment and sample selection. These two sections provide valuable guidance regarding how these two functions should be performed.

The self-assessment section of the protocol contains information that can be applied to audit design. Self-assessment is an internal financial assessment to determine the monetary impact of the matter. The approach of a review can include reviewing either all claims affected or a statistically valid sample of the claims.

Sample selection must include several elements. These elements are drawn from the Government sampling program known as RAT–STATS. All of these elements are set forth in more detail in the Provider Self-Disclosure Protocol, but the elements are (1) Sampling unit, (2) sampling frame, (3) probe, (4) sample size, (5) random numbers, (6) sample design and (7) missing sample items. All of these sampling items should be clearly documented by the physician practice and compiled in the format set forth in the Provider Self-Disclosure Protocol. Use of the format set forth in the Provider Self-Disclosure Protocol will help physician practices to ensure that the elements of their internal audits are in conformance with OIG standards.

TOOLKIT FOR ASSESSING HEALTH-SYSTEM CAPACITY FOR CRISIS MANAGEMENT

INTRODUCTION

Disasters and crises are highly unpredictable. They can hit communities at any time, causing substantial human suffering and loss of life. If national and local systems, particularly health systems, are ill prepared to deal with a crisis, the vulnerability of both individuals and communities becomes even more pronounced. The sudden increase in demand for essential health services brought on by a crisis often overwhelms health systems and their institutions, rendering them unable to provide the necessary life-saving interventions.

Preparing a health system for crises is no trivial task. Strengthening stewardship, implementing preparedness planning as a continuous process with a multihazard approach and establishing sustainable crisis-management and health-related risk-reduction programs require a clear understanding of the situation of a country. Unfortunately, until now, no standard formal methodology for assessing the preparedness of a health system for crises has been established.

In 2008, with the support of the Directorate-General for Health and Consumers (DG SANCO), WHO launched the project, "Support to health security, preparedness planning and crises management in European Union (EU), EU accession and neighboring (ENP) countries," with the aim of improving preparedness for public health emergencies in EU Member States and selected EU accession and ENP countries in the WHO European Region. One of the goals was to refine the assessment tool for health-sector crisis-preparedness developed on the basis of experience gained through the joint European Community (EC)–WHO project, "Support to health security and preparedness planning in EU neighboring (ENP) countries (2007–2008)," within which assessments on crises planning and management were carried out in Armenia, Azerbaijan and the Republic of Moldova. Further experience gained during a second round of assessments conducted in Kazakhstan, Kyrgyzstan, Poland, Turkey and Ukraine enabled finalization of the assessment tool. The WHO health-system framework *(1)* was the conceptual basis used for describing and analyzing health systems during all country assessments. The following documents provided inspiration for the structure and development of the toolkit:

> *Hospital safety index. Guide for evaluators (2), Health-sector self-assessment tool for disaster risk reduction (3)* and *Protocol for assessing national surveillance and response capacities for the International Health Regulations (2005) (4).*

It is our firm belief that by accurately anticipating the health needs of the population and effectively preparing for those needs, health systems can respond promptly in the event of a crisis, thus saving lives and alleviating suffering. In developing this toolkit, it has been our intention to provide ministries of health, and other relevant authorities, with a guide for use in evaluating the capacity of health systems for crisis management and in addressing any identified gaps.

BACKGROUND

Health crises are often unpredictable, occurring at any place or time. They can cause significant human suffering and loss of life and can have serious economic repercussions. Communities are particularly vulnerable when national and local systems, particularly health systems, are unable to cope with the consequences of a crisis, often because a sudden increase in demand overwhelms the institutions involved.

In this document, the terms *health emergencies* and *health crises* refer to the health threats associated with new or newly emerging diseases, the accidental release or deliberate use of biological, chemical or radionuclear agents, natural disasters, human-made disasters, complex emergencies, conflicts and other events with a potentially catastrophic impact on human health, including the potential implications of climate change.

In a changing global environment, preparing for and preventing a health crisis is becoming more complex. The increasing number of weather-related events (floods, storms, extreme temperatures, etc.) and the increasing threat of a human influenza pandemic have highlighted the need for worldwide cooperation in strengthening public health defenses to respond to emerging international health problems. The spate of declarations and agreements made by the global community in recent years underlines the need for all countries to be prepared to meet these and other emerging threats to public health (Table 1 ■).

Within the framework of its medium-term strategic plan for 2008–2013, WHO is committed to collaborating with Member States to strengthen their capacity and overall preparedness for health crises and ensure the interoperability and coherence of their health-system crisis-management plans. To this end, WHO recommends establishing comprehensive programs based on an all-hazards approach. The all-hazards concept acknowledges that, while hazards vary in source (natural, technological, societal), they often challenge health systems in similar ways. Thus, usually, the model used as a basis for action to reduce risk and to prepare for and respond to emergencies,

TABLE 1 **Declarations and Agreements Relating to Strengthening Health-System Capacity for Disaster Preparedness**

Declarations/Agreements	Notes
WHO eleventh general program of work (2006–2015)	Identifies the need to strengthen health systems as a key priority.
World Health Assembly resolutions WHA58.1 (2005) and WHA59.22 (2006) *(5, 6)*	These resolutions reinforce the WHO mandate to support Member States in preparing their health systems for crises and to strengthen its own institutional readiness.
The Millennium Development Goals (MDG)	MDG are directly and/or indirectly health-related; their achievement is crucial to strengthening health systems.
The Hyogo Framework (2005–2015) *(7)*	Adopted by 168 countries, the Hyogo Framework is a comprehensive action-oriented response to the growing impact of disasters on individuals, communities and national development. It stresses five priorities for action, one of which is to strengthen disaster preparedness at all levels.
EC communication on strengthening coordination on generic preparedness planning for public health emergencies at EU level and EU technical guidance on generic preparedness planning (2005) *(8, 9)*	The action recommended in these documents is being implemented at the political and technical levels in WHO European Member States with the support of the European Center for Disease Prevention and Control (ECDC), which provides scientific advice, technical assistance and training.
World Health Assembly resolution WHA58.5 (2005) *(10)* acknowledging the serious threat to human health represented by outbreaks of avian influenza and associated human cases.	Stresses the need for all countries to collaborate with WHO and each other to reduce the risk of a human pandemic of avian influenza A (H5N1).
International Health Regulations (IHR) (2005) *(11)*	Approved by WHO Member States during the 58th session of the World Health Assembly in June 2007, IHR (2005) came into force as international law. The Regulations specifically target the need to respond to "public health emergencies of international concern," calling for the strengthening of health systems by improving national core capacity and mobilizing collective global action to deal with public health crises of international concern.

regardless of cause, is the same. Experience shows that, to a large degree, the various elements of essential response action are generic (health information in crises, an emergency operations center, coordination activities, logistics, public communications, etc.) irrespective of the hazard, and that prioritizing them generates synergies that benefit action.

WHO advocates for cross-border cooperation aimed at developing mutual assistance agreements between countries and improving health-related crisis preparedness and management. The capability of each country to respond will thus be strengthened and international ties improved. IHR (2005) *(11)* requires States Parties to "prevent, protect against, control and provide a public health response to the international spread of disease so as to avoid unnecessary interference with international traffic and trade," emphasizing the importance of international collaboration.

PURPOSE OF THE TOOLKIT

The overall goal of the toolkit is to help countries minimize the impact of future health crises by assessing the capacity of their health systems to respond to various threats and identify gaps.

The toolkit does not enter into technical detail, nor is it intended to replace the preexisting planning process. It is an instrument, which breaks down the complex crisis-preparedness process into manageable units and functions as an aide-memoire, thus enabling a ministry of health to:

- record and classify information regarding its capacity to manage crises;
- establish responsibility for specific tasks;
- determine the relationship between those involved in these tasks (partners, sectors, disciplines) with the aim of synergizing resources;
- identify shortcomings and gaps; and
- monitor progress.

The toolkit can be used to stimulate communication and coordination at all stages of preparing for and managing a health crisis. Although ministries of health should take the lead in strengthening their national health systems, there is much to be gained from multisectoral collaboration with national and international agencies to ensure the mobilization of all resources available in the case of a threat. Health-sector crisis preparedness is a process that needs to be updated continuously in the light of changes in the health system and the identification of new threats and gaps. Involving the stakeholders and sharing information with them enhances this process.

In carrying out assessments of health-system preparedness, it may be necessary to adapt the toolkit to accommodate national specifics. Assessments can be supported by WHO at the request of the country.

STRUCTURE OF THE TOOLKIT

The toolkit comprises the user manual (Part 1) and the assessment form (Part 2).

User manual

In addition to information on the general background and objectives of the assessment, the user manual includes:

- a glossary of the main technical terms used in the document;
- the procedures for and recommendations on using the toolkit, including instructions on how to complete the assessment form and suggestions on the selection of assessment sites;
- recommendations on follow-up of the assessment and development of a plan of action;
- information about the essential attributes and indicator-related questions contained in the assessment form;
- a list of possible sources of the information required for assessment of the essential attributes; and
- recommendations on relevant additional reading.

Assessment form

The assessment form is sectioned according to the six functions (building blocks) of the WHO health-system framework (Table 2 ■).

TABLE 2   The WHO Health-System Framework

Functions	Overall Goals/Outcomes
Leadership and governance	Improved health (level and equity)
Health workforce	Responsiveness
Medical products, vaccines and technology	Social and financial risk protection
	Improved efficiency
Health information	
Health financing	
Service delivery	

WHO defines **health systems** as comprising all the resources, organizations, and institutions that are devoted to producing interdependent actions aimed principally at improving, maintaining or restoring health. Further information on health systems can be found in the following documents: *The world health report 2000 (12)*, *Everybody's business: Strengthening health systems to improve health outcomes (1)* and the report of the European Ministerial Conference on Health Systems, which includes *The Tallinn Charter: Health systems for health and wealth (13)*.

Leadership and governance (also called stewardship) is arguably the most complex function of any health system; it is also the most critical *(12)*. Successful leadership and governance require strategic policy frameworks that are combined with oversight, coalition-building, accountability and appropriate regulations and incentives *(14)*. In relation to crisis management, this means ensuring that national policies provide for a health-sector crisis-management program. Effective coordination structures, partnerships and advocacy are also needed, as well as relevant, up-to-date information for decision making, public-information strategies and monitoring and evaluation.

Health workforce (human resources for health) includes all health workers engaged in action to protect and improve the health of a population. "A well-performing health workforce is one, which works in ways that are responsive, fair and efficient, to achieve the best health outcomes possible, given available resources and circumstances" *(14)*. This necessitates the fair distribution of a sufficient number and mix of competent, responsive and productive staff. A preparedness program aims to ensure that such staff represents an integral part of the health workforce by conducting training-needs assessments, developing curricula and training material and organizing training courses.

A well-functioning health system ensures equitable access to essential **medical products, vaccines and technologies** of assured quality, safety, efficacy and cost–effectiveness, and their scientifically sound and cost-effective use *(14)*. Medical equipment and supplies for prehospital activities, hospitals, temporary health facilities, public health pharmaceutical services, laboratory services and reserve blood services needed in case of a crisis also fall under "medical products, vaccines and technologies".

A well-functioning **health information system** is one that ensures the production, analysis, dissemination and use of reliable and timely information on health determinants, health-system performance and health status *(14)*. A health information system also covers the collection, analysis and reporting of data. This includes data gathered through risk and needs assessments (hazard, vulnerability and capacity) and those relating to early-warning systems and the overall management of information.

A good **health-financing system** ensures the availability of adequate funds for the health system, and its financial protection in case of a crisis. In addition to providing funds for essential health-sector crisis-management programs, it ensures that crisis victims have access to essential services and that health facilities and equipment are adequately insured for damage or loss.

Service delivery is the process of delivering safe and effective health interventions of high quality, both equitably and with a minimum waste of resources, to individuals or communities in need of them. The crisis-preparedness process provided by the WHO health-system framework *(4)* makes it possible to review the organization and management of services, ensure the resilience of health care facilities and safeguard the quality, safety and continuity of care across health facilities during a crisis.

The six sections of the assessment form (structured according to the functions of the WHO health-system framework *(4)*) are broken down into the "key components" of a health-sector crisis-preparedness program (Table 3 ■).

Certain attributes are considered essential for the successful implementation of each key component. There are 51 essential attributes; they are listed according to the key components of each of the six WHO health-system framework functions blocks.

The assessment is facilitated by questions relating to each of the essential attributes. Assessors are required to answer each indicator-related question by choosing "yes," "partially,"

or "no," and to justify the answer given. This information forms the basis of a detailed narrative assessment report, which can be used to develop a plan of action to address gaps identified and monitor progress during follow-up assessments. Table 4 ■ exemplifies the structure of the assessment form.

PROCEDURES FOR AND RECOMMENDATIONS ON USING THE TOOLKIT

General coordination and pre-assessment activities

The assessment process is initiated by a coordination group comprising professionals from the decision-making level of the ministry of health and other relevant institutions responsible for health-sector crisis management. It is the responsibility of

---

TABLE 3   Key Components of the WHO Health-System Framework, by Function

Functions	Key Components
Leadership and governance	Legal framework for national multisectoral emergency management Legal framework for health-sector emergency management National multisectoral institutional framework for multisectoral emergency management Institutional framework for health-sector emergency management Health-sector emergency-management program components
Health workforce	Human resources for health-sector emergency management
Medical products, vaccines and technology	Medical supplies and equipment for emergency-response operations
Heath information	Information-management systems for risk-reduction and emergency-preparedness programs Information-management systems for emergency response and recovery Risk communication
Health financing	National and subnational strategies for financing health-sector emergency management
Service delivery	Response capacity and capability Emergency-medical-services (EMS) system and mass-casualty management Management of hospitals in mass-casualty incidents Continuity of essential health programs and services Logistics and operational support functions in emergencies

---

TABLE 4   Structure of the Assessment Form

Function	Leadership and Governance			
Key component	**1.1.** Legal framework for national multisectoral emergency management			
Essential attribute	**1.** Laws, policies, plans and procedures relevant to national multisectoral emergency management			

	Answer (enter X where applicable)			
Indicator-related questions	Yes	Partly	No	Justification
(a) Does the legislation follow an all-hazard approach?	○	○	○	
(b) Does the legislation consider all phases of emergency management?	○	○	○	
(c) Is the legislation reviewed and revised regularly?	○	○	○	
(d) Are procedures for declaring and terminating a state of emergency at both the national and subnational levels defined in the legislation?	○	○	○	

the coordination group to set up the assessment team, select the assessment sites and ensure the preparation of a report on the findings and recommendations of the team. On the basis of this report, the coordination group is responsible for and/or supervises the development of a national plan of action to address identified gaps in the crisis-management program of the health sector. If such a program does not yet exist, the plan of action should define steps to be taken to establish one. With a view to obtaining the necessary governmental support to implement the plan of action, it is of the utmost importance that the senior decision makers appointed as members of the coordination group by the ministry of health participate in all steps of the assessment.

Activities leading to the assessment include the establishment of an assessment team, the selection of assessment sites and the compilation of relevant background information, such as country risk profiles, policy and legislation documents, and organigrams of existing crisis-management structures.

If requested by the country, the WHO Country Office and/ or the WHO Regional Office can provide technical support for the preparation and conduct of the assessment, including introductory training on its methodology.

Composition of the assessment team

TEAM LEADER
The team leader should be a representative of the ministry of health, responsible for health-sector crisis preparedness and management. The team leader is responsible for organizing and implementing the mission (including field visits), following up on the assessment and ensuring that all team members are briefed on the objectives of the assessment and on how it is to be conducted.

TEAM MEMBERS
Members of the assessment team should be drawn from the various disciplines involved in health-system crisis preparedness and management (Table 5 ■). As it might not be possible to gather experts in all of the below-mentioned areas, professionals with less experience, or advanced-level students in these areas, may be selected to collect the data. These individuals should be closely supervised and should consult experts at

all times regarding the interpretation of their findings. Team members' evaluations should be limited to their own areas of expertise.

Selection of sites for assessment

Assessments should be carried out through field visits at the national and subnational[1] levels. The coordination group, in collaboration with the assessment team leader, select the sites to be assessed. Annex 2 lists potential sources of information required for the assessment of the essential attributes and can be used in connection with the selection of the assessment sites.

At the national level, field visits should be arranged with the relevant stakeholders of health-sector crisis management. Though the focus of the assessment is on the health sector, interviews should be held with representatives of relevant stakeholders in other sectors (including private institutions), as well as nongovernmental organizations (NGOs) and international organizations. A schedule for the assessment should be set up in table format and should include details relating to each field visit and interview (site to be assessed, names of assessors, timing, etc.).

A general sampling strategy is followed (which entails collecting information from health facilities, laboratories, blood banks, public health institutes, etc.) at the national and subnational (provincial and municipal) levels. Precision sampling requiring evaluation across all functions of the health system throughout the country is not required. Rather than conducting a scientific study, the aim is to identify the strengths and weaknesses of health-system management capacity and develop a plan of action to address identified gaps. In addition, financial and time constraints may not permit precision sampling.

At the subnational level, health-sector crisis-management systems can be categorized as: (i) particularly well-functioning; (ii) functioning at an average level; and (iii) poorly functioning. It is important that each of these categories be represented in the sample, as well as areas at particular risk, such as those prone to specific natural hazards and vulnerable communities.

---

[1]The subnational level is defined in this document as any administrative level below the national level, such as the provincial or municipal levels.

TABLE 5   Assessment-Team Expertise, by Health-System Function

Health-System Function	Required Expertise of Assessment-Team Members
Leadership and governance	Policy-makers at national level
Health workforce	Health-sector professionals with knowledge of human resources' management
Medical products, vaccines and technologies	Health professionals involved in management of medical equipment, medical supplies, pharmaceuticals and laboratory services
Health information	Experts in surveillance, risk assessment and mapping
	Professionals responsible for IHR implementation
	Professionals with knowledge of information management and communication in crises
Health financing	An economist or other professional with knowledge of health financing
Service delivery	Health professionals with expertise in crisis management at the subnational level, experience in emergency medical services and hospital management in mass-casualty situations, and/or knowledge of logistics

ASSESSMENT ACTIVITIES
Site visits

The main purpose of the site visits is to determine the capacity of the health system for crisis management by gathering relevant information using the assessment form in Part 2 of the toolkit.

In order for the visit to be successful, thorough planning is critical. To this end, the ministry of health, the coordination group and the leader of the assessment team should agree on the timetable prior to the arrival of the assessment team. The essential attributes to be assessed at each site should be identified in advance. On-site evaluation will involve asking questions, observing practices and gathering documentation concerning site activities.

The approach at each site should be to:

* hold an initial meeting between the main stakeholders at the site and the assessment team to explain the objectives of the assessment and clarify related questions;
* visit the health facility (or facilities), if applicable;
* obtain informal feedback on pre-identified problems and issues regarding health-sector crisis management;
* complete the assessment form in relation to the site.

During site visits, a high level of ethical behavior is expected from the team members. In visiting facilities, they should not interfere with the daily work.

The assessment team should meet to document findings, discuss challenges, strengths and weaknesses that are encountered at the sites visited, and formulate possible recommendations. A field assessment communication checklist has been compiled to this end. The preliminary results of the assessment should be treated as confidential and must not be discussed with outside parties.

Completion of the assessment form

Before using the assessment form during a site visit, it is of the utmost importance that the assessors familiarize themselves with the essential attributes related to that site and their underlying principles. (See also the chapter entitled, "Guidance for the assessment process," below).

(a) *Essential attributes and indicator-related questions*
The absence or presence of the essential attributes is evaluated through a set of indicator-related questions related to each attribute (see also Table 4 above). Taking the local context into account, the assessor needs to decide whether the answer to the question is "yes," "partially," or "no," using the appropriate color code (see *(b)* below).

(b) *Color coding*
The color-code matrix illustrated in Annex 5 enables visualization of the evaluation results whereby green means "yes," red means "no," and yellow means "partially."

(c) *Justification for answers to indicator-related questions*
To enable optimal compilation of the assessment report, it is important to elaborate on the answers given. This is done in the space allocated for this purpose alongside each indicator-related question. If more room is required, a separate log may be used.

(d) *Summary of findings*
When all the indicator-related questions relating to the essential attribute(s) of a key component have been answered, the assessor is required to summarize the findings on that key component.

(e) *Recommendations for priority action*
When the assessment of all the key components of a health-system function has been completed, the assessors make their recommendations for priority action in the dedicated box at the end of the section on that particular health-system function.

Finalization of the assessment and development of plan of action

On completion of the assessment, the team meets to discuss its findings and formulate preliminary recommendations of priority action to address identified gaps. These are then discussed with the main stakeholders involved in the assessment process and health-sector crisis management. Thereafter, the team triangulates the findings and agrees on the final recommendations, on the basis of which it develops the first draft of a plan of action. A template for structuring the plan is included in the assessment form.

Writing the assessment report

This is a team activity. The main content of the report is based on the summaries of findings relating to the individual key components and the recommendations for priority action with respect to each health-system function. The outline of an assessment report can be found in Annex 7. The report may include a draft plan of action.

PLANNING FOR THE FUTURE
Plan of action

One of the main objectives of the assessment is to identify gaps in the overall capacity for health management during crises with the aim of developing a plan of action to address these gaps and strengthen capacity. Existing national structures, resources for the implementation of action, existing emergency-preparedness and/or emergency-response plans and the importance of linking with other sectors involved in crisis management should be taken into account when developing the plan. It should encompass the whole of the health sector and aim at building the capacity required to anticipate and prevent health crises and to prepare for, respond to, recover from and mitigate their effects. The outline of a plan of action is annexed to the assessment form (Part 2 of the toolkit).

The plan of action should be developed by the coordination group, based on a draft prepared by the assessment team. It is important that all the relevant senior decision makers and stakeholders are consulted during the process of developing the action plan. Eventually, the action plan should be formally endorsed.

Follow-up assessments

To monitor the implementation of the action plan and measure changes over time, follow-up assessments should be conducted periodically (e.g., every two years). Consideration might also be given to carrying out additional follow-up assessments that are limited to those health-system functions where major gaps have been identified. However, such partial assessments should not replace the periodic follow-up assessments since the different components of health-sector crisis management are normally closely intertwined.

GUIDANCE FOR THE ASSESSMENT PROCESS

The next six sections represent the six functions (building blocks) of the WHO health-system framework *(4)*. Each is sectioned according to the key components of each function and the 51 attributes considered essential for the achievement of the key components. To facilitate assessment, a list of indicator-related questions has been compiled for each of the essential attributes.

Regarding the essential attributes, possible sources of the information are listed in Annex 2; for some, keynotes have been added.

Most of the indicator-related questions are followed by explanatory text. In some cases, the explanations follow two or more closely related questions. If a question is considered self-evident, no explanation is included.

Recommended reading is listed for each of the essential attributes.

◗ SECTION 1. LEADERSHIP AND GOVERNANCE

Leadership and governance pertain to the careful and responsible management of the health system, which reflects the policies and action of all sectors involved in population health. Good governance is reflected, for example, in the existence of relevant policy, the allocation of the necessary resources to implement it, the enforcement of its implementation, the assignment of accountability and the involvement of civil society.

> **Key component 1.1** Legal framework for national multisectoral emergency management
>
> **Essential attribute 1** Laws, policies, plans and procedures relevant to national multisectoral emergency management

KEYNOTES

Recent experience related to crises, such as the H1N1 pandemic, has demonstrated that the legal aspects of emergency management are critical to the comprehensiveness of preparedness for public health emergencies. It is, therefore, important that the assessment include a review of the legal framework for managing emergencies at both the national and subnational levels.

A legal framework for multisectoral emergency management encompasses all the laws, policies, guidelines, plans and/or process descriptions related to this area. It should define emergency-management structures, the roles, responsibilities and authority of those involved and the rights and responsibilities of citizens and non-citizens. It should also define the procedures for and standards of program implementation, including, for example, those relevant to data availability, compatibility and sharing, and the interoperability of the information system. The framework should also provide for the resources required to ensure the functioning of the structure. A regulatory framework for public health includes the laws, polices, administrative rules and regulations, executive orders, memoranda of understanding and mutual-aid agreements pertinent to public health.

Assessors need to determine the hierarchy of the legal documents. The provisions of high-ranking documents, such as the constitution and parliamentary laws, may override the contradictory provisions of executive regulations of a more inferior standing.

National policy on emergency management should be supported by legislation, which guides all aspects of this area, using an all-hazards approach based on the recognition that, regardless of the type of emergency, all responses have common elements of management.

INDICATOR-RELATED QUESTIONS

a.   *Does the legislation follow an all-hazards approach?*

b.   *Does the legislation consider all phases of emergency management?*

c.   *Is the legislation reviewed and revised regularly?*
     The legislation should seek to institutionalize an all-hazards, whole-health approach and should require that all phases of emergency management be given due consideration. These phases include anticipation, prevention, risk reduction, mitigation, preparedness, response and recovery, and post-event evaluation and revision. The legislation should establish the minimum standards required for emergency-management programs at the national and subnational levels.

     Assessors should bear in mind that certain information, especially at the national level, is considered confidential in some countries (for example, the location and content of stockpiles) and may not be accessible to them.

d.   *Are procedures for declaring and terminating a state of emergency at both the national and subnational levels defined in the legislation?*
     The legislation should clearly define how and by whom a state of emergency is declared and terminated, the criteria for doing so, as well as the process for informing the authorities and the public of the situation. It should also clarify the precise roles, rights and obligations of authorities, organizations and individuals during a state of emergency, and distinguish between local, regional and national states of emergency.

e.   *Does the legislation recognize, and is it consistent with, legally binding international agreements and conventions to which the country is a party and/or which it has ratified (in particular, IHR 2005 (11) and the Hyogo Framework for Action, 2005–2015) (7)?*

Assessors should review the national legislation in the context of international treaties and conventions to which the country is a party and highlight possible contradictions.

f. *Does a formal arrangement exist for the protection and identification of infrastructures and personnel?*
    The legal framework should incorporate the protection and identification of infrastructures and personnel. According to the *Protocol additional to the Geneva Conventions of 12 August 1949, and relating to the protection of victims of international armed conflicts (Protocol I), 8 June 1977 (15)*, measures for identifying persons are closely connected with the concept of protection, which constitutes the very basis of international humanitarian law. These measures provide the individuals concerned with a means of proving their status and claiming their rightful protection, particularly in conflict situations (including internal conflicts).

RECOMMENDED READING

European Commission. *Technical guidance on generic preparedness planning—interim document—April 2005.* Brussels, European Commission, 2005 (http://ec.europa.eu /health/ph_threats/Bioterrorisme/keydo_bio_01_en.pdf, accessed 7 April 2011).

Guidelines for assessing disaster preparedness in the health sector. Washington, DC, Pan American Health Organization, 1995 (http://helid.digicollection.org/en/d/J060/, accessed 7 April 2011).

Jackson BA et al. *Protecting emergency responders. Volume 3. Safety management in disaster and terrorism response.* Atlanta, The National Institute for Occupational Safety and Health, 2004 (http://www.rand.org/content/dam/rand/pubs /monographs/2004/RAND_MG170.pdf, accessed 7 April 2011).

Koob, P. *Health sector emergency preparedness guide.* Geneva, World Health Organization, 1998 (http://www .who.int/disasters/repo/5814.doc, accessed 7 April 2011).

Marshall, LW. International Disaster Response Law: An Introduction. *American Journal of Disaster Medicine.* 2008 May–June, 3(3):181–4.

Protocol additional to the Geneva Conventions of 12 August 1949, and relating to the protection of victims of non-international armed conflicts (Protocol II), 8 June 1977. Geneva, International Committee of the Red Cross, 1977 (http://www.icrc.org/ihl.nsf/INTRO/475?OpenDocument, accessed 5 August 2011).

Protocol additional to the Geneva Conventions of 12 August 1949, and relating to the Adoption of an Additional Distinctive Emblem (Protocol III), 8 December 2005. Geneva, International Committee of the Red Cross, 1977 (http:// www.icrc.org/ihl.nsf/INTRO/615?OpenDocument, accessed 5 August 2011).

Essential attribute 2 National structure for multisectoral emergency management and coordination

KEYNOTES

The assessment should reveal the scope of authority (including delegated authority) of the partners within the national structure for multisectoral emergency management and coordination, as well as the level of interaction within the structure. The assessor may consider developing an organigram of the structure with special emphasis on the health sector.

INDICATOR-RELATED QUESTIONS

a. *Does the national structure for emergency management and coordination consist of a high-level multisectoral committee?*

b. *Is it supported by an operational entity and relevant subcommittees on specific technical issues?*

c. *Are the roles and responsibilities of the various partners clearly defined?*

d. *Is health on board of this committee and have resources been allocated for health-sector disaster risk reduction, emergency preparedness and response?*
    The legislation should ensure the existence of: (i) a high-level multisectoral committee to steer and coordinate emergency procedures; (ii) an operational crisis-management entity responsible for implementing action related to emergencies and reporting to the high-level multisectoral committee; and (iii) sufficient resources to implement action, based on risk assessments.

    Depending on the social context, the focus of the national policy and strategy in this area must be clearly directed at enabling the coordinating entities at all administrative levels to prepare for, respond to and facilitate recovery from an emergency. In reviewing the legal documents, the assessors should specifically evaluate the role and responsibilities of the ministry of health in relation to health emergencies.

    The legal framework should specify the roles of partners, such as governmental departments, defense forces, public and private agencies and institutions, civil-society organizations and international partners, and their interaction in the emergency-management process, particularly during the response phase.

    Provisions for the registration of foreign and domestic humanitarian agencies, the establishment of humanitarian operations and logistics mechanisms (including the importation, storage and distribution of humanitarian aid), and the sharing of information and resources, should also be considered.

RECOMMENDED READING

Baker D, Refsgaard K. Institutional development and scale matching in disaster response management. *Ecological Economics*, 2007, 63:331–343.

Koob P. *Health sector emergency preparedness guide.* Geneva, World Health Organization, 1998 (http://www.who.int /disasters/repo/5814.doc, accessed 9 April 2011).

Key component 1.2 Legal framework for health-sector emergency management

Essential attribute 3 Laws, policies, plans, and procedures relevant to health-sector emergency management

KEYNOTE

The legal framework for the health sector establishes the structure, procedures and dedicated resources for emergency management and defines the roles, responsibilities and authority of those involved in managing the health aspects of a crisis.

INDICATOR-RELATED QUESTIONS

a. *Does the legislation follow a whole-health, all-hazards approach to emergency management?*

b. *Does it cover all phases of emergency management?*

c. *Is it reviewed and revised regularly?*

d. *Does it define the conditions and procedures for quarantine and isolation relevant to emergencies?*
   The legislation pertaining to health-sector emergency management should provide for a whole-health, all-hazards approach and cover all phases of emergency management, including the following: prevention (including risk assessment); risk reduction; mitigation; preparedness; response and recovery; regular evaluation; and updating. The whole-health approach recommends that emergency-preparedness planning include—in addition to the cross-cutting topics of coordination and information and support services—the following areas: environment and health (including water safety, sanitation and hygiene); chronic diseases (including mental health); maternal, newborn and child health; communicable diseases; nutrition; pharmaceutical and biological products; and health care delivery (including health infrastructure). Specialized services may be included for the management of specific risks and, at the planning stage, investigations should be made into capacity available in health institutions, government institutions, the private sector, the military medical services, the national Red Cross and Red Crescent Societies and NGOs.
   The legislation should require that all government material, especially at the national level, be considered confidential (for example, the location and content of stockpiles) and, therefore, inaccessible to assessors.
   In relation to work carried out within the emergency-preparedness program, relevant legislation should require participating agencies to develop expertise in and capacity for risk assessment, risk reduction, coordination and partnerships, public information and risk communication, institutional capacity-building and monitoring and evaluation. It should also define the conditions and requirements for and the authority of health workers with regard to the decontamination, isolation or quarantine of individuals,

groups, areas, buildings, vehicles, etc., and the tracing and protection of exposed contacts.
   The legislation should establish the minimum standards required for health-related emergency-management programs at the national and subnational levels. It should support the requirement that such programs be based on risk assessments and include a regulation on the protection and identification of personnel and infrastructures. It is possible that the latter is included in a national document relating to one of the other key components.
   In reviewing the national and, if relevant, subnational legal bases for managing health emergencies, assessors should verify that the authority and responsibilities of the health sector are defined at both levels.

RECOMMENDED READING

International Health Regulations (2005). Geneva, World Health Organization, 2008 (http://www.who.int/entity/csr /ihr/IHR_2005_en.pdf, accessed 7 April 2011).

Hyogo Framework for Action 2005–2015. Geneva, United Nations International Strategy for Disaster Reduction, 2005 (http://www.unisdr.org/wcdr/intergover/official-doc/L-docs /Hyogo-framework-for-action-english.pdf, accessed 7 April 2011).

Technical guidance on generic preparedness planning— interim document—April 2005. Brussels, European Union, 2005 (http://ec.europa.eu/health/ph_threats/Bioterrorisme /keydo_bio_01_en.pdf, accessed 7 April 2011).

Strengthening health systems' response to crises. Towards a new focus on disaster preparedness. Report on a WHO workshop, Skopje, The former Yugoslav Republic of Macedonia, 13–15 July 2004. Copenhagen, WHO Regional Office for Europe, 2006 (http://www.euro.who.int/__data/assets /pdf_file/0004/79006/E87920.pdf, accessed 7 April 2011).

Stier DD, Goodman RA. Mutual aid agreements: essential legal tools for public health preparedness and response. *American Journal of Public Health,* 2007, 97(Supplement 1): 62–68 (http://www.ncbi.nlm.nih.gov/pmc/articles /PMC1854975/pdf/0970062.pdf, accessed 7 April 2011).

Essential attribute 4 Structure for health-sector emergency management and coordination

KEYNOTES

The legislation should describe the structure for health-sector emergency management and how the coordination of medical activities and training programs, and the prioritization of needs identified through vulnerability and needs assessments, are incorporated.

INDICATOR-RELATED QUESTIONS

a. *Does the structure for health-sector emergency management consist of a high-level multidisciplinary committee?*

b. *Is it linked at all levels to similar structures in other sectors?*

c. *Is it supported by an operational entity and relevant subcommittees on specific technical issues?*

d. *Does it specify the roles and responsibilities of key health-sector stakeholders?*

e. *Does it promote mechanisms to ensure the allocation of resources for disaster risk reduction, emergency preparedness and response?*
Legislation should exist mandating the establishment—at both the national and subnational levels—of a dedicated high-level, multidisciplinary health-sector committee, which may be supported by an operational entity. Furthermore, it should define the roles, responsibilities and authority of key stakeholders in the health sector and provide the legal basis for the allocation of sufficient resources for action related to risk reduction, emergency preparedness and response, based on risk and needs assessments. (Regarding resources, see also essential attributes 15, 30, 31, 32, 33, 36, and 38).

Assessors should review the legal documents to clarify whether the ministry of health has the lead role in health emergencies or whether, depending on the social context, this function has been delegated to one or more health-sector organizations.

There should also be legislation specifying the roles of health partners, such as government departments, defense forces, public and private agencies and institutions, civil-society organizations, and international partners. This should include provisions for the registration of humanitarian agencies, the establishment of humanitarian operations and logistics mechanisms (including the importation, storage and distribution of humanitarian aid) and the standardization and sharing of data, information and resources (see also essential attribute 2).

RECOMMENDED READING

Johns Hopkins School of Hygiene and Public Health, International Federation of the Red Cross and Red Crescent Societies. *Public health guide for emergencies. First edition.* Geneva, IFRC, 2004 (http://pdf.usaid.gov/pdf_docs /PNACU086.pdf, accessed 16 July 2011).

Baker D, Refsgaard K. Institutional development and scale matching in disaster response management. *Ecological Economics*, 2007, 63(2–3):331–343.

Essential attribute 5 Regulation of external health-related emergency assistance

INDICATOR-RELATED QUESTIONS

a. *Are there any regulations relating to the entry of foreign health workers to provide emergency relief services?*
Assessors should review the regulations on international relief activities to determine whether they include provisions relating to foreign medical teams, disaster victim identification teams, and so on, and the importation of medicines, other medical supplies, field hospitals, and medical equipment.

b. *Are medical relief items exempt from import tax?*

c. *Are there any regulations relating to donations of health and medical items?*

RECOMMENDED READING

Guidelines for drug donations. Geneva, World Health Organization, 1999 (http://whqlibdoc.who.int/hq/1999/WHO_ EDM_PAR_99.4.pdf, accessed 7 April 2011).

Pan American Health Organization, WHO Regional Office for the Western Pacific. *Guidelines for the use of foreign field hospitals in the aftermath sudden-impact disasters.* Washington, DC, Pan American Health Organization, 2003 (http://www.paho.org/english/dd/ped/FieldHospitalsFolleto .pdf, accessed 7 April 2011).

Stier DD, Goodman RA. Mutual aid agreements: essential legal tools for public health preparedness and response. *American Journal of Public Health,* 2007, 97(Suppl. 1): 62–68 (http://www.ncbi.nlm.nih.gov/pmc/articles /PMC1854975/pdf/0970062.pdf, accessed 7 April 2011).

Key component 1.3 National institutional framework for multisectoral emergency management

Essential attribute 6 National committee for multisectoral emergency management

KEYNOTES

The institutional framework is the overarching emergency-management mechanism at the national level. Usually, a multisectoral steering committee is established at the highest political level (e.g., the prime minister's office or the cabinet of ministers), supported by an operational entity (essential attribute 7). A similar set-up is frequently found in the health sector (see essential attribute 8).

INDICATOR-RELATED QUESTIONS

a. *Has a national committee for multisectoral emergency management been established?*

b. *If so, does the committee include high-level representatives of all relevant sectors?*

c. *Are the responsibilities and authority of the committee members and secretariat defined?*

d. *Are procedures for convening meetings defined?*

e. *Is the committee supported by an operational entity?*
The national committee for multisectoral emergency management should be responsible for providing overall political and strategic leadership on the key aspects of processes related to crisis management. Members of the committee should be high-level decision makers from relevant ministries and institutions. The mandate, responsibilities and authority of the committee and its link to the national operational entity for multisectoral emergency management (essential attribute 7) should be formally specified. Procedures for including ad hoc, temporary members should be defined.

As emergencies in most countries are dealt with primarily at the local level, the national structure for multisectoral emergency management and coordination (essential attribute 2) will only be properly effective if complementary emergency-management arrangements exist at all levels of government administration, particularly at the local level.

f.   *Is the committee linked to similar structures at all levels?*

RECOMMENDED READING

Briggs SM. Regional interoperability: making systems connect in complex disasters. *The Journal of Trauma Injury, Infection and Critical Care,* 2009, 67:88–90.

Oloruntoba R. An analysis of the Cyclone Larry emergency relief chain: Some key success factors. *International Journal of Production Economics,* 2010, 126:85–101.

Essential attribute 7   National operational entity for multisectoral emergency management

INDICATOR-RELATED QUESTIONS

a.   *Does the national operational entity for multisectoral emergency management possess sufficient resources and support systems to enable it to fulfill its mandate?*

b.   *Are the responsibilities and authority of the entity defined?*

c.   *Does the entity coordinate and supervise national preparedness planning involving all relevant stakeholders?*

d.   *Are similar structures in place at all administrative levels?*
The national operational entity for multisectoral emergency management could be a ministry, an agency, a service or the like, with a mandate to provide the overall technical leadership of processes and tasks related to emergency management and responsibility for coordinating and supervising them. In many countries, the ministry for emergencies acts as the operational arm of the national multisectoral management committee and has links to similar structures at lower administrative levels. The entity should receive sufficient resources (staff, equipment and funding) to enable it to fulfill its mandate.

RECOMMENDED READING

Briggs SM. Regional interoperability: making systems connect in complex disasters. *The Journal of Trauma Injury, Infection and Critical Care,* 2009, 67:88–90.

Koh HK et al. Regionalization of local public health systems in the era of preparedness. *Annual Review of Public Health,* 2008, 29:205–218.

Key component 1.4   National institutional framework for health-sector emergency management

Essential attribute 8   National committee for health-sector emergency management

KEYNOTES

The institutional framework of the health sector is the overarching mechanism for managing health emergencies at the national level. Often, a multidisciplinary steering committee exists at the highest political level in the ministry of health. It may be supported by an operational entity (see essential attribute 9) and represented by a similar structure at the subnational level.

INDICATOR-RELATED QUESTIONS

a.   *Has a national committee for health-sector emergency management been established?*

b.   *If so, does the committee include high-level representatives of all relevant sectors and disciplines?*

c.   *Are the responsibilities and authority of the members of the committee and its secretariat defined?*

d.   *Are procedures for convening meetings of the committee defined?*

e.   *Is the committee supported by an operational entity?*

f.   *Is the committee linked to complementary structures at all levels?*
The national committee for health-sector emergency management should provide the overall strategic leadership and supervision of the health-related aspects of emergency management. Formal documents should exist specifying the mandate, responsibilities and authority of the committee and its links to other national and subnational committees and operational entities.

The national committee for health-sector emergency management should supervise and direct the health-sector emergency-preparedness program (essential attribute 12) and lead emergency response and recovery operations (essential attribute 13). Regular meetings should be held, chaired by a health-sector crisis coordinator. Committee members should be senior managers from operational departments within the ministry of health and from public and private health entities. Committee members should be capable of contributing substantively (both technically and operationally) to planning health-sector emergency preparedness and coordinating the implementation of action. They should be authorized by their organizations and departments to commit to decisions made by the committee. The roles, responsibilities and authority of each committee member must be clearly delineated to ensure operational effectiveness in the event of a health emergency.

Although policy and technical frameworks for health-sector emergency management are set up at the national level, they are executed at the local level. Therefore, detailed, regularly updated plans should exist at this level and they should be disseminated to all relevant stakeholders.

RECOMMENDED READING

Briggs SM. Regional interoperability: making systems connect in complex disasters. *The Journal of Trauma Injury, Infection and Critical Care,* 2009, 67:88–90.

Koh HK et al. Regionalization of local public health systems in the era of preparedness. *Annual Review of Public Health,* 2008, 29:205–218.

Koob P. *Health sector emergency preparedness guide.* Geneva, World Health Organization, 1998 (http://www.who.int /disasters/repo/5814.doc, accessed 11 April 2011).

Essential attribute 9 National operational entity for health-sector emergency management

INDICATOR-RELATED QUESTIONS

a. Are the available resources (staff, equipment, finances) and systems (emergency- operations centers, transport and communications systems) considered sufficient to allow the operational entity for health-sector emergency management to fulfill its mandate?

b. Are the responsibilities and authority of the national operational entity for health-sector management defined?
The national operational entity for health-sector emergency management could be a unit or focal point in the ministry of health or, for example, a center or institution. In this connection, WHO understands the focal point to be an entity responsible for overseeing the emergency-preparedness efforts of the ministry of health (such as the development of guidelines for hospital preparedness). The operational entity should report to the national committee for health-sector emergency management (essential attribute 8) and take action in accordance with the decisions of the committee. The head of the operational entity should be a member of the national committee for health-sector emergency management.

c. Does the operational entity coordinate and supervise the planning of the national health-sector emergency-preparedness program and, if so, are all the relevant stakeholders involved?
Coordination is the key responsibility of the national operational entity for health-sector management and requires the following action: convening meetings of the different actors; ensuring information-exchange; facilitating agreement on strategies developed in response to assessments and on follow-up mechanisms; planning joint action; assigning tasks and responsibilities; evaluating actions taken; and readjusting plans.

d. Are there similar entities in place at all administrative levels?
The national operational entity for health-sector emergency management should be replicated at the subnational level. It should be authorized by the ministry of health and/or local authorities to coordinate all aspects of the national

health-sector program on risk-reduction and emergency-management programs (essential attributes 11 and 12).

RECOMMENDED READING

Briggs SM. Regional interoperability: making systems connect in complex disasters. *The Journal of Trauma Injury, Infection and Critical Care,* 2009, 67:88–90.

Koh HK et al. Regionalization of local public health systems in the era of preparedness. *Annual Review of Public Health,* 2008, 29:205–218.

Koob P. *Health sector emergency preparedness guide.* Geneva, World Health Organization, 1998 (http://www.who.int /disasters/repo/5814.doc, accessed 11 April 2011).

Essential attribute 10 Mechanisms of coordination and partnership-building

INDICATOR-RELATED QUESTIONS

a. Do existing mechanisms of emergency coordination and partnership-building include agreements with entities in the public and private sectors and civil society?
The coordination framework should include regular partnership-mapping. Since the roles and operational responsibilities of each partner must be clearly established before an eventual health emergency, it is possible that mutual-aid agreements have been established with organizations, such as the International Federation of Red Cross and Red Crescent Societies (IFRC) and WHO, as well as NGOs and other regional and national entities.

b. Are the health authorities at all levels involved in governmental and nongovernmental coordination mechanisms?

c. Do existing coordination mechanisms include regular planning meetings on disaster-risk reduction and preparedness during emergency operations?

d. Do existing mechanisms of coordination and partnership-building promote the documentation and follow-up of decisions made at the planning meetings?
Mechanisms should exist for the coordination of all activities related to health-sector emergency preparedness, response and recovery. Information-sharing procedures should be agreed upon by the partners involved to ensure compatibility of information flow and analysis.
Assessors should consult the minutes of recent coordination meetings to establish their frequency before or during a crisis, as well as the level of participation in, and follow-up on, decisions made at the meetings.

e. Does the institutional framework promote joint planning procedures (to identify and deal with duplications and gaps in program implementation)?

f. Do existing mechanisms of coordination and partnership-building promote the joint mobilization of, and access to, resources?

The health-sector institutional framework for emergency management should identify resource providers and promote joint planning. For example, ministries and government departments can provide the necessary human resources, services and supplies and the military, police, fire, and utility services can provide essential logistical support (mobile hospitals, ambulances, vehicles, and fuel), security and emergency services.

The institutional framework should also create an environment that allows the intervention of foreign and/or international agencies in an emergency situation, as well as agreement protocols between neighboring countries. These can be more specific than international standards or conventions and include operational details and information on procedures and mechanisms for prompt and effective intercountry communication and mandatory national-health standards.

RECOMMENDED READING

Global assessment of health sector emergency preparedness and response. Geneva, World Health Organization, 2008 (http://www.who.int/hac/about/Global_survey_inside.pdf, accessed 11 April 2011).

Keim M. Using a community-based approach for prevention and mitigation of national health emergencies. *Pacific Health Dialog*, 2002, 9(1):93–96.

Koob P. *Health sector emergency preparedness guide*. Geneva, World Health Organization, 1998 (http://www.who.int/disasters/repo/5814.doc, accessed 11 April 2011).

Stier DD, Goodman RA. Mutual aid agreements: essential legal tools for public health preparedness and response. *American Journal of Public Health*, 2007, 97:62–68.

> **Key component 1.5**   Components of national program on health-sector emergency management
>
> **Essential attribute 11**   National health-sector program on risk reduction

KEYNOTES

A program on health-sector emergency management is one of long-term, integrated, multidisciplinary developmental activities, with goals of strengthening the overall capacity of the health sector to manage the health aspects of all types of hazards in an efficient manner. The core components of such a program are disaster risk reduction, emergency preparedness, and response and recovery.

A risk-reduction program should be developed on the basis of regularly updated risk assessments (see essential attribute 21). The results of these assessments are combined into a national profile, which is used by planners to identify the factors that put communities at risk for various hazards and prevent them from becoming emergencies. Once a risk has been defined and the capacity of services required to deal with it assessed, programs can be adjusted to focus on reducing the risk and increasing capacity, if necessary.

Assessing and reducing disaster risk requires all stakeholders to be on board and to place high priority on the provision of sufficient resources to this end.

INDICATOR-RELATED QUESTIONS

a. *Has a national health-sector risk-reduction program been established?*

b. *If so, does it, in collaboration with the national operational entity for multisectoral emergency management, identify risk-prone populations on the basis of risk analyses?*

c. *Does the program identify risk-prone health facilities on the basis of risk analyses?*
Assessors should establish whether a national profile of health risks, based on risk analyses, exists and is updated regularly. They should ensure that both the profile and the risk maps refer not only to hazards but also to risks (bearing the risk formula in mind: *risk* is proportional to *hazard* times *vulnerability* divided by *capacity*).

A national profile of health risks is a comprehensive record of assets, liabilities, and emergency threats at both the national and subnational levels covering a particular period of time.

d. *Does the program have the resources to address vulnerabilities and reduce risks?*
Assessors should look into whether the national risk-reduction program systematically uses available information to determine the likelihood of certain events and the magnitude of their possible consequences. The program should define acceptable levels of risk on the basis of risk assessments and assess whether the capacity and resources available are sufficient to address or manage unacceptable risks.

Resources should be allocated and available for the mitigation of identified vulnerabilities to reduce risks.

RECOMMENDED READING

Arnold JL. Risk and risk assessment in health emergency management. *Prehospital and Disaster Medicine*, 2005, 20:143–154.

Boroschek Krauskopf R, Retamales Saavedra R. *Guidelines for vulnerability reduction in the design of new health facilities*. Washington, DC, Pan American Health Organization, 2004 (http://www.unisdr.org/eng/library/Literature/7760.pdf, accessed 11 April 2011).

Global assessment of health sector emergency preparedness and response. Geneva, World Health Organization, 2008 (http://www.who.int/hac/about/Global_survey_inside.pdf, accessed 11 April 2011).

United Nations International Strategy for Disaster Reduction. *Living with risk. A global review of disaster reduction initiatives*. Geneva, United Nations Publications, 2004 (http://www.unisdr.org/publications/v.php?id=657.accessed 11 April 2011).

United Nations International Strategy for Disaster Reduction, World Health Organization, World Bank. *Hospitals safe from disasters. Reduce risk, protect health facilities, save lives.* Geneva, United Nations International Strategy for Disaster Reduction, 2009 (http://www.unisdr.org /eng/public_aware/world_camp/2008-2009/pdf/wdrc-2008-2009-information-kit.pdf, accessed 11 April 2011).

Koob P. *Health sector emergency preparedness guide.* Geneva, World Health Organization, 1998, (http://www.who.int /disasters/repo/5814.doc, accessed 11 April 2011).

Thomalla F et al. Reducing hazard vulnerability: towards a common approach between disaster risk reduction and climate adaptation. *Disasters*, 2006, 30:39–48.

Essential attribute 12 Multisectoral and health-sector programs on emergency preparedness

KEYNOTES

Emergency preparedness relates to measures taken to build and maintain the generic capacity required to enable anticipation of, response to and recovery from emergencies, regardless of cause.

Preparedness is not the same as preparation. Preparedness is not event-focused (as preparation is) but systems-focused. Preparedness builds and maintains the generic platforms and operating systems necessary to ensure that event-specific alerts, preparation, response and recovery can and do happen. Emergency preparedness is a continuous iterative process, integral to the development process. Preparedness cannot be just a plan; it must be based on a program with its own financial and human resources and annual work plans. Building effective preparedness programs involves effort at all levels of government and coordination between government sectors, the private sector and NGOs to determine threats and vulnerabilities and identify required resources.

The principle work domains of an emergency-preparedness program are regulation (laws, authorities), direction (policies, procedures, guidelines) and execution (plans, resources, knowledge, skills, awareness, and attitudes). The quality of work carried out in each of these domains determines the level of readiness of a country, agency or institution to manage an emergency.

The coordination of emergency-preparedness planning and response activities (including research, training and education, disaster-related drills and public information) is usually designated to one main agency (such as the ministry for emergencies). The health sector may have a similar entity responsible for the health aspects of an emergency or it may be represented on the main agency's team. On a day-today basis, the emergency-preparedness program carries out research, planning, training and education activities related to emergency response. These include: conducting risk analyses to determine the effects of real or possible hazards; working with appropriate departments on risk-mitigation programs; developing inventories of resources; identifying resource deficiencies and recommending corrective action; establishing and maintaining protocols for communications and alert systems; and continually seeking resources to enhance the quality of the emergency-preparedness program itself.

Assessors should establish whether emergency-preparedness programs exist at the national and/or subnational levels and whether they include most or all of the necessary components.

INDICATOR-RELATED QUESTIONS

a. *Do emergency-preparedness programs existing at the national and/or subnational levels promote and conduct research? (See also essential attribute 14.)*

b. *Do they include the development and dissemination of emergency-management guidelines?*
The program should be based on hazard, vulnerability and risk assessments. Simple, flexible emergency-management guidelines specific to the local risk profile should be developed by those expected to implement them, taking best practices into consideration.
Assessors should establish whether emergency-management guidelines on developing exercises and drills exist and whether they provide for feedback and recommendations after each exercise or drill with a view to improving them.

c. *Do they foresee reviews and revisions of emergency-management policies?*
Policies and guidelines should be reviewed and amended regularly (which, in many countries, means annually) or after each event. Assessors should establish whether the program promotes mechanisms to this end.

d. *Do they include the development, organization and delivery of emergency-management training programs?*
The emergency-preparedness program should ensure that health-sector staff at all levels has the opportunity to participate in accredited education, training, drills and exercises in emergency management (see also essential attribute 16). It should also ensure the development and implementation of public-education programs.

e. *Do they include the promotion of a participatory emergency-management planning process?*
A preparedness and response plan is an agreed and approved set of arrangements for responding to and recovering from crises. It delineates responsibilities, management structures, strategies and resources (see also essential attribute 10).

f. *Do they mobilize and allocate resources for preparedness? (See also essential attributes 15, 17–20, 31 and 33.)*

g. *Do they include the development and maintenance of information systems and databases? (See also essential attributes 21–25.)*

h. *Do they include the development of risk-communication, health-promotion and education strategies? (See also essential attributes 28 and 29.)*

i. *Do they foresee the development and evaluation of exercises and drills?*

j. Do they include the development and maintenance of standards for emergency-management plans?
Emergency-management plans (on risk reduction, emergency response and business continuity) should exist at the national, subnational and facilities' levels and should all follow a similar structure and format.

k. Do they provide for the coordination and monitoring of, and the regular reporting on, program implementation?
A built-in feedback loop should allow for the regular monitoring and evaluation of program implementation.

Assessors should verify whether plans for the implementation of emergency-program activities and reports on their results are published regularly and disseminated to relevant stakeholders.

RECOMMENDED READING

Adini B et al. Assessing levels of hospital emergency preparedness. *Prehospital and Disaster Medicine,* 2006, 21:451–457.

Ginter PM, Duncan WJ, Abdolrasulnia M. Hospital strategic preparedness planning: the new imperative. *Prehospital and Disaster Medicine,* 2007, 22(6):529– 536.

Glik DC. Risk communication for public health emergencies. *Annual Review of Public Health,* 2007, 28:33–54.

Global assessment of health sector emergency preparedness and response. Geneva, World Health Organization, 2008 (http://www.who.int/hac/about/Global_survey_inside.pdf, accessed 11 April 2011).

Koob P. *Health sector emergency preparedness guide.* Geneva, World Health Organization, 1998 (http://www.who.int /disasters/repo/5814.doc, accessed 11 April 2011).

State health emergency response plan (SHERP Victoria). Melbourne, Department of Health, 2009 (http://www .dhs.vic.gov.au/__data/assets/pdf_file/0005/400883 /SHERP_2nd_edition_web.pdf, accessed 11 April 2011).

Stier DD, Goodman RA. Mutual aid agreements: essential legal tools for public health preparedness and response. *American Journal of Public Health,* 2007, 97(1):62–68 (http://ajph.aphapublications.org/cgi/content/short/97 /Supplement_1/S62, accessed 11 April 2011).

> **Essential attribute 13** National health-sector plan for emergency response and recovery

KEYNOTES

An emergency-response plan is an agreed set of arrangements for responding to and facilitating recovery from emergencies. Its objectives are to protect life, property and the environment, and to safeguard the basic functions of lifelines and essential services. To be able to plan emergency response, it is necessary that decision makers at the government and community levels recognize the existence of risks and vulnerabilities, the possibility that emergencies will occur, and the benefits of planning to deal with them. A national health-sector plan for emergency response is essentially an umbrella instrument that facilitates collaboration among response agencies and relevant sectors and levels of government, all of which have their own plans. The government's responsibility at national level is not to provide direct services but to support response agencies and local government in their operations. Thus, the national focus is on resource mobilization, logistics, communications, coordination between different jurisdictions and agencies, technical assistance and public information. Areas of responsibility specific to the national level include national security, foreign assistance, immigration and border control, customs and excise, donor coordination, refugees and cross-border coordination.

The implementation of a national health-sector emergency-response plan is guaranteed through appropriate legislation (see also essential attributes 1 and 3) and the designation of an organization responsible for coordinating the planning of action related to response and recovery in the event of an emergency (see also essential attributes 6–9).

INDICATOR-RELATED QUESTIONS

a. Is the national emergency-response plan based on an all-hazards approach and risk assessment?

b. Does the plan include contingency measures?

c. Is it compatible with relevant intersectoral and subnational health plans?

d. Does it define activation, coordination and incident-command mechanisms?

e. Is it based on available resources?

f. Is it disseminated to key stakeholders after each revision?

g. Is it regularly tested through exercises, drills and simulations?

h. Has it been disseminated to the public?
In developing the national emergency-response plan, account should be taken of plans existing at lower administrative levels, other national-level plans and plans developed for specific hazards. All plans should be disseminated to stakeholders. They should be updated annually or after any emergency event.

RECOMMENDED READING

Perry RW, Lindell MK. Preparedness for emergency response: guidelines for the emergency planning process. *Disasters,* 2003, 27(4):336–350.

State Health Emergency Response Plan (SHERP Victoria). Melbourne, Department of Health, 2009 (http://www.dhs.vic.gov.au/__data/assets /pdf_file/0005/400883/SHERP_2nd_edition_web.pdf, accessed 11 April 2011).

Essential attribute 14   Research and evidence base

INDICATOR-RELATED QUESTIONS

a. *Is the research agenda defined?*

b. *Have resources been allocated for research?*

c. *Have research results been applied?*
A research agenda should be defined by the ministry of health with the focus on supporting and effective decision making. Drills and exercises generate evidence about what works and what does not; disseminating this knowledge should be institutionalized. Monitoring and evaluation exercises should be carried out for all aspects of health-sector emergency preparedness; the experience gained will benefit planning, programming and policy development.

Assessors should verify that the ministry of health supports the improvement of scientific and technical methods of, and capacity for, risk assessment, monitoring and early warning through research, partnerships and training, and by building technical capacity. The ministry of health should promote the application of in situ and space-based earth observations, space technologies, remote sensing, geographic information systems, hazard modeling and prediction, weather and climate modeling and forecasting, communication tools and studies of the costs and benefits of risk assessment and early warning.

RECOMMENDED READING

A *methodological approach to monitoring and assessing scientific advice provision and impact: a test case analysis of the mechanism by which scientific advice catalyzes interactions among societal actors. Framework contract no. RTD–JRC/00–06 June* 2003. *Final report* for *the European Commission.* Twickenham, The Evaluation Partnership, 2003 (ec.europa.eu/research/science-society/pdf /bioterrorism_report_en.pdf, accessed 7 August 2011).

Nelson CD et al. How can we strengthen the evidence base in public health preparedness? *Disaster Medicine and Public Health Preparedness,* 2008, 2:247–249.

◗ SECTION 2. HEALTH WORKFORCE

Health workers are the cornerstone of the health care delivery system. They influence accessibility to and the quality and cost of health care, and the delivery of interventions to improve health outcomes, including progress towards attaining the health-related MDG and achieving health for all.

Key component 2.1   Human resources for health-sector emergency management

Essential attribute 15   Development of human resources

KEYNOTE

The emergency-preparedness program is responsible for ensuring that, taking the given circumstances and available resources (e.g., finances, hospital capacity for mass-casualties) into account, a sufficient number of qualified staff with an appropriate mix of skills is available to respond to any crisis and that relevant continuous education and training programs are in place.

INDICATOR-RELATED QUESTIONS

a. *Does a human-resources plan for emergency management exist and, if so, is it based on defined competencies?*
Assessors should determine whether the ministry of health has a strategy for the development of human resources. It should be based on an assessment of available human resources at the national level, including a gap analysis, and define the required competencies of emergency-management staff.

Furthermore, assessors should verify that:

- the roles, responsibilities and authority of each person identified as a responder in case of a crisis are clearly defined and that there are written terms of reference for each function;
- measures exist for identifying gaps vis-à-vis skilled staff and that critical positions are filled through recruitment procedures and/or on the basis of education and training.

It is necessary to plan surge capacity and identify a sufficient number of suitable staff to ensure the capacity required to respond to an emergency at short notice.

The procedures to be followed for mobilizing staff, and information about the roles, responsibilities, and authority of those involved, should be circulated to relevant departments and organizations.

b. *Is there a database of staff trained in emergency management and is it maintained?*
The ministry of health should have a database of the workforce available at the national level, as well as details of the roles of staff in an eventual crisis. The database should include, for example, doctors, nurses, paramedics, drivers, administrative staff, laboratory technicians, dispatchers, media and communications specialists, and relevant staff of public and private health organizations, IFRC, NGOs, civil society, international organizations, the military, the police force and civil defense.

This information should be accessible to the national operational entity for health-sector emergency management to enable the organization of resources for effective delivery, when necessary.

c. *Do procedures exist for integrating national and international volunteers into service delivery in emergency situations?*
A volunteer policy includes procedures for coordinating volunteers to ensure consistency in the quality of service delivery. Training courses to improve the effectiveness of volunteers should be identified and available.

RECOMMENDED READING

Hsu EB et al. Healthcare worker competencies for disaster training. *BMC Medical Education*, 2006, 6:19 (http://www.ncbi.nlm.nih.gov/pmc/articles/PMC1471784/, accessed 12 April 2011).

Reilly, M., Markenson, D. S. Education and training of hospital workers: who are essential personnel during a disaster? *Prehospital and Disaster Medicine*, 2009, 24:239–245.

Schultz, C. H., Stratton, S. J. Improving hospital surge capacity: a new concept for emergency credentialing of volunteers. *Annals of Emergency Medicine*, 2007, 49(5):602–609 (http://www.annemergmed.com/article/S0196-0644(06)02349-3/abstract, accessed 12 April 2011).

Stier DD, Goodman RA. Mutual aid agreements: essential legal tools for public health preparedness and response. *American Journal of Public Health*, 2007, 97:62–68 (http://www.ncbi.nlm.nih.gov/pmc/articles/PMC1854975/, accessed 12 April 2011).

Williams J, Nocera M, Casteel C. The effectiveness of disaster training for health care workers: a systematic review. *Annals of Emergency Medicine*, 2008, 52(3):211–222.e2 (http://www.annemergmed.com/article/S0196-0644(07)01624-1/abstract, accessed 12 April 2011).

> **Essential attribute 16** Training and education

KEYNOTES

One of the key objectives of an emergency-preparedness program is to ensure that training and education programs in emergency management are available, accessible, appropriate and effective. This involves determining the managerial, technical and administrative competencies required by conducting periodic needs assessments involving all health staff and ensuring that these are reflected in job descriptions and that a range of effective training courses is available and accessible to all staff members.

Assessors should verify the roles and responsibilities of the ministry of health and other actors, such as the ministries for emergencies and education and NGOs working in the area of health education. They should also determine the availability of training in competency-building for the management of public health services and the delivery of health care.

Nurses comprise the largest portion of the health workforce in most countries. They deliver core services at all levels of the health system and across the continuum of care to promote health, improve patient care, deliver services and contribute to positive health outcomes. Therefore, special emphasis should be placed on training nurses in emergency management.

INDICATOR-RELATED QUESTIONS

a. *Do needs assessments determine the frequency and content of training, as well as the number of participants?*

b. *Does a needs-based training plan exist?*

c. *Do the curricula cater for the different competencies required?*

National programs should ensure the availability of education and training programs that cater for the various categories of health staff (nurses, paramedics, doctors, hospital managers). The training programs should be academically supported, accredited and available in the national language(s). The curricula and format of the courses should be reviewed on a regular basis and adapted to the local needs (e.g., required staffing skills, capacity for training institutions). Complementary training opportunities, such as on-the-job training and pre- and postgraduate courses, should also be available.

Assessors should ascertain whether the emergency-management competencies required for the key ministry-of-health posts have been determined and are reflected in the job descriptions. They should also ensure that assessments of training needs are carried out periodically and that the design and delivery of training and education programs are competency-based.

Some or all of the following topics should be included in the training programs: risk management; risk assessment; rapid post-disaster needs assessment; mass-casualty management; hospital preparedness; search and rescue; control of communicable diseases and pandemics; chemical incidents; food and nutrition; management of supplies; noncommunicable diseases in emergencies.

All disaster-response plans must be tested and staff trained in using them.

d. *Are the curricula and training materials harmonized across stakeholders?*
Operational guidelines and technical publications relating to health-sector emergency management should be distributed widely among partners to ensure commonality of response.

e. *Does a formal mechanism exist for reviewing and revising curricula?*

f. *Does training include exercises and drills?*

g. *Are opportunities provided for emergency-management training?*
All health-sector crisis-management courses, as well as drills and exercises, should be accessible to all relevant partners to ensure the use of a common methodology and harmonized standard operating procedures. International training courses (e.g., those hosted by the Regional Office and/or the European Center for Disease Prevention and Control [ECDC]) should be available to key response staff.

h. *Have sufficient resources been allocated for training programs?*
Assessors should verify that the annual budgets of emergency-preparedness programs include sufficient funds for training and education activities.

RECOMMENDED READING

Core public health worker competencies for emergency preparedness and response. Columbia, Center for Health

Policy, Columbia University School of Nursing, 2001 (http://www.nnepi.org/pdf/IC_Public_Health1.pdf, accessed 17 July 2011).

Ghori, Uddin S. et al. Emergency preparedness: addressing a residency training gap. *Academic Medicine*, 2008, 83:298–304.

Hsu, E. B. et al. Effectiveness of hospital staff mass-casualty incident training methods: a systematic literature review. *Prehospital and Disaster Medicine*, 2004, 19:192–200.

SECTION 3. MEDICAL PRODUCTS, VACCINES AND TECHNOLOGY

Appropriate and cost-effective diagnostic and therapeutic medical products are essential for the provision of quality health care and the mitigation of human mortality and morbidity in an emergency.

Key component 3.1 Medical supplies and equipment for emergency-response operations

Essential attribute 17 Medical equipment and supplies for prehospital and hospital (including temporary health facilities) activities and other public health interventions

INDICATOR-RELATED QUESTIONS

a. *Are essential medical supplies and equipment for emergency operations determined on the basis of risk assessments and analyses?*

b. *Are they readily available in sufficient quantities?*

c. *Are medical supplies periodically tested, and are expired or inappropriate items disposed of in accordance with established guidelines?*

Assessors need to verify that standardized lists of emergency medical supplies and equipment exist, that they were developed according to the needs identified through risk assessments, that they are comprehensive and include the appropriate items (i.e., that they reflect the policies and guidelines of the ministry of health accurately and do not conflict with international best practices), and that mechanisms exist to ensure the timely delivery of such items to the local level when requested. Stockpiles should be stored at secure and easily accessible locations.

The national repository should be organized with a focus on flexible response and include, for example, antibiotics, chemical antidotes, antitoxins, life-support medications, intravenous equipment, airway maintenance supplies and medical/surgical items. The repository should be designed to supplement and supply national and subnational health facilities in the event of an emergency. In the same way, supplies and equipment should be stored for influenza pandemics (e.g., antiviral drugs, vaccines, personal protective equipment (PPE) for medical staff and laboratory diagnostics equipment). The appropriate quantities of supplies should be determined by data projecting the annual national needs.

An inventory process should be in place to ensure that a minimum stock of essential medical supplies and equipment is maintained. The repository should be replicated at the subnational and facility levels.

d. *Are maintenance of the inventory and the rotation and safe stockpiling of medical supplies and equipment executed in accordance with established guidelines?*

e. *Is there a system in place, including cold chain, for the distribution of medical supplies and equipment in the event of a health-sector emergency?*

f. *Do procedures exist for the exceptional procurement of medical supplies that are not on the list of basic equipment?*

Assessors should verify that procedures exist for the periodic testing, replacement and/or disposal of stockpile medical supplies and equipment. There should also be procedures for drawing up contracts for the delivery of supplies and services during emergencies, including technical specifications and information about the prices, delivery times and reliability of the goods. A method of tracking deliveries and reporting discrepancies must be in place.

Assessors also need to establish whether there are procedures for requesting, accepting and refusing medicines, personnel, field hospitals and other services (donations) provided by international partners and whether provision has been made for import-tax exemption for, and the speedy clearance of, medical supplies.

RECOMMENDED READING

Emergency response and recovery. Non statutory guidance accompanying the civil contingencies act, 2004. London, HM Government, 2010 (http://www.worcestershire.gov.uk/cms/pdf/EmergencyResponse&Recovery%20April%202010.pdf, accessed 15 April 2011).

Balcik B et al. Coordination in humanitarian relief chains: practices, challenges and opportunities. *International Journal of Production Economics*, 2010, 126(1):22–34.

Brown DW et al. Evidence-based approach for disaster preparedness authorities to inform the contents of repositories for prescription medications for chronic disease management and control. *Prehospital and Disaster Medicine*, 2008, 23(5):447–457.

Pan American Health Organization. *Guidelines for the use of foreign field hospital in the aftermath of sudden-impact disasters.* Washington, DC, Pan American Health Organization, 2003 (http://helid.digicollection.org/en/p/printable.html, accessed 15 April 2011).

Pan American Health Organization. *Humanitarian assistance in disaster situations. A guide for effective aid.* Washington, DC, Pan American Health Organization,

1999 (http://www.paho.org/english/ped/pedhumen.pdf, accessed 15 April 2011).

Pan American Health Organization. *Humanitarian supply management and logistics in the health sector.* Washington, DC, Pan American Health Organization, 2001 (http://www .paho.org/english/ped/HumanitarianSupply-part1.pdf, accessed 15 April 2011).

Structural, non-structural and functional indicators. Manila, WHO Regional Office for the Western Pacific, 2009 (http:// www.wpro.who.int/NR/rdonlyres/E554CC53-4C8C-4340- 9CCC-47EE5727BB0C/0/IndicatorsforSafeHospitals DRAFTApril2009.pdf, accessed 15 April 2011).

Essential attribute 18   Pharmaceutical services

INDICATOR QUESTIONS

a.   *Are essential pharmaceutical supplies for emergency operations determined on the basis of risk analyses?*

b.   *Are they readily available in sufficient quantities?*

c.   *Are pharmaceutical supplies periodically tested, and are expired or inappropriate items disposed of in accordance with established guidelines?*

d.   *Are maintenance of the inventory and the rotation and safe stockpiling of pharmaceutical supplies executed in accordance with established guidelines?*

e.   *Is there a system in place, including cold chain, for the distribution of pharmaceutical supplies in the event of a health-sector emergency?*

f.   *Do procedures exist for the exceptional procurement of pharmaceutical supplies that are not on the list of essential drugs?*
     Assessors should verify that procedures exist for the periodic testing, replacement and/or disposal of stockpile pharmaceuticals. There should also be procedures for drawing up contracts for the delivery of pharmaceutical supplies in emergencies, including technical specifications and information about the prices, delivery times and reliability of the goods. A method of tracking deliveries and reporting discrepancies must be in place.

     Assessors also need to establish whether procedures are in place for requesting, accepting and refusing medicines, personnel, field hospitals and other services (donations) provided by international partners, and whether provision has been made for import-tax exemption for, and the speedy clearance of, pharmaceutical supplies.

RECOMMENDED READING

Pan American Health Organization, WHO Regional Office for the Western Pacific. *Humanitarian supply management and logistics in the health sector.* Washington, DC, Pan American Health Organization, 2001 (http://www.paho.org /english/ped/HumanitarianSupply-part1.pdf. accessed 15 April 2011).

World Health Organization et al. *The interagency emergency health kit 2006. Medicines and medical devices for 10 000 people for approximately 3 months. An interagency document.* Geneva, World Health Organization, 2006 (WHO/ PSM/PAR/2006.4) (http://apps.who.int/medicinedocs/en/d /Js13486e/6.10.5.html, accessed 8 May 2011).

Essential attribute 19   Laboratory services

INDICATOR-RELATED QUESTIONS

a.   *Are essential laboratory supplies and equipment for emergency operations determined on the basis of risk analyses?*

b.   *Are they readily available in sufficient quantities?*

c.   *Are laboratory supplies and equipment periodically tested, and are expired or inappropriate items disposed of in accordance with established guidelines?*

d.   *Do procedures exist for the exceptional procurement of laboratory supplies and equipment?*

e.   *Are the safe transport and export of biological and environmental specimens for testing and/or confirmation by national and international reference laboratories assured?*
     Assessors should verify that procedures exist for the periodic testing, replacement and/or disposal of stockpile laboratory supplies and equipment. There should also be procedures for drawing up contracts for the delivery of supplies and services in emergencies, including technical specifications and information about the prices, delivery times and reliability of the goods. A method of tracking deliveries and reporting discrepancies must be in place.

     Assessors also need to establish whether there are procedures for requesting, accepting and refusing medicines, personnel, field hospitals and other services (donations) provided by international partners and whether provision has been made for import-tax exemption for, and the speedy clearance of, laboratory supplies.

     Procedures for diagnosing samples quickly must be in place and regularly tested. Essential laboratory services and basic laboratory testing, such as complete blood count, chemistry profile, electrolysis, blood-gas analysis, blood culture and sputum examination, should be maintained. Protocols should be established with national and reference laboratories on the rapid sharing of information and specimens, including cross-border transport to international reference laboratories.

RECOMMENDED READING

Guidelines for the collection of clinical specimens during field investigation of outbreaks. Geneva, World Health Organization, 2000 (WHO/CDS/CSR/EDC/2000.4) (http://www .who.int/entity/csr/resources/publications/surveillance /whocdscsredc2004.pdf, assessed 15 April 2011).

Pan American Health Organization, WHO Regional Office for the Western Pacific. *Humanitarian supply management and logistics in the health sector.* Washington, DC, Pan American Health Organization, 2001 (http://www.paho.org /english/ped/HumanitarianSupply-part1.pdf. accessed 15 April 2011).

State health emergency response plan (SHERP Victoria). Second edition. Melbourne, Department of Health, 2009 (http:// www.dhs.vic.gov.au/_data/assets/pdf_file/0005/400883 /SHERP_2nd_edition_web.pdf, accessed 15 April 2011).

World Health Organization et al. *The interagency emergency health kit 2006. Medicines and medical devices for 10 000 people for approximately 3 months. An interagency document.* Geneva, World Health Organization, 2006 (WHO/ PSM/PAR/2006.4) (http://apps.who.int/medicinedocs/en/d /Js13486e/6.10.5.html, accessed 8 May 2011).

Essential attribute 20   Blood services

INDICATOR-RELATED QUESTIONS

a. *Are essential supplies and equipment for blood services determined on the basis of risk analyses?*

b. *Are blood supplies readily available in sufficient quantities?*

c. *Are arrangements in place (including public campaigns) for the rapid and exceptional collection, storage and distribution of blood and are these in accordance with established guidelines?*

d. *Do procedures exist for the exceptional procurement of supplies and equipment for blood services?*

e. *Is the safety of blood and blood products (and their safe disposal) ensured in accordance with established guidelines?*

Assessors should verify that procedures exist for the periodic testing, replacement and/or disposal of stockpile supplies and equipment for blood services. There should also be procedures for drawing up contracts for the delivery of supplies and services in emergencies, including technical specifications and information on the prices, delivery times and reliability of the goods. A method of tracking deliveries and reporting discrepancies must be in place.

Assessors also need to establish whether procedures exist for requesting, accepting and refusing medicines, personnel, field hospitals and other services (donations) provided by international partners and whether provision has been made for import-tax exemption for, and the speedy clearance of, blood and blood products.

As the most important factor in the initial response to a disaster, assessors should determine whether an adequate blood inventory is being maintained. A seven-day supply of all blood types should be available at all times unless risk analyses demonstrate different needs.

RECOMMENDED READING

Blood safety and laboratory technology [web site]. New Delhi, WHO Regional Office for South East Asia, 2011 (http:// www.searo.who.int/EN/Section10/Section17.htm, accessed 15 April 2011).

Pan American Health Organization, WHO Regional Office for the Western Pacific. *Humanitarian supply management and logistics in the health sector.* Washington, DC, Pan American Health Organization, 2001 (http://www.paho.org /english/ped/HumanitarianSupply-part1.pdf, accessed 15 April 2011).

World Health Organization et al. *The interagency emergency health kit 2006. Medicines and medical devices for 10 000 people for approximately 3 months. An interagency document.* Geneva, World Health Organization, 2006 (WHO /PSM/PAR/2006.4) (http://apps.who.int/medicinedocs/en/d /Js13486e/6.10.5.html, accessed 15 April 2011).

SECTION 4. HEALTH INFORMATION

Key component 4.1   Information-management systems for risk-reduction and emergency-preparedness programs

Essential attribute 21   Information system for risk assessment and emergency-preparedness planning

KEYNOTES

Up-to-date, reliable data and information are required to conduct risk assessments and carry out the emergency-preparedness planning necessary to ensure appropriate decision making. These data and information should be available through a distributed, interoperable and reliable information system that connects institutions (including the ministry of health) with the necessary mandate to collect and maintain them. At the same time, the data coming from these different institutions need to be compatible and documented if they are to be combined in the context of risk assessment and emergency planning. Finally, the use of geography and the geographic information system (GIS) as a neutral platform for the integration of these data to visualize and analyze risk calls for an information system that combines the geographical and time dimensions properly.

All the aforementioned elements are generally handled through the National Spatial Data Infrastructure (NSDI), a forum that groups partners according to their agreement on and implementation of the policies, standards and procedures necessary to ensure data compatibility and system interoperability in general, and to support emergency management in particular.

Once the above is in place, the necessary technical capacity and resources need to be available for conducting the risk assessments and using their results as a basis for planning action towards risk reduction and emergency preparedness.

A risk assessment starts with the identification of hazards that are prevalent at the national, subnational (community and municipal), or infrastructure levels. The vulnerabilities and capacities of the exposed populations, health infrastructures and services at these levels are then assessed on the basis of available data and information and combined with the aforementioned hazards profile to obtain the geographical distribution of risks.

Since planning for emergencies is based on risk-assessment analyses, its quality ultimately depends on the quality of the assessment.

INDICATOR-RELATED QUESTIONS

a.   *Are the responsibilities and authority related to the information system defined?*

b.   *Do protocols and procedures exist for the collection, management, analysis and dissemination of the necessary data for conducting risk assessments and performing emergency-preparedness planning?*

c.   *Does a national profile of health risks exist and, if so, is it based on disaggregated risk, hazard and vulnerability data?*
     Conducting a geographically based risk assessment to develop a national profile of health risks is a data-intensive exercise.

     Assessors should investigate when the latest national population census was conducted and check whether GIS was used and whether the demographic data are readily available in a format that could be used in a risk assessment.

     Assessors should also look into finding an up-to-date list of administrative divisions down to the local level (e.g., district, municipality) and determine whether the delimitation of these units exists in GIS format.

d.   *Are reports on the activities of the emergency-preparedness program published and disseminated regularly?*

RECOMMENDED READING

Communicable disease control in emergencies. A field manual. Geneva, World Health Organization, 2005 (http://www.who.int/infectious-disease-news/IDdocs/whocds200527/ISBN_9241546166.pdf, accessed 16 April 2011).

Framework and standards for country health information systems. Second edition. Geneva, World Health Organization, 2008 (http://www.who.int/healthmetrics/documents/hmn_framework200803.pdf, accessed 16 April 2011).

Essential attribute 22   National health information system

KEYNOTES

A national health information system collects data from the health sector and, in combination with data from other relevant sectors, analyses them, ensures their overall quality, relevance and timeliness, and converts them into information for use in health-related decision making. Reliable and timely health information is essential to public health action, including that related to strengthening health systems. The need for sound information is especially critical in connection with emergent diseases and other acute health threats in that rapid awareness, investigation and response can save lives and prevent national outbreaks and even global pandemics.

One of the key elements of a health information system is public health surveillance (see also essential attribute 24). This element is especially relevant when the need for timely reporting and response (as in the case of epidemic diseases), and effective links to those responsible for disease control, impose additional requirements on the health information system.

The responsibility for health data is often divided among different ministries or institutions and coordination may be difficult because of financial and administrative constraints. However, health information systems should be responsive to the needs and requirements of all those concerned and this should be assured through a single, comprehensive plan developed through widespread collaboration. The control of major diseases should also be approached in a comprehensive and coherent manner.

Good management of health information requires the capacity to gather, process and disseminate information to all relevant stakeholders on a 24/7 basis. Ideally, there should be a health information center, which:

*   is accessible 24/7;
*   is linked to multiple information sources (ambulance-dispatch centers, the meteorological Office, ministries, etc.) (see also essential attribute 27) to ensure the constant flow and sharing of information on any potential crises (also at the international level), as appropriate;
*   is autonomous (equipped to operate independent of any outside source, for example, of electricity and telecommunications, that may be impacted in a crisis);
*   has standard operating procedures to ensure commonality of information management across partners; and
*   generates reports to stakeholders, as needed, using standard formats and templates.

Assessors should verify whether this capacity has been developed as part of the responsibilities of the country to facilitate a rapid exchange of information nationally and internationally in the event of a crisis.

INDICATOR-RELATED QUESTIONS

a.   *Does the national health information system provide disaggregated data for health-related emergency management at the national and subnational levels?*
     A national health information system contributes significantly to health-related emergency management at all levels. Relevant data on the pre-crisis situation provide the baseline for comparison that enables meaningful conclusions to be drawn about the effects of the crisis and priority responses.

     Assessors should, therefore, first verify whether complete, up-to-date registries are available for and enable the mapping of the following assets:

*   health facilities (public and private);
*   pharmacies and medical stores;
*   cold stores;
*   laboratories;
*   blood banks;
*   human (health-related) resources;
*   medical supplies and equipment for emergency-response operations.

Assessors should then identify the health indicators for which data are available through the health information system and ascertain their level of disaggregation.

Finally, assessors should verify whether mechanisms exist to ensure the timely provision of the above-mentioned disaggregated baseline data relevant to health-related emergency management at the national and subnational levels, if needed.

b. Are the triggers for switching from routine to emergency reporting defined?
The elements of reporting (e.g., frequency, content) during emergencies differ significantly from those of routine reporting.

Assessors should verify that triggers are defined for switching from routine to emergency reporting.

RECOMMENDED READING

Framework and standards for country health information systems. Geneva, World Health Organization, 2008 (http://www.who.int/healthmetrics/documents/hmn_framework200803.pdf, accessed 18 April 2010).

Health information systems development and strengthening: guidance on needs assessment for national health information systems development. Brazzaville, WHO Regional Office for Africa, 2000.

Measuring health systems strengthening and trends: a toolkit for countries. Geneva, World Health Organization, 2010 (http://www.who.int/entity/healthinfo/HSS_MandE_framework_Oct_2010.pdf, accessed 6 August 2010).

Essential attribute 23 National and international information-sharing

(See also essential attribute 40 on prevention and control of communicable diseases and immunization.)

KEYNOTES

Information-sharing and strategies on how to communicate information within and beyond a country's border are an integral component of national emergency planning. Detailed plans on what is to be communicated by whom, to whom and how in case of an emergency must be prepared in advance and repeatedly revised. Communication strategies for dealing with possible scenarios should define their objectives, target audiences, key messages, communication channels and action plans.

Assessors should verify whether mechanisms exist to facilitate communication and information-sharing among stakeholders and partners, including those in the non-health sector, at the national and international levels. In the case of an emergency, information must flow both ways. The objective of carrying out surveillance, surveys and outbreak investigations is not simply to collect data and distribute health information but also to evaluate the response of the health system to the emergency and provide feedback to data collectors. Strong links between health care facility-based surveillance systems and public health surveillance systems are essential. Mechanisms should exist that facilitate the immediate reporting of all available information about possible public health threats of potential concern to the (local) public health authorities and, through them, to the national and international levels.

INDICATOR-RELATED QUESTIONS

a. Have information mechanisms for use in emergency situations been established at the community level and is trained staff available?
It is essential that populations at risk have the information they need to make well-informed decisions and take the appropriate action to protect their health and safety during an emergency.

Assessors should verify whether relevant information mechanisms exist at the community level. Communication channels should be clearly defined and the staff involved trained and readily available.

b. Does the information-management system facilitate reporting according to IHR and other mandatory reporting requirements?
States Parties to IHR (2005) have agreed to meet their requirements and obligations concerning the reporting, verification, and assessment of public health events of international concern, the implementation of WHO-recommended control measures and the development of core capacities for surveillance and response. IHR (2005) also require that States Parties collaborate with each other, as well as with WHO and other partners, in assessing and responding to significant public health events.

Assessors should verify that the information-management system is capable of meeting the IHR and other reporting requirements and that it is being used for this purpose.

RECOMMENDED READING

Abdallah, S., Burnham, G., eds. *The Johns Hopkins and IFRC public health guide for emergencies. First edition.* Geneva, International Federation of the Red Cross and Red Crescent Societies, 2004 (http://www.terzomondo.org/library /essentials/IFRC_Public_Health_Guide.pdf, accessed 18 April 2004).

Early recognition, reporting and infection control management of acute respiratory diseases of potential international concern. Aide memoire. Geneva, World Health Organization, 2008 (http://www.who.int/entity/csr/disease/avian_influenza/guidelines/EPR_AM4_E3.pdf, accessed 18 April 2011).

International Health Regulations (2005). *Second edition.* Geneva, World Health Organization, 2008 (http:// whqlibdoc.who.int/publications/2008/9789241580410_eng .pdf, accessed 18 April 2011).

World Health Organization outbreak communication planning guide. Geneva, World Health Organization, 2008 (http:// www.who.int/ihr/elibrary/WHOOutbreakComms PlanngGuide.pdf, accessed 18 April 2011).

Essential attribute 24 Surveillance systems

(See also essential attribute 22.)

KEYNOTES

Surveillance is the ongoing, systematic collection, analysis and interpretation of health data. The information generated from these data is used to plan and implement priority public health interventions and to monitor and evaluate the effectiveness of these interventions. Thus, surveillance data facilitate decision making and contribute to assessing program implementation. Surveillance is essential for monitoring disease or nutritional trends and for identifying high-risk groups or high-risk situations. The application of a surveillance system in emergency situations requires the timely collection, analysis and dissemination of information.

In emergency situations, rapid and informed decision making is a priority. Sensitivity is more important than specificity in the early stages and the surveillance system needs to be adapted accordingly. Epidemiologists tend to follow routine reporting protocols to ensure accuracy of the analysis of health data. Specific training in conducting epidemiological investigations during emergencies can facilitate an understanding of the slightly different approaches to data collection that are required in emergencies (such as the introduction of syndromic surveillance). Assessors should check whether such training is available.

In protracted emergencies, data are needed on injuries, communicable diseases, vectors, food safety, nutrition, disability, some priority noncommunicable diseases, blood safety, mental health, etc. The emergency surveillance system needs to gather these data from communities, hospitals, laboratories and blood banks in both the public and the private sectors, and to ensure that they are integrated in surveillance reports.

Surveillance of a situation according to certain key indicators makes it possible to monitor and document its evolution and progress. The monitoring of short-term trends, especially the incidence of excess cases, is of paramount importance after a disaster. Because the time and resources available for collecting, analyzing and reporting data are limited, particularly in the acute phase of an emergency, only the most essential indicators should be selected. These should be determined in advance on the basis of known risks. Relevant case definitions, case-confirmation criteria, reporting thresholds, reporting schedules and reporting formats should be carefully reviewed once an emergency occurs and temporary, situation-specific revisions should be made whenever necessary.

When setting up surveillance systems, it is important to be aware of the local distribution of health conditions and include these in the surveillance program.

Assessors should verify that all stakeholders involved in the collection of health data are identified and that their input is coordinated with and integrated in the surveillance process. For the sake of consistency, all authorities and institutions reporting through the surveillance system should use standardized case definitions. The system should be based on mandatory "zero reporting," which means that each site shall report for each reporting period even if it means reporting zero cases. This avoids the confusion of equating "no report" and "no cases." The system should also be time calibrated (e.g., daily zero reporting at first) and should define the criteria for changing reporting periods (e.g., from daily to weekly) and for returning to routine surveillance.

INDICATOR-RELATED QUESTIONS

a. *Do emergency managers have access to relevant data (including data on trauma and injuries, communicable diseases, vector-borne diseases, water quality, nutrition, noncommunicable diseases, and food safety)?*

b. *Are epidemic-related intelligence activities being carried out (baseline estimates, definition of trends and thresholds for alert and action defined at the primary-response level, regular analysis of epidemic-prone diseases, etc.)?*

c. *Is early-warning capacity in place to enable recognition of and reporting on any event of potential public health concern within 24 hours?*
The early-warning system is an important component of surveillance. It is aimed at predicting, detecting and confirming public health events in a timely fashion, and at disseminating information appropriately so that effective public health action can be taken.

Assessors should verify the existence of mechanisms to facilitate the early recognition of events of potential public health concern and the reporting of these events within 24 hours.

d. *Is the surveillance system able to provide sufficiently trained staff?*

e. *Is there a network infrastructure, including surge capacity, to enable adequate response to an event?*

f. *Does the surveillance system have standardized protocols defining roles, responsibilities and procedures related to the standardization, collection, management, analysis and dissemination of data?*

g. *Does the surveillance system provide for data-sharing with agricultural, veterinary and environmental-disease surveillance systems?*

RECOMMENDED READING

Abdallah S, Burnham G, eds. *The Johns Hopkins and IFRC public health guide for emergencies. First edition.* Geneva, International Federation of the Red Cross and Red Crescent Societies, 2004 (http://www.terzomondo.org/library/essentials/IFRC_Public_Health_Guide.pdf, accessed 18 April 2004).

Handbook for participants, management of public health risks in disasters. Regional training course on management of public health risks in disasters (MPHR). Cairo, WHO Regional Office for the Eastern Mediterranean, 2008.

> **Key component 4.2** Information-management systems for emergency response and recovery
>
> **Essential attribute 25** Rapid health-needs assessment

KEYNOTES

A rapid health-needs assessment[2] is a collection of subjective and objective information that can be used to measure the damage caused, identify the basic needs of an affected population, and determine the level and type of response needed. Its main steps are: to define the assessment priorities; to collect the data (by reviewing existing information, inspecting the affected area, interviewing key people and carrying out a rapid survey); to analyze and interpret the findings; and to present the results and conclusions. A rapid health-needs assessment is not an end in itself but the first step in a continuous process. In addition to providing initial, action-oriented information as clearly as possible, it forms the basis of more comprehensive follow-up assessments.

The objectives of a health-related humanitarian intervention during the acute phase of an emergency situation are to reduce excess mortality and morbidity and stabilize the population's health situation as rapidly as possible. In a situation marked by confusion, disruption and, often, danger, managers need access to a continuous flow of information, which—as a result of the circumstances—may not always be precise.

In most emergencies, timeliness must take precedence over accuracy, which means that life-saving decisions are taken on the basis of incomplete data. While the objective of a rapid health-needs assessment is to avoid making decisions without solid information, equally, "paralysis by analysis" must be avoided as the cost of more accurate and comprehensive information can be very high. Information in the early stages of an emergency does not need to be precise. The health sector is often overly concerned with accuracy and loses much time in pursuing it. For example, it is enough to know that about 1000 people depend on a water source, rather than to waste time in confirming that the exact number of people is 992.

There are several kinds of rapid health-needs assessment. Those carried out at the local level by local staff are required in any event. They should be based on a standardized method and format, as well as on agreed denominators, so that information from multiple sources can be usefully collated. Assessments carried out by national-level health staff, international agencies or NGOs should be conducted as joint assessments.

---

[2] The key questions to be answered in a rapid health-needs assessment are the following. Is there an emergency or not? What are the type, impact and possible evolution of the emergency? What are the most severely affected geographic area and catchment population? What is the main health problem? What is the existing response capacity? What are the critical information gaps (for follow-up assessments)? What response action is recommended as priority? What resources are needed to implement priority action? *(17)*

INDICATOR-RELATED QUESTIONS

a. *Do mechanisms exist for carrying out rapid health-needs assessments?*

b. *Are the necessary resources and trained staff available for doing so?*
   Assessors should verify that the following elements are in place:

   • clearly defined criteria for rapid health-needs assessment, i.e., when and when not to carry out an assessment, how to do so and which data to collect;
   • agreement with the sub-national authorities on the authority of the assessment team;
   • information on support for assessment teams (security, transport, communications, funding);
   • agreed and reliable denominators extracted from the different registries maintained by the health information system (see essential attribute 22), as well as the most recent population figures (see essential attribute 21);
   • adequate training for the staff and mechanisms to ensure that those involved are experienced;
   • a balanced team (vis-à-vis expertise, representation of different entities, etc.).

   Since a rapid health-needs assessment requires a broad analysis, public health generalists, rather than specialists, should be included in the team.

   Assessors should also verify that all possible avenues are explored to find the capacity required for carrying out rapid health-needs assessments. One example could be to identify potential institutions and agencies that could provide the necessary resources and integrate their input.

c. *Do data resulting from rapid health-needs assessments determine resources' allocation and priority action?*
   Assessors should verify that mechanisms exist for allocating resources and setting priorities on the basis of data resulting from rapid health-needs assessments. This requires that assessment reports are clear, standardized, action-oriented, timely and widely distributed.

d. *Do these data reflect the needs in terms of the population and health services' delivery?*
   A common mistake in carrying out rapid health-needs assessments is to determine health needs according to the presence or absence of health services without considering the health status of the population and the risks to which it is exposed. Systemic links should be established between health needs associated with: (i) current and future health risks; (ii) the capacity to deliver priority health care services; and (iii) the current health status. Addressing the determinants of the health status is necessary to improve the health of the affected population; systematic ways of doing so need to be found.

   The data do not need to be collected by external teams. A well-designed local emergency reporting system that continues to function in a crisis can provide all this information just as effectively and at considerably less cost both in time and resources.

RECOMMENDED READING

Darcy J, Hofmann C A. *According to need? Needs assessment and decision-making in the humanitarian sector. HPG Report 15, September 2003*. London, Overseas Development Institute, 2003 (http://www.odi.org.uk/resources /download/239.pdf, accessed 28 October 2011).

Inter-Agency Standing Committee, Global Health Cluster. *Health Cluster guide. A practical guide for country-level implementation of the Health Cluster*. Geneva, World Health Organization, 2009 (http://whqlibdoc.who.int /hq/2009/WHO_HAC_MAN_2009.7_eng.pdf, accessed 18 April 2011).

Rapid health assessment guidelines. Regional training course on rapid health assessment, 27–30 November 2007, Ha Noi, Viet Nam. Manila, WHO Regional Office for the Western Pacific, 2007 (http://www.wpro.who.int/internet /files/eha/dir/Regional%20Training%20Course%20on%20 Rapid%20Health%20Assessment/RHA%20global%20 health%20cluster.pdf, accessed 18 April 2011).

Thieren M. Health information systems in humanitarian emergencies. *Bulletin of the World Health Organization*, 2005, 83(8):584–589 (http://www.who.int/bulletin /volumes/83/8/584.pdf, accessed 18 April 2011).

> **Essential attribute 26** Multisectoral initial rapid assessment (IRA)

KEYNOTES

The purpose of a multisectoral IRA is to quickly provide an overview of an emergency situation based on essential multisectoral data, identify its immediate impacts of the crisis, estimate the needs and vulnerabilities of the affected population, and define the priorities for humanitarian action *(18)*. The areas assessed are security, infrastructure, shelter, sanitation and access to food and water. Frequently, health is not included, usually because the health sector has the reputation of collecting data efficiently through its own reporting systems. Other sectors do not have this capacity built in to their normal working methods. However, it is important for the health sector to be represented on an IRA team. This provides health staff with the opportunity to access data on important determinants of health at an early stage, which facilitates the prediction and prevention of future health risks. In addition, the IRA team can benefit from the information and comments provided by the health staff, which will improve the quality and usefulness of their report.

An IRA team should comprise generalists from various sectors rather than specialists only. However, although the use of generalists increases flexibility and reduces the expenses and time required, it does not eliminate the need for specialists. While junior staff members can participate effectively in the data-gathering process, the overall coordination and management of IRAs requires significant experience in emergency-related assessment and monitoring activities.

Data provided by means of IRAs are preliminary and their quality is limited by constraints in time and opportunity to structure their sampling and collection during the onset of an emergency. The exercise is limited to an approximate assessment of damage and immediate needs and cannot provide comprehensive, statistically sound or in-depth qualitative data. However, the IRA is the first step in a continuous process and, therefore, identifies needs to be considered in more comprehensive follow-up assessments (see also essential attribute 25).

One of the most common errors made in carrying out IRAs is to collect too much data and/or irrelevant information. It is important that the information needed at the different stages of emergency management is clearly defined (see also essential attribute 12).

INDICATOR-RELATED QUESTIONS

a. *Is the health sector fully involved in the planning, preparation and implementation of IRAs?*

b. *Do health professionals receive appropriate training in carrying out IRAs?*
    Although the health sector is not responsible for the overall IRA process, it should be fully involved and contribute actively. The assessment of health-sector damages (loss of staff, loss of services, lack of water for health care facilities, etc.) is a critical issue.

    Assessors should verify that participants in IRAs are adequately trained and significantly experienced in emergency-related assessment and monitoring activities and that they have a full understanding of the methodology, practical options and limitations of the exercise.

c. *Do mechanisms exist for allocating resources and initiating priority action based on IRA data?*
    Assessors should verify that mechanisms exist for allocating resources and setting priorities on the basis of IRA data. This requires that IRA reports are clear, standardized, action-oriented, timely and widely distributed.

RECOMMENDED READING

Checchi F, Roberts L. *Interpreting and using mortality data in humanitarian emergencies: A primer for non-epidemiologists. Humanitarian Practice Network (HPN) paper no. 52, September 2005*. London, Overseas Development Institute, 2005 (http://www.odihpn.org/documents/networkpaper052 .pdf, accessed 19 April 2011).

Guidelines for emergency assessment. Geneva, International Federation of Red Cross and Red Crescent Societies, 2005 (http:// www.proventionconsortium.org/themes/default/pdfs/71600- Guidelines-for-emergency-en.pdf, accessed 19 April 2011).

Handbook for participants, management of public health risks in disasters. Regional training course on management of public health risks in disasters (MPHR). Cairo, WHO Regional Office for the Eastern Mediterranean, 2008.

Initial rapid assessment (IRA): guidance notes for country level. Version for field testing. Geneva, Inter-Agency Standing Committee, 2007 (www.humanitarianreform.org /humanitarianreform/Portals/1/cluster%20approach%20page /clusters%20pages/health%20cluster/RT/IRA_Guidance_ Country%20Level_field_test.doc, accessed 19 April 2011).

Essential attribute 27 Emergency reporting system

KEYNOTES

An emergency reporting system provides information on all health-sector activities with the exception of surveillance, which usually has its own system. It furnishes decision makers with an overview of the daily activities of the office, program, hospital, service or institution in question and the problems or constraints they are encountering. It also provides the latest status reports on functionality (damages and repairs), staffing, supplies, security, and other factors, as well as information on workload (e.g., number of patients seen or specimens processed per day), meetings held and decisions taken.

Routine data reporting takes place weekly or monthly. The data, which are collected and processed regularly, are usually based on a set of indicators. However, a routine reporting system, which requires the collection of large quantities of data, is not efficient in emergencies. It does not include reporting on damaged or destroyed facilities, or on missing staff and supplies and, thus, cannot provide all the relevant information needed for rapid decision making in emergencies. In addition, it is very slow and cannot capture the onset of severe emergencies (e.g., an outbreak of disease) early enough.

In emergency situations, only data that are necessary for decision making should be collected and processed. These data must be reported on a more frequent basis (daily) from the onset of an emergency. Indicators for new events might not exist in the routine reporting system and in emergency situations investigations might have to be made without them. This implies that surveillance should be based not only on a set of indicators but also on the actual emergency event.

Assessors should verify that mechanisms exist for reporting emergency events in a timely manner.

INDICATOR-RELATED QUESTIONS

a. *Does an emergency reporting system exist?*

b. *Are resources and trained staff available ?*
   Assessors should verify that an emergency reporting system exists, that there are activating and de-activating trigger mechanisms, and that staff have been trained in using the system.

c. *Does the emergency reporting system provide information on critical human resources, health infrastructure, etc.?*
   Assessors should verify whether there are mechanisms for collating the reports of all the programs and services of the ministry of health and ensuring that they reach decision makers in a timely manner.

d. *Are data from all relevant stakeholders collected through the emergency reporting system?*
   Assessors should verify the existence of mechanisms to ensure that data from various stakeholders can be collected and processed if needed.

KEY REFERENCE DOCUMENT

Connolly MA, ed. *Communicable disease control in emergencies. A field manual.* Geneva, World Health Organization, 2005 (WHO/CDS/2005.27) (http://www .who.int/infectious-disease-news/IDdocs/whocds200527/ ISBN_9241546166.pdf, accessed 19 April 2011).

Key component 4.3 Risk communication

Essential attribute 28 Strategies for risk communication with the public and the media

KEYNOTES

During an emergency, communication with the public and the media needs to be carefully planned and executed. It also needs to be properly integrated with emergency-management activities.[3] To communicate effectively through the media[4], response managers must plan their communication strategies accordingly and be ready promptly to provide transparent messages addressing public concerns. Doing so strengthens public confidence, minimizes secondary damage (such as adverse economic or political impact) and maintains the credibility of the health sector.

INDICATOR-RELATED QUESTIONS

a. *Are the communication strategies based on risk assessment?*

b. *Are there coordination mechanisms in place for involving stakeholders in the formulation of information for the public and the media to ensure consistency?*
   To ensure the timely delivery of accurate and consistent information, coordination mechanisms should be in place to streamline information-sharing among various stakeholders.

c. *Do procedures exist for the dissemination of information?*
   Assessors should determine whether channels have been identified for the dissemination of messages (e.g., radio, television, World Wide Web, telephone and information services, social networks) and whether documented plans and procedures exist for interacting with the media and the public during an emergency.

d. *Is information regarding ongoing emergency-preparedness activities systematically communicated to the public and the media?*

e. *Do the communication strategies also target minority and vulnerable populations?*

---

[3]The WHO outbreak communication principles are: 1. trust; 2. early announcement; 3. transparency; 4. listening; and planning *(19)*.

[4]WHO recommends seven steps to effective media communication during public health emergencies: (1) assessment of media needs, media constraints and internal media-relations' capabilities; (2) development of goals, plans and strategies; (3) training of communicators; (4) preparation of messages; (5) identification of media outlets and media activities; (6) delivery of messages; and (7) evaluation of messages and performance *(20)*.

Assessors should verify whether mechanisms for reaching vulnerable, isolated and minority populations exist—including ways of overcoming challenges related to technology, language and culture—and whether representatives of these groups are included in the planning process.

f. Is the function of spokesperson defined?
A well-trained, lead spokesperson and a media communication team are necessary to ensure effective media communications during public health emergencies.

Assessors should verify whether a spokesperson with the necessary training in risk communication and public health has been designated. The spokesperson should have excellent communication skills and sufficient experience to be able to simplify information flow and promote the consistency of message content. Several trained persons should be available to act as backup in different scenarios, if needed.

RECOMMENDED READING

Effective media communication during public health emergencies. A WHO handbook. Geneva, World Health Organization, 2005 (WHO/CDS/2005.31) (http://www.who.int /entity/csr/resources/publications/WHO%20MEDIA%20 HANDBOOK.pdf, accessed 19 April 2011).

Effective media communication during public health emergencies. A WHO field guide. Geneva, World Health Organization, 2005 (WHO/CDS/2005.31a) (http://www.who.int /entity/csr/resources/publications/WHO%20MEDIA%20 FIELD%20GUIDE.pdf, accessed 19 April 2011).

Pan American Health Organization, WHO Regional Office for the Western Pacific. *Creating a communication strategy for pandemic influenza.* Washington, DC, Pan American Health Organization, 2009 (http://www.paho.org/english/ad /PAHO_CommStrategy_Eng.pdf, accessed 19 April 2011).

World Health Organization outbreak communication planning guide. Geneva, World Health Organization, 2008 (http://www .who.int/ihr/elibrary/WHOOutbreakCommsPlanngGuide.pdf, accessed 19 April 2011).

> **Essential attribute 29**   Strategies for risk communication with staff involved in emergency operations

KEYNOTES

Although the degree of risk varies in emergency-response operations, security incidents can occur that sometimes result in the death of responders. Although security risks cannot be completely eliminated during these operations, they can be kept to an absolute minimum. One way of doing so is to ensure that responders are aware of the risks and immediately provided with the necessary support (transport, protection, etc.) to enable them to fulfill their roles. All responders should participate in security-related courses on, for example, radio communication, the local language and culture and how to deal with checkpoints, road-traffic accidents, criminal activity or open-conflict situations.

The health sector is responsible for ensuring that all emergency responders have access to accurate and reliable information about the health risks they could face while carrying out their duties during an emergency and for providing them with advice on how to protect themselves. It is important that mechanisms exist for the rapid development of event-specific information for emergency-response agencies and the dissemination of this information to all stakeholders.

As regards telecommunications equipment (see also essential attribute 48), it is of vital importance that the communications system enables constant and direct communication among stakeholders, between stakeholders and responders, and among the responders themselves. It is important that responders from all sectors involved in telecommunications receive adequate training in how to set up and use the telecommunications equipment. They should also verify the existence of basic security regulations.

Standard procedures should be established for the systematic and immediate reporting of all security incidents affecting responders. Reports should include only facts and avoid assumptions or conclusions. At the same time, it should be possible for responders to report any observations of danger. A developing risk—such as renewed movement of terrain after a landslide or mudflow caused by floods or an earthquake—might be discovered by a responder at a location some distance from the place in which its consequences will endanger the lives of relief workers.

INDICATOR-RELATED QUESTIONS

a. Do coordination mechanisms exist to ensure the consistency of information supplied by stakeholders to responders?
During operations, responders might receive conflicting information, attributable often to the fact that the various reporting parties assess risks differently, which could undermine the security of the responders. In addition, if responders receive information that is inconsistent with their observations, they might start to doubt any of the information provided.

Assessors should determine whether stakeholders have mechanisms for ensuring the consistency of risk information provided to responders, as well as the accuracy and reliability of advice on how to protect themselves.

b. Do procedures exist for the communication of risk information by stakeholders to responders?
It is important that responders involved in emergency operations be provided with timely and reliable health and safety information.

Assessors should verify the existence of procedures to be followed by stakeholders in doing so.

c. Has information on specific risks and self-protection measures for responders involved in emergency operations been prepared and, if so, is it regularly updated and disseminated?
Mechanisms must be in place to enable the prompt communication of information on possible risks and self-protection measures to responders. For example, PPE,

vaccinations, prophylactic medication and other such factors may need to be addressed in the midst of a rapidly evolving emergency. Information of this kind must be regularly updated and disseminated. Furthermore, it is important for team members to recognize that the action taken by one team member can affect the security of others, sometimes in ways that are not obvious. Hence, responders need to take charge of their own security and try to minimize not only their own security risks but also those of the team as a whole[5].

RECOMMENDED READING

Emergency response and recovery. Non statutory guidance accompanying the Civil Contingencies Act 2004. London, Her Majesty's Government, 2010 (http://www.worcestershire.gov.uk/cms/pdf/EmergencyResponse&Recovery%20April%202010.pdf, accessed 19 April 2011).

Resilient telecommunications. In: *Emergency response and recovery. Non statutory guidance accompanying the Civil Contingencies Act 2004. Third edition.* London, Her Majesty's Government, 2010 (http://www.cabinetoffice.gov.uk/sites/default/files/resources/emergency-response-recovery_0.pdf, accessed 19 April 2011).

● SECTION 5. HEALTH FINANCING

This chapter evaluates the health financing strategies and mechanisms required to ensure the funding and financial protection necessary to enable the health system to reduce existing risks and avoid generating new ones.

Key component 5.1 National and subnational strategies for financing health-sector emergency management

Essential attribute 30 Multisectoral mechanisms of financing emergency preparedness and management

INDICATOR-RELATED QUESTIONS

a. *Are funds available for the multisectoral preparedness for, and management of, emergencies at the national and subnational levels?*

b. *Do multisectoral financing mechanisms include contingency funding for response and recovery at the national and subnational levels?*

---

[5]The following "seven pillars of security" may be useful in strengthening individual responsibility: (1) acceptance (accepting that normal personal freedom may be restricted); (2) identification (always carrying proper identification for operations, vehicles, staff, etc.); (3) information (taking responsibility for updating oneself about the security situation); (4) regulations (following appropriate security rules and regulations (with respect, for example, to travel, curfews, etc.); (5) behavior (being honest, practicing self-discipline and showing respect for the local culture and social habits); communication (observing the security rules about promptly communicating one's whereabouts) (6) protection (taking simple precautions to protect oneself and other team members and understanding the evacuation procedures) *(21).*

c. *Are multisectoral financing procedures available for the request, acceptance and utilization of international financial assistance?*
Assessors should verify whether funds are dedicated in the national budget for emergency-management and preparedness planning, more specifically for human resources, coordination, staff training, information management, simulation exercises, public awareness, supplies and equipment, and monitoring and evaluation. There should be a fast-track mechanism for requests from the ministry of health for national emergency contingency funds.

RECOMMENDED READING

Langabeer JR et al. Investment, managerial capacity, and bias in public health preparedness. *American Journal of Disaster Medicine*, 2009, 4(4):207–215.

De Lorenzo RA. Financing hospital disaster preparedness. *Prehospital and Disaster Medicine*, 2007, 22(5):436–439.

Essential attribute 31 Health-sector financing mechanisms

KEYNOTE

The financing strategy of the ministry of health should provide for emergency-management activities, including operations for risk reduction and emergency preparedness and response. This also means funding action to determine the resilience of critical medical facilities (hospitals, laboratories, blood banks, warehouses, etc.) and to make necessary improvements according to a plan based on risk assessment and the level of importance of the facility. Funding to reduce the structural and nonstructural vulnerability of health facilities should be a budgetary priority.

INDICATOR-RELATED QUESTIONS

a. *Do the health-sector financing mechanisms include a budget for a risk-reduction program?*

b. *Are funds designated for a health-sector emergency-preparedness program?*
Assessors should verify that funds for emergency preparedness are allocated in the budget of the ministry of health.

c. *Do mechanisms exist for accessing contingency funds for health-sector emergency-response and recovery operations?*
Assessors should determine whether the ministry of health has contingency funds and, if so, whether they are easily accessible when a crisis situation demands a rapid response necessitating an increase in health expenditure that is not provided for in the normal budget. Contingency funds should be sufficient to meet most needs in the short-term (staffing, procurement of essential supplies and services) according to the scenarios outlined in the risk assessment. The administrative procedures for accessing and allocating contingency funds in a crisis should be flexible and transparent and they should cater for fast-tracking.

d. *Do health-sector financing mechanisms include effective and rapid recovery for loss and damage (e.g., damage to health facilities)?*

Critical facilities should be insured for damage in the event of a natural or human-made disaster. Insurance should be comprehensive and a fast-tracking mechanism should be in place for the dealing with claims connected with the restoration of the facility.

Health staff operating in crises at the national and international levels should be insured for accidents, illness and death while performing their duties. Catastrophe bonds should be available to assist insurance companies to meet their commitments in the event of a major catastrophe, the impact of which exceeds their absorption capacity.

RECOMMENDED READING

Hanfling D. Equipment, supplies and pharmaceuticals: how much might it cost to achieve basic surge capacity? *Academic Emergency Medicine*, 2006, 13:1232–1237.

SECTION 6. SERVICE DELIVERY

Key component 6.1 Response capacity and capability

Essential attribute 32 Subnational health-sector emergency-response plans

(See also essential attribute 13.)

INDICATOR-RELATED QUESTIONS

a. *Are subnational emergency-response plans based on national policy?*

Subnational health-related emergency-response plans should ensure safe, effective and coordinated health and medical response in an emergency by:

- establishing a health-sector incident management structure at the subnational level that both interfaces and works with the national incident management structure;
- coordinating health resources (from those at the incident site to those at the receiving health care facilities);
- managing prehospital resources and ensuring hospital interaction.

Emergency-response plans should follow an all-hazards approach, the concept of which acknowledges that, while hazards vary in source (natural, technological, social), they often challenge health systems in similar ways. Thus, the principles outlined in emergency-response plans should apply in any type of emergency. Experience shows that a substantial part of essential response action is generic (dissemination of health information, establishment of an emergency-operations center, coordination of activities, logistics, communication with the public, etc.), irrespective

of the hazard. Prioritizing these generic response measures generates synergies that benefit overall response operations and results. Assessors should verify that subnational emergency-response plans follow national policy and involve all relevant stakeholders, which would ensure the effective management and coordination of the whole-health response.

b. *Are these plans compatible with the relevant subnational multisectoral emergency plan?*

Evaluators should verify that health-sector emergency-response plans are compatible with and linked to the relevant subnational multisectoral emergency plan.

c. *Do the plans define mechanisms for activation, coordination, command, and control?*

To ensure appropriate mechanisms for the activation, coordination, command and control of an emergency response, the existence of an integrated incident-management system (IMS) is essential. IMS (also referred to as "incident-command system") involves personnel, policies, procedures, facilities and equipment combined in a common organizational structure designed to improve emergency-response operations of all types and levels of complexity. An emergency operation in response to an incident, the nature and scale of which could have an impact on the health and well-being of the population, typically involves multiple agencies and requires the integration of their emergency plans.

d. *Are the plans based on available resources?*

e. *Are the plans tested, validated, exercised, and maintained?*

f. *Are the plans revised on the basis of lessons learned?*

Assessors should verify that subnational plans are: (i) based on available resources; (ii) regularly tested, validated, exercised and maintained; and (iii) revised on the basis of lessons learned. They should also establish whether key staff with responsibilities in health-sector response receives regular training as part of the process to ensure functionality of the plan.

g. *Are the plans disseminated to key stakeholders after each revision?*

Planning a health-sector emergency-response plan at the subnational level requires the involvement of many stakeholders to ensure that it is managed and coordinated according to the whole-health approach. Therefore, it is important to disseminate the emergency-response plan to the key stakeholders every time it is revised.

N.B. In general, key stakeholders are required, in consultation with partner agencies, to develop standard operating procedures (SOPs) consistent with the principles of the emergency-response plan. SOPs form a major component of the plan and should be clearly formulated, regularly reviewed, and distributed to all concerned after every revision.

RECOMMENDED READING

Mass casualty management systems. Strategies and guidelines for building health sector capacity. Geneva, World Health Organization, 2007 (http://www.who.int/hac/techguidance /MCM_guidelines_inside_final.pdf, accessed 25 April 2011).

State health emergency response plan. SHERP Victoria. Second edition—2009. Melbourne, Department of Health, 2009 (http://www.dhs.vic.gov.au/__data/assets/pdf_ file/0005/400883/SHERP_2nd_edition_web.pdf, accessed 25 April 2011).

Wahle T, Beatty G. *Emergency management guide for business & industry: a step-by-step approach to emergency planning, response and recovery for companies of all sizes.* Washington, DC, Federal Emergency Management Agency, 1993 (http://www.fema.gov/pdf/business/guide/bizindst .pdf, accessed 25 April 2011).

Essential attribute 33 Surge capacity for subnational health-sector response

---

(See also key component 2.1.)

KEYNOTES

The concept of medical surge forms the cornerstone of preparedness planning for major incidents of medical concern. *Surge* can be defined as "a demand for health services in a mass-casualty incident where additional capacities (in terms of the amount of personnel, equipment or supplies) and/or capabilities (in terms of specialized expertise) are required" *(22)*.

Medical surge has two components, capacity and capability. Medical surge *capacity* refers to the ability to evaluate and care for a markedly increased volume of patients (i.e., exceeding normal operating capacity). The surge requirements may extend beyond direct patient care to include such tasks as extensive laboratory studies or epidemiological investigations.

Medical surge *capability* refers to the ability of the health care infrastructure to manage patients (e.g., those infected with highly contagious pathogens) requiring unusual or specialized medical evaluation and care (i.e., specialized medical and health services) that are not normally available at the location at which they are needed. Surge capability also includes special interventions to safeguard those providing medical care to these patients and to protect other patients in the health care facility concerned.

Staff training is a key element of both the surge capacity and the surge capability of the health sector.

A mass-casualty incident has been defined as an event which generates more patients at one time than locally available resources can manage using routine procedures. It requires exceptional emergency arrangements and additional or extraordinary assistance *(23)*. It has also been defined as any event resulting in a number of victims large enough to disrupt the normal course of emergency and health care services *(24)*.

Although national policy on managing mass-casualty incidents is essential, preparedness at the subnational (provincial and municipal) levels is crucial to the success of the national emergency plan. Strategies for enhancing medical surge capacity and capability require a systems-based approach rooted in interdisciplinary coordination at the local level. Ideally, this approach should be tiered to link hospitals, hospital networks and management systems at the national and subnational levels, and comprise: management of individual health care assets (tier 1); management of a hospitals' network (tier 2); management of municipal response (tier 3); management of provincial response (tier 4); and national coordination and support to lower-level tiers (tier 5) *(22)*. Larger countries might be able to apply all five tiers but constraints in smaller countries could exclude this possibility. To make the tier approach more flexible, it might be useful to consider scaling the response.

The tiers of a mass-casualty management system do not operate in a vacuum. To assure maximum response in a mass-casualty incident, there should be coordination among the different tiers and between these and the non-medical incident response. At the same time, it is important to use resources and services as far as possible and to strengthen and develop them when necessary.

INDICATOR-RELATED QUESTIONS

a. *Do mechanisms exist for the rapid mobilization of additional resources (personnel, equipment and materials) to and between the subnational levels?*

A scalable approach to assuring the necessary medical surge capacity for mass-casualty management requires the integration of stakeholders' efforts and relevant available resources (field hospitals, mobile hubs, military transport capacity, etc.), at both the national and subnational levels, including the private sector, NGOs, the military, and others (see also essential attribute 4).

b. *Are there procedures in place for the pre-positioning of essential supplies and for their release to high-risk areas?*

In order to supplement health-sector resources, private health services (including ambulance services, private hospitals and health professionals) and NGOs should be included as part of the surge capacity. The local emergency-management authorities should have access to an inventory of available services and resources (including human resources). Procedures for pre-positioning various supplies (e.g., medicines, disaster stockpiles) and an adequate management system should be in place. The private sector, NGOs and other stakeholders should participate in planning the response to mass-casualty incidents, as well as in relevant training exercises. Private companies and businesses may also be able to contribute significantly to planning and response. In this context, standardized procedures and risk communication are the key elements in enhancing cooperation and coordination among the actors.

c. *Do mechanisms of hospital networking exist?*

In emergency situations, public, diagnostic, and curative health facilities can become overwhelmed, and it is of paramount importance that they can share the increased demand for medical intervention. To this end, hospital networking might be included in subnational (provincial and municipal) emergency-response plans.

d. *Do procedures and the required capacity (ventilators, incubators, etc.) exist for providing life support and critical care during patient dispatch to hospitals outside the affected area?*

RECOMMENDED READING

American Red Cross et al. *Emergency management guide for business and industry. A step-by-step approach to emergency planning, response and recovery for companies of all sizes.* Washington, DC, Federal Emergency Management Agency, 1993 (http://www.fema.gov/pdf/business/guide /bizindst.pdf, accessed 26 April 2011).

Knebel A, Trabert E, eds. *Medical surge capacity and capability: a management system for integrating medical and health resources during large-scale emergencies.* Washington, DC, Department of Health and Human Services, 2007 (http://www.phe.gov/preparedness/planning/mscc /handbook/pages/default.aspx, accessed 20 July 2011).

Mass casualty management systems. Strategies and guidelines for building health sector capacity. Geneva, World Health Organization, 2007 (http://www.who.int/hac/techguidance /MCM_guidelines_inside_final.pdf, accessed 26 April 2011).

Essential attribute 34 Management of prehospital medical operations

---

INDICATOR-RELATED QUESTIONS

a. *Is there a system in place for managing medical activities at the scene?*
    Prehospital medical operations include the medical evacuation and triage of patients and their dispatch to and receipt by health care facilities. In terms of space, prehospital medical care starts at the disaster site and continues to the triage or reception area of the receiving hospital; in terms of time, from when the alarm is heard (or the pre-alert, when there is warning time) until the admission of the last casualty. Each country has its own prehospital system, also for medical operations, and its ministry of health should issue policy and application guidelines within the framework of that system at the multisectoral level (see also key components 5 and 6).
    Regardless of the policy being followed on alerting the different emergency services (e.g., the use of a single national emergency number), assessors should verify whether efficient communication systems and clear procedures for doing so are in place and in accordance with the multisectoral emergency plan.
    The management of prehospital medical operations involves considering the following broad spectrum of components during assessments:

- integrated incident-management and command system (see also essential attribute 32);
- medical surge capacity (see also essential attribute 33);
- pre-positioning of disaster stocks;
- on-site organization of medical activities;
- activity types, services to be delivered and services-delivery agencies;
- triage (different types and algorithms; medical-disaster triage teams, etc.);
- emergency communications;
- logistics for prehospital medical operations (see also essential attribute 50);
- evacuation process;
- intersectoral coordination;
- coordination between prehospital and hospital components;
- health-sector preparedness (e.g., disaster and trauma teams);
- different types of training;
- community preparedness.

Assessors should determine whether all seven steps of the prehospital chain[6] are in place and whether the system is compatible with the different characteristics of disasters (type, magnitude, scope, accessibility of disaster site, etc.). The fundamental prerequisites for success are the following: an intersectoral emergency-management strategy based on broad health-sector policy; the designation and clear definition of overall authority and responsibilities (also in relation to the disaster site); regular training programs in emergency management; and medical teams trained and ready to operate in special environments.

b. *Is a standardized triage system in place?*
    When the number of casualties in an emergency exceeds the capacity of the individual medical teams to cope, it is necessary to organize the emergency-management triage process as quickly as possible. Although the goal of triage is to provide the greatest chance of survival to the largest possible number of casualties, assessors should bear in mind that triage is an ongoing process, which includes continuous evaluation and re-evaluation at each level of the chain over time. Triage protocols are of limited value unless triage is viewed as a process including: assessment of the medical condition of the patients; provision of immediate, basic, life-saving care; decision making on the degree of priority for further medical care; and/or evacuation of patients. Therefore, it is necessary to integrate triage protocols into the broader framework of a mass-casualty management system.
    The triage system should be standardized, taking protocols, methodology (forms and tags), staff education and resources into account. There are many different triage protocols in use in the countries. In some, trained laypersons and emergency and rescue personnel (e.g., firefighters) participate in a non-medical triage "system."

---

[6]The seven steps of the prehospital chain are (1) alert (in some situations warning); (2) reconnaissance; (3) setting up front medical organization; (4) triage and emergency care; (5) medical care during relief and rescue operations; (6) medical evacuation; (7) hospital reception (unloading of patients) *(25).*

In others, where physicians actively contribute to the delivery of prehospital medical care in mass-casualty incidents, the protocols are based on medical triage, which is handled by medical personnel with clinical experience (mainly, but not limited to, emergency medical technicians, emergency physicians and trauma surgeons). All countries would benefit from developing their own triage protocols based on medical triage rather than on non-medical protocols.

The triage process itself does not guarantee the efficient management of prehospital activities and use of scarce resources. The delivery of basic life-saving care and the appropriate dispatch of patients are of primary importance if the management of a mass-casualty incident is to result in a positive health outcome.[7]

c. *Is there a system in place for medical evacuation and dispatch to appropriate health care facilities?*
Assessors should check whether procedures for the evacuation and dispatch of patients to receiving hospitals are in place. This is a major element of response management.

Dispatch and transport are not the same. It is important to carry out patient dispatch according to pre-established criteria, such as the capacity and capability of the receiving hospitals.

Assessors should also verify whether there are provisions for the implementation of an advanced medical post (AMP) in emergencies for the registration, triage, medical care, discharge or evacuation of all casualties. An AMP might consist of several sections (e.g., for command, evacuation, care delivery, and administration), all of which carry out duties assigned to them in an emergency. However, not all situations require the establishment of a formal AMP. In some cases, other quality health care facilities with resources for patient transport might carry out AMP activities, or it may be decided to transfer victims to hospitals immediately (especially if the total number of severe cases is low).

d. *Do search and rescue operations include a medical component?*
Assessors should verify whether a medical component is included in search-and-rescue operations. The aim of including medical staff in a search and rescue task force is to assure health care and emergency medical treatment for members of the task force and advanced life support for victims. It is not the intention that these medical staff should act as a free-standing medical resource at the disaster site. Capable local medical systems are considered to be the primary providers of general medical care for disaster victims.

e. *Are there specific arrangements in place for the prehospital handling of patients with diseases with epidemic*

potential and victims of chemical, biological, radiological, and nuclear (CBRN) incidents?
Assessors should verify that prehospital management plans and procedures incorporate the following: management of diseases with epidemic potential[8] and CBRN incidents, such as adequate resources (e.g., PPE, life-saving antidotes, personnel); training; protection of the health transport system; contribution to communicable-diseases surveillance and response to outbreaks; sentinel and warning system for unusual events (CBRN); mass decontamination of casualties; and waste management. Arrangements with stakeholders outside the health sector (police, firefighters, etc.) should also be in place.

RECOMMENDED READING

Mass casualty management system. Strategies and guidelines for building health sector capacity. Geneva, World Health Organization, 2007 (http://www.who.int/hac/techguidance /MCM_guidelines_inside_final.pdf, accessed 26 April 2011).
Urban search and rescue capability guidelines for structural collapse response. Canberra, Emergency Management Australia, 2002 (http://www.ema.gov.au/www/emaweb/rwpattach.nsf /VAP/(3273BD3F76A7A5DEDAE36942A54D7D90) ~Manual16-UARCapabilityGuidelinesforStructuralCollapse Response.pdf/$file/Manual16-USARCapabilityGuidelines-forStructuralCollapseResponse.pdf, accessed 26 April 2011).

Essential attribute 35 Management of situations involving mass fatality and missing persons

KEYNOTE

Assessors need to verify whether there are mechanisms and procedures in place for the management of victims and missing persons. Governments have a critical role to play in standardizing procedures to guide the process, ensure compliance with legal norms, and guarantee respect for the deceased and their families (see also essential attribute 1).

The management of victims involves several activities: the search for corpses; their transfer to the facility serving as a morgue; identification procedures, if required; the delivery of bodies to family members; and disposal of the bodies (in accordance with the wishes of the families and the religious and cultural norms of the community). This process requires the involvement of different stakeholders, including rescue personnel, experts in forensic medicine, public prosecutors, police, administrative personnel, psychologists, support teams, representatives of NGOs and international organizations, community volunteers and religious representatives.

Assessors should identify the leading agency for the management of victims and missing persons. Normally, the health sector would take the leading role in addressing public health concerns related to corpses (e.g., presumed epidemiological risks) and in providing medical and psychological assistance to

---

[7]Dispatch in disasters has two components: quantitative (capacity for transport, types of vehicles, etc.); and qualitative (types of medical care, medical staff and health care facility needed for patient care and evacuation).

[8]It is important to note that communicable diseases with epidemic potential pose a different challenge regardless of whether or not there is human-to-human transmission.

victims' families. To avoid duplication of effort, it is of primary importance to coordinate all action taken. When foreign aid is involved, the work becomes even more complex. In such cases, it is necessary to include embassies and the ministry of foreign affairs. Early coordination is vital at the subnational (provincial and municipal) levels and national disaster-preparedness plans should address this. (See also essential attributes 10, 12, and 13.)

INDICATOR-RELATED QUESTIONS

a. *Are there mechanisms in place for identifying victims and tracking missing persons?*

b. *Are there mechanisms in place for the storage and release of corpses?*
The mobilization of forensic resources may be delayed for days, resulting in lost opportunities of early identification as the bodies decompose. Visual recognition (although there is a risk of error by the observer) or photographs of fresh bodies are the simplest forms of identification and can maximize the early non-forensic identification process. Visual recognition should be confirmed by the identification of other material, such as clothing or personal effects.

Assessors should verify that identification procedures include: *unique referencing* (sequentially assigning unique references to each body or body part); *labeling* (entering each unique reference on a body tag); *taking photographs* (ensuring that each unique reference is visible in a photograph); *recording* (documenting data relating to the body, e.g., sex, age, personal belongings); and *securing* (securely packaging personal belongings labeled with body tags with the same unique reference as the body or body part and stored with the body or body part).

The responsible authority should not release a body until identification is certain. It must also provide release documentation (a letter or death certificate).

The recovery and storage of bodies are also issues that need special consideration. In emergencies, body recovery can take from a few days to several weeks; however, in the case of a very large disaster (such as an earthquake), the period necessary for this action may be longer. Without cold storage, decomposition advances rapidly. Burial preserves evidence for possible future forensic investigation and is thus the most practical method of disposing of dead bodies.

However, the cremation of unidentified bodies should be avoided.

c. *Are there mechanisms in place for informing the public about the dead?*
In the event of mass fatalities, the way in which information about dead bodies and their release is conveyed to the public is important. The commonly held belief that human and animal corpses pose a public health threat confuses the authorities and the general public alike. In past crises, confusion of this kind has frequently led to incorrect prioritization and misuse of scarce resources.

d. *Are there mechanisms in place for assisting international disaster victim identification (DVI) teams, if needed?*

e. *Has surge capacity been provided for with respect to forensics and mortuaries?*
In an emergency situation, forensic institutes and mortuaries might become overwhelmed. Close collaboration is needed among professionals and experts carrying out medicolegal work[9] and stakeholders that are able to provide these services. The composition of a medicolegal working group for managing mass fatalities will vary according to the conditions at the disaster site, the human resources available on site and the preparedness plan. When faced with a disaster, a community must incorporate resources, including scientists and professionals with specific roles in the community, such as those related to family support, logistics, dissemination of information and communication. Agreements should be made with the appropriate individuals or groups regarding the necessary personnel, work areas, transport, instruments, communications equipment and other material. Consideration needs to be given to potential temporary locations for medicolegal tasks, which in an emergency might include sites usually used for other purposes (for example, warehouses, sheds, farms, meat-packing plants, or sports fields). DVI teams are more and more frequently used in many countries where the teams and the equipment they require are prepared in advance.

Assessors should verify whether mechanisms exist for enhancing forensics and mortuary capacity to meet an increased demand (see also essential attribute 33).

RECOMMENDED READING

Disaster victim guide. Lyon, Interpol, 1997 (http://www.interpol.int/public/DisasterVictim/guide/default.asp, accessed 1 May 2011).

Guidance on dealing with fatalities in emergencies. London, Home Office and Cabinet Office, 2004 (http://www.kenyoninternational.com/useful_info/UK%20Home%20Office%20Guidance%20on%20Dealing%20with%20Fatalities%20in%20Emergencies,%202004.pdf, accessed 1 May 2011).

Morgan O, Tidball-Binz M, van Alphen D. *Management of dead bodies after disasters: A field manual for first responders.* Washington, DC, Pan American Health Organization, 2006 (http://www.paho.org/english/dd/ped/deadbodiesfieldmanual.htm, accessed 1 May 2011).

Pan American Health Organization, WHO Regional Office for the Western Pacific. *Management of dead bodies in disaster situations.* Washington, DC, Pan American Health

---

[9]The objectives of medicolegal work are to: legally determine or pronounce death; recover the remains of the dead; establish the identity of the dead; estimate the time of death; determine the cause of death; explain the possible circumstances of death; prepare the remains for final disposal; and study the event with a view to prevention in the future.

Organization, 2004 (Disaster management and guidelines series, No. 5; http://www.paho.org/english/dd/ped /DeadBodiesBook.pdf, accessed 1 May 2011).

> **Key component 6.2** EMS system and mass-casualty management
>
> **Essential attribute 36** Capacity for mass-casualty management

KEYNOTES

Since there is no internationally agreed definition of an EMS system (components, stakeholders, service-delivery mechanisms, management structures), each country must have its own definition of this concept. One definition commonly encountered is:

> " … *a community-based system, which provides for the utilization of available personnel, equipment, transportation and communication to ensure effective and coordinated delivery of medical care (such as, first aid and basic life support (BLS)) in emergency situations resulting from accidents, illnesses or other emergency situations from the site up to hospital-care delivery, and to contribute to mass-casualty management (including disasters)" (26).*

An EMS system should deliver community-based health services that are fully integrated with the overall health care system (providers of public and other health care) and public safety agencies (first responders; community-level first-aid volunteers).

EMS must also contribute to the identification and modification of illness and injury risks, the provision of care in the case of acute illness and injury, the monitoring of community health and the efficient management of mass-casualty incidents.

Whatever the definition, the goal of those who plan and implement EMS should be to provide total care from the scene of the emergency through the delivery of hospital care and rehabilitation. An EMS system must have strong, continuous medical leadership. The use of all existing community-level resources (including private-sector and NGO assets) is essential if public safety services and emergency medical care are to be provided. This implies the creation of an EMS council or committee at the national level (covering policy, regulations, norms, standards, etc.) and a similar body at the local-government level (covering decisions, operations and funding). An advisory function is needed at both levels. There should be laws and regulations on the liability, accountability, sustainability and professionalism of the EMS system. Norms and standards should ensure the quality of the services and the efficient use of existing resources. In order to avoid duplication and ensure effectiveness, the activities of all stakeholders in the EMS system should be integrated and coordinated in a functional network. The integration of prehospital and hospital components is of paramount importance both in general and in times of major emergencies (see also essential attribute 34). The standardization of EMS elements (ambulance equipment; staff training; accreditation) is also critical.

INDICATOR-RELATED QUESTIONS

a. *Are EMS plans (for dispatch, on-site management, transportation and evacuation) adaptable to mass-casualty incidents and other similar crises?*

b. *Do the plans include the simultaneous management of day-to-day emergencies?*
To ensure EMS has the flexibility not only to manage daily emergencies but also to adapt to mass-casualty incidents if necessary, the geographical area covered by the EMS system must be well defined. Each region of the country should have EMS systems, which together could guarantee EMS access at the national level. In rural areas especially, EMS coverage might be low and here the concept of the community emergency-response team (CERT) should be adopted and fully integrated as part of the overall EMS system. CERT is a flexible service-delivery model that provides a solution to the problem of prolonged ambulance response times in rural and remote communities. Through a collaborative partnership between the EMS and the local community, CERT provides BLS and first aid to the sick and injured until the ambulance arrives.

One of the essential components of an EMS system is a reliable communications system, which can be simple or complex depending upon the number of agencies involved. The area covered by the communications system (catchment area) should be well defined. It is of vital importance that it allows for permanent interoperability between the main EMS stakeholders (i.e., direct radio communication among all providers and health care facilities) to ensure that the receiving facilities are ready and able to accept patients and maintain patient and provider safety.

A communications system is not limited to material means of communication (e.g., radio) but includes information management (see also essential attribute 48).

Since dispatch, and the medical regulation of patient transfer to receiving hospitals in the catchment area, when applicable, are key functions in any EMS system each agency is responsible for using a communications system that is compatible with those of their local dispatch centers and hospitals. Protocols must be established defining minimum standards both for the dispatch centers (to ensure uniformity of dispatch) and for the training and certification of the dispatchers.

A mechanism should be in place for monitoring the quality of the communication system (e.g., age and reliability of equipment and the quality of the dispatching process).

c. *Are there mechanisms in place for accessing local, regional, and national EMS resources?*
Assessors should verify that mechanisms are in place for accessing local EMS resources in a timely manner when needed.

It is essential that stakeholders in the EMS system (such as the police, hospitals and ambulance services) are efficiently coordinated and that its resources are used effectively. Hence, each stakeholder, as well as the EMS system as a whole, should be assessed on a regular basis with a view to managing community needs and maintaining the services offered as efficiently and effectively as possible with the resources available.

The EMS stakeholders must have sufficient resources (including staff) to coordinate responses and carry out the activities for which they are responsible. Standardization is of paramount importance and the data-collection systems developed by the different stakeholders should be capable of monitoring resources and fully intercompatible. The data collected must be readily available for use in determining the quantity, quality, and utilization of resources and should include information on existing formal programs for recruiting and retaining EMS personnel, including volunteers.

d. Is the role of EMS in identifying and reporting unusual public health events clearly defined?
Among other responsibilities, EMS have public health responsibilities, such as contributing to surveillance for outbreaks of communicable diseases and to the sentinel and early-warning systems for unusual events (CBRN).

e. Are EMS providers included in coordination meetings, joint exercises, drills and training exercises?
Periodic disaster drills and exercises serve to assess performance, refine management and educate personnel and the community.

Assessors should verify that drills and exercises take place regularly, that all EMS providers are included in coordination meetings, joint exercises, drills and training, and that they receive feedback on their performances.

RECOMMENDED READING

De Boer J, Dubouloz M, eds. *Handbook of disaster medicine. Emergency medicine in mass casualty situations.* Zeist, VSP International Science Publishers, 2000.

Mass casualty management systems. Strategies and guidelines for building health sector capacity. Geneva, World Health Organization, 2007 (http://www.who.int/hac/techguidance /MCM_guidelines_inside_final.pdf, accessed 1 May 2011).

Strategy & recommendations in organizing & managing emergency medical services (EMS) in developing countries in managing daily emergencies & disasters. An ADPC perspective. Bangkok, Asian Disaster Preparedness Center, 2003 (http://www.adpc.net/v2007/ikm/ONLINE%20 DOCUMENTS/downloads/ADUMP/EMS%20Paper%20 FINAL.pdf, accessed 1 May 2011).

Key component 6.3 Management of hospitals in mass-casualty incidents

Essential attribute 37 Hospital emergency-preparedness program

INDICATOR-RELATED QUESTIONS

a. Does a formal hospital emergency-preparedness program exist?

b. If so, is staff assigned to the program?

c. Are funds allocated to the program?

d. Are resources available for the program?

e. Does the program fully incorporate the concept of safer hospitals?
The ability of a hospital to manage its resources optimally in an emergency and to integrate with the community-level response is dependent on its emergency-preparedness program. Preparedness is a continuous process; thus, a hospital emergency-preparedness program should cover all hospital activities, i.e., not only those aimed at response but also at mitigation, rehabilitation, etc., taking all potential hazards into consideration (an all-hazards approach). This involves planning (especially for hospital response and contingency measures in emergencies), exercises, training, community education, information management, communication and warning systems. It is crucial in preparedness planning to define the system (the way in which resources are organized) and the process (action and interaction). Staff should receive education and training in how the system works to be able to fulfill their assigned roles.

An integral component of the hospital emergency-preparedness program is the hospital emergency-response plan. It defines the management structure of the hospital and the methodology to be used by the hospital during an emergency response or in preparing the hospital for response if there is warning time (see also essential attribute 38). Surge capacity (to enhance the capacity for care delivery) is one of the key elements of hospital preparedness, as is the networking of hospitals and referral systems at the subnational levels (and, in certain scenarios, at the national level). Thus, the compatibility, complementarities and/or synergism of the individual hospital emergency-response plans, as well as any cross-border cooperation, also need to be considered by the hospital emergency-preparedness program (see also essential attribute 33). Other health care facilities, including public and private institutions, should be included in the networking and referral process.

RECOMMENDED READING

Hospital emergency response checklist. An all-hazards tool for hospital administrators and emergency managers. Copenhagen, WHO Regional Office for Europe, 2011 (http:// www.euro.who.int/__data/assets/pdf_file/0020/148214 /Hospital_emerg_checklist.pdf, accessed 29 October 2011).

United Nations International Strategy for Disaster Reduction, The World Bank, World Health Organization. *Hospitals safe from disasters. Reduce risk, protect health facilities, save lives. 2008–2009 world disaster reduction campaign.*

Geneva, United Nations International Strategy for Disaster Reduction, 2009 (http://www.unisdr.org/eng/public_aware /world_camp/2008-2009/pdf/wdrc-2008-2009-information-kit.pdf, accessed 2 May 2011).

Mass casualty management hospital emergency response plan. Regional training course on mass casualty management and hospital preparedness. Manila, WHO Regional Office for the Western Pacific, 2008 (http://acilafet.org/upload /dosyalar/Hospital_emergency_response_plan_Toolkit_ .pdf, accessed 2 May 2011).

Safe hospitals. A collective responsibility. A global measure of disaster reduction. Washington, DC, Pan American Health Organization, 2008 (http://www.paho.org/english/dd/ped /SafeHospitalsBooklet.pdf, accessed 2 May 2011).

Essential attribute 38 Hospital plans for emergency response and recovery

KEYNOTES

Plans for emergency response and recovery are an integral component of a hospital-preparedness program and represent the output defining the management structure and methodology to be used by a hospital during an emergency response (or in preparing a hospital for response if there is warning time), as well as the management arrangements for returning to normal operations as quickly as possible after the recovery phase (see also essential attribute 37).

Common reasons for the failure of hospital plans for emergency response and recovery are that:

- they were developed in isolation by a very limited group of experts;
- the end-users (staff) were not included in the development process, nor did they receive appropriate training;
- there was a breakdown in communication;
- the plans were neither validated nor maintained;
- the plans lacked mechanisms for coordinating with outside partners, including the prehospital component, and other health care facilities.

Assessors should look specifically for such gaps when evaluating hospital emergency-response and recovery plans.

A hospital plan for emergency *response* defines the management structure of and the methodology to be used by a hospital during an emergency response (or to prepare the hospital for response, if there is warning time). The plan is of critical importance in defining the management processes that enable the hospital to coordinate its actions with other health care facilities and responders.

When the hospital plan for emergency response is activated, an incident-command group decides on the priority action to be taken within its framework. In an emergency situation, each specific assignment of the emergency-management system is positioned on an organizational chart and is allocated a job action sheet (checklist) designed to direct those involved. The organizational chart and job action sheets form the backbone of the plan. The chart needs to be revised regularly and adapted to the actual management of service lines and departments.

A hospital plan for emergency *recovery* aims to facilitate the recovery of affected individuals, communities and infrastructures as quickly and practicably as possible. This is best achieved through effective and efficient management arrangements. As in the case of response plans, it is crucial that recovery-management arrangements are reviewed on a regular basis, particularly after the occurrence of major events.

The training of those who actively contribute to the development of hospital plans for emergency response and recovery is a key activity.

INDICATOR-RELATED QUESTIONS

a. *Do hospitals have planning committees for emergency response and recovery?*

The development of emergency plans for response and recovery is a fundamental activity of hospital management in mass-casualty incidents, requiring the full attention and strong support of the health authorities and the local community. Hospital planning committees for response and recovery comprise people trained in developing these plans.

Assessors should check whether such a committee exists and, if so, whether it has a clear mandate and the full authority to develop plans for emergency response and recovery. They should request a list of committee members that includes their functions and disciplines.

b. *Do hospitals have plans for emergency response and recovery?*

c. *If so, were these plans developed through a continuous planning process involving a planning committee?*

d. *Are they in accordance with national policy?*

Assessors should verify whether the plans were developed through an on-going planning process. Hospital plans for emergency response and recovery comprise only one of the outputs of the emergency-planning process and serve as a basis for allocating resources for hospital emergency preparedness. Other important outputs are: awareness-raising among hospital staff; promotion of a risk-management culture within the health care facility; conducting a vulnerability analysis resulting in possible recommendations for action towards mitigation, prevention and correction; motivating key staff to become active partners in assisting the hospital managerial team in risk management; developing partnerships with other key stakeholders; developing exercises; and improving the management of daily emergencies.

In addition, assessors should establish whether the plans were developed by a planning committee through a process to integrate them with already existing strategies, plans and resources, and whether they are in accordance with national policy.

e. *Is a plan for emergency response and recovery a requirement for hospital accreditation?*

f. *Are hospital plans for emergency response and recovery validated and accredited in accordance with national criteria?*

g. *Are the plans reviewed, exercised, revised, and updated regularly?*

Assessors must verify that hospital plans for emergency response and recovery are not merely copies of other plans, that they were developed through an interactive process and meet the national planning criteria, and that they were tested and validated according to the national criteria. In addition, they should look into whether key staff is familiar with the details of the plans, which would imply that they receive regular training. Exercises and drills must take place regularly and lessons learned must be incorporated in the revision process, which should occur on a regular basis. To this end, assessors should interview not only the medical director or members of the planning committee but also key staff working in the different departments.

h. *Are the plans linked to subnational multisectoral emergency-response plans?*

Assessors should verify that the hospital plans are not isolated subnational health-sector or multisectoral emergency-response plans. It is important that the hospital plans reflect the role of the hospital with respect to subnational emergency-response operations and that they are linked to the respective provincial and municipal health-sector or multisectoral hospital emergency-response plans.

i. *Are the plans complemented by contingency procedures for internal incidents and local threats?*

Assessors should verify whether the planning process and the plans per se follow an all-hazards approach, implying that the response would be applicable to all kinds of hazard events. The generic plan serves as the basis for developing contingency plans or procedures to be followed in the case of local threats and internal incidents (such as the outbreak of an infectious disease or an internal fire).

j. *Do the plans include mechanisms for switching to emergency mode?*

Mechanisms for activating emergency-response plans and contingency plans related to internal emergencies, as well as level of activation, must be well described in the plans to enable activation at any time on the basis of validating criteria. These criteria should not be based on trauma and injuries alone; the hospital surveillance system must be capable of detecting clusters of conditions, which are unexpected in relation to time and place (e.g., pandemic cases of disease, clusters of cases of communicable diseases, and chemical subchronic intoxication). The plans must also clearly indicate who is responsible for activating the plan, how it should be done and when (who, how, and when). During exercises and drills, such procedures should be regularly tested and updated if necessary.

RECOMMENDED READING

Hospital preparedness checklist for pandemic influenza. Focus on pandemic (H1N1) 2009. Copenhagen, WHO Regional Office for Europe, 2009 (http://www.euro.who.int/__data /assets/pdf_file/0004/78988/E93006.pdf, accessed 1 May 2011).

Hospital emergency response checklist. An all-hazards tool for hospital administrators and emergency managers. Copenhagen, WHO Regional Office for Europe, 2011 (http://www .euro.who.int/__data/assets/pdf_file/0020/148214/Hospital_ emerg_checklist.pdf, accessed on 29 October 2011).

Mass casualty management hospital emergency response plan. Regional training course on mass casualty management and hospital preparedness. Manila, WHO Regional Office for the Western Pacific, 2008 (http://acilafet.org/upload /dosyalar/Hospital_emergency_response_plan_Toolkit_ .pdf, accessed 2 May 2011).

Mass casualty management systems, strategies and guidelines for building health sector capacity. Geneva, World Health Organization, 2007 (http://whqlibdoc.who.int/publica- tions/2007/9789241596053_eng.pdf, accessed 2 May 2011).

> **Key component 6.4** Continuity of essential health programs and services
>
> **Essential attribute 39** Continuous delivery of essential health and hospital services

KEYNOTES

Disasters often affect hospitals and with serious consequences. To optimize patient care during emergencies, it is necessary to identify and maintain essential health services. Activities, such as maintaining essential equipment, ensuring the availability of electrical power and water supplies, and contributing to damage assessment and rehabilitating lifelines, are essential to the continuity of business operations and the delivery of essential services.

INDICATOR-RELATED QUESTIONS

a. *Does capacity exist for the immediate assessment of structural, nonstructural and functional safety after any incident?*

Assessing the damage to and safety of hospital buildings is the first step to be taken after a disaster, when applicable. Staff responsible for damage assessment should be and a list of potential staff kept up to date. The expertise of engineers and architects, usually from outside the hospital, will also be needed. Therefore, hospital emergency-response plans should include procedures for coordinating and working with other main stakeholders and for identifying any extra technical expertise needed from outside the hospital. The plans should also identify mechanisms for restoring critical equipment and lifelines, in cooperation with the relevant community services.

b. *Do procedures exist for ensuring back-up of critical resources (e.g., water, electricity, heating etc.)?*

Assessors should verify that procedures exist for ensuring back-up for critical resources (power, oxygen, water, etc.)

and essential lifelines in health care facilities. Mechanisms should be in place for determining the operational level of critical equipment and for setting up a monitoring system to facilitate the anticipation of problems, such as shortage or overuse (see also essential attribute 51).

c. *Do plans exist for ensuring the continuous delivery of essential hospital services (e.g., maternal care, dialysis, etc.)?*
In any kind of emergency, hospitals must ensure the continuous delivery of essential services (i.e., services that must be provided at all times) in parallel to carrying out the emergency response. Plans should list all hospital services in priority order and identify those that are essential. Coordination with the health authorities and neighboring hospitals is crucial to the continuity of essential hospital services. The roles and responsibilities of each member of the local health care network must be clearly defined.

RECOMMENDED READING

Hospital preparedness checklist for pandemic influenza. Focus on pandemic (H1N1) 2009. Copenhagen, WHO Regional Office for Europe, 2009 (http://www.euro.who.int/__data /assets/pdf_file/0004/78988/E93006.pdf, accessed 1 May 2011).

Hospital emergency response checklist. An all-hazards tool for hospital administrators and emergency managers. Copenhagen, WHO Regional Office for Europe, 2011 (http:// www.euro.who.int/__data/assets/pdf_file/0020/148214 /Hospital_emerg_checklist.pdf, accessed 29 October 2011).

Pandemic flu: managing demand and capacity in health care organisations. (Surge). London, Department of Health, 2009 (http://www.dh.gov.uk/prod_consum_dh/groups /dh_digitalassets/documents/digitalasset/dh_098750.pdf, accessed 1 May 2011).

Safe hospital in emergencies and disasters. Structural, non-structural and functional indicators. Manila, WHO Regional Office for the Western Pacific, 2009 (http://www .wpro.who.int/NR/rdonlyres/390133EC-089F-4C77-902D- DFEE8532F558/0/SafeHospitalsinEmergenciesand Disasters160709.pdf, accessed 1 May 2011).

Essential attribute 40 Prevention and control of communicable diseases and immunization

KEYNOTES

Health care facilities should have a clear policy on the early detection of contagious patients, especially those with communicable diseases with a human-to-human mode of transmission, as well as practical guidelines on and procedures for prehospital and hospital triage, admission, treatment, isolation and reporting (in accordance with the policies and guidelines recommended by the health authorities) (see also essential attribute 27).

In a pandemic, for instance, there should be coordination between the hospital and alternative treatment sites. An infection control program or relevant procedures should cover standard precautions, contact precautions, droplet precautions, environmental and engineering control and administrative control.

Assessors should verify that facility-level environmental control systems (e.g., ventilation systems) are in place and that individual protective equipment is available in health care facilities for staff, patients, and visitors. They should also evaluate the level of readiness (competence, knowledge, skills, and abilities) of the staff for taking infection-control measures, both routine and special, and urgently establishing the training activities required for different scenarios. The staff should be capable of managing health problems, from prevention to care delivery and follow-up. Standard precautions should be fully established and routinely practiced; examples of these are: hand hygiene; use of PPE (including gloves, facial protection, and gowns); respiratory hygiene and cough etiquette, if relevant; prevention of needlestick and injuries from other sharp instruments; environmental cleaning; linen and waste disposal, if relevant; and disinfection of equipment for patient care.

At the local (hospital) level, assessors should check whether the emergency-response plans include the following contingency measures and/or whether others exist:

*   appointment of a hospital epidemiologist with overall responsibility for activities related to early warning and monitoring in the hospital;
*   of the information to be collected routinely and in emergencies and instructions on how it is to be used;
*   establishment of communication channels within health care facilities and with public health authorities for the reporting of unusual health events by health workers;
*   establishment of data collection and reporting mechanisms in accordance with national health policy and directives, tailored to the local context;
*   establishment of procedures for immediate investigation into reports by health care workers of unusual health events and/or signals detected through monitoring activities;
*   prompt distribution to hospital clinicians and other relevant decision makers of information obtained through monitoring activities and/or the investigation of unusual health events and/or signals;
*   establishment of procedures to facilitate access to health care facilities by suspected or confirmed epidemic or pandemic patients, such as information-sharing (including that for the public, the staff and key stakeholders) with other stakeholders, especially EMS, the dispatch center and private doctors;
*   establishment of special procedures related to infection prevention and control, including patient arrival at the health care facilities' reception areas for epidemic or pandemic patients, physical examination, triage, general nursing care and the flow of epidemic, pandemic and non-epidemic patients outside and inside the hospital;
*   establishment of procedures for locating a well-ventilated isolation room in the hospital, cohorting epidemic and

pandemic patients, and ensuring adherence to requirements relating to minimum distance between beds (particularly important for droplet diseases);

- establishment of procedures for referral and follow-up of epidemic and pandemic patients not admitted to hospital;
- staff training for different functions with a focus on infection-control measures;
- establishment of procedures for logistics planning, e.g., for procurement of PPE, equipment and supplies;
- establishment of ambulatory-care arrangements, including location, functional aspects, procedures, staffing, equipment and management;
- establishment of procedures for implementing standardized treatment protocols on providing care to patients with suspected and confirmed communicable diseases with a view to preventing spread and protecting staff;
- establishment of procedures for communicating information to patients, visitors, staff, and the public;
- introduction of mechanisms for providing continued care for communicable diseases patients in emergencies (e.g., treatment for HIV patients).

INDICATOR-RELATED QUESTIONS

a. *Is an active health-surveillance system with early-warning capacity in place?*

Assessors should verify the existence of a routine, ongoing infection-control program and a surveillance system that can act as an early-warning system for communicable diseases. This should be the basis for building further management capacity for major epidemics (see also the section entitled "health information" and key components 8, 9, and 10). The surveillance system must be capable of detecting clusters, atypical clinical presentations, and the like, at the earliest possible stage. Initial cases of communicable diseases with epidemic potential should immediately elicit a reaction from the health care facility (see also essential attribute 1).

For instance, during an influenza pandemic, unusual health events might signal the emergence of novel influenza viruses or changes in the characteristics of circulating influenza viruses (increased virulence, resistance to antivirals, increased transmissibility), which warrant investigation. In addition to serving as an early-warning function, the laboratory and epidemiological data obtained through systematic collection and analysis will allow the public health authorities to monitor the progress of severe influenza-related diseases and inform interventions aimed at dealing with those at the highest risk of severe outcome.

b. *Is there sufficient capacity for setting up special immunization programs to meet needs?*

Following an emergency, the affected population is often displaced and temporarily resettled. Resettlement may entail high population densities, inadequate shelter, insufficient water supplies and sanitation, and a lack of even basic health care. In such situations, there is an increased threat of communicable diseases and a high risk of epidemics.

A systematic approach to the control of communicable diseases is a key component of humanitarian response and crucial in protecting the health of affected populations. Cooperation among the agencies working at the local, national and international levels is required, as well as collaboration among all sectors involved in emergency response (see also essential attribute 47).

One of the key components of prevention is mass vaccination against diseases. A successful campaign involves the community, the health authorities, international and nongovernmental organizations and private practitioners. Involving all stakeholders in planning a campaign will ensure that everyone is aware of its purpose and of the target population.

Assessors should verify that: the necessary capacity for immunization programs exists; all relevant staff is informed of the purpose of vaccination campaigns and the technical issues pertinent to the specific vaccine(s); stocks are available and can be deployed when needed; and cold chain is ensured.

RECOMMENDED READING

Connolly MA, et al. Communicable diseases in complex emergencies: impact and challenges. *Lancet,* 2004, 364(9449):1974–1983.

Hospital preparedness checklist for pandemic influenza. Focus on pandemic (H1N1) 2009. Copenhagen, WHO Regional Office for Europe, 2009 (http://www.euro.who.int/__data /assets/pdf_file/0004/78988/E93006.pdf, accessed 1 May 2011).

Infection prevention and control of epidemic- and pandemic-prone acute respiratory diseases in health care. WHO interim guidelines, June 2007. Geneva, World Health Organization, 2007 (WHO/CDS/EPR/2007.6; http://www .who.int/entity/csr/resources/publications/WHO_CDS_ EPR_2007_6c.pdf, accessed 1 May 2011).

Prevention of hospital-acquired infection. A practical guide. Second edition. Geneva, World Health Organization, 2002 (WHO/CDS/CSR/EPH/2002.12; http://www.who.int/csr /resources/publications/whocdscsreph200212.pdf, accessed 1 May 2011).

Essential attribute 41 Mother-and-child health care and reproductive health

KEYNOTES

Poor reproductive health is a significant cause of death and disease in emergency situations. In an emergency, the priority should be to restore the services for mother-and-child health care and reproductive health as quickly as possible, and to equip local staff with guidance on the management of individuals whose treatment has been disrupted or delayed. Emergency care in the area of reproductive health is necessary for the physical, mental and social well-being of those affected. It should be delivered in a timely manner, integrated with primary health care (PHC) and coordinated with the efforts of other sectors and institutions (see essential attribute 46). The affected community must be involved in program planning so that religious and cultural sensitivities are taken into consideration.

INDICATOR-RELATED QUESTIONS

a. *Are there mechanisms in place to ensure the continued delivery of core components of reproductive-health programs in an emergency situation?*

Assessors should verify that mechanisms are in place to safeguard the core components of programs on reproductive health and mother-and-child health care during an emergency.

The minimum initial service package (MISP)[10], developed by several international agencies addresses this need during the acute phase. MISP has five objectives: (1) to identify a lead organization for MISP implementation; (2) to prevent and manage the consequences of sexual violence; (3) to reduce HIV transmission; (4) to prevent excess maternal and newborn morbidity and mortality; and (5) to plan for comprehensive sexual- and reproductive-health services that are integrated in PHC as far as the situation permits. MISP focuses mainly on internally displaced people (IDP) and complex emergencies and outlines priority life-saving strategies and activities to be implemented at the onset of every humanitarian crisis. The package forms the starting point for sexual- and reproductive-health programming, which should aim at building comprehensive sexual- and reproductive-health services.

While MISP outlines priority strategies and activities, the United Nations Population Fund (UNFPA) reproductive health kit for emergency situations provides the actual material resources needed for implementing them. The UNFPA has organized 12 self-contained reproductive health kits that conform with the new WHO emergency health kit.

Assessors should verify that the objectives of MISP are represented in preparedness and response plans and that there are procedures for accessing reproductive health kits in case of emergency.

b. *Are there mechanisms in place to ensure the continued delivery of care for newborn and emergency obstetrical patients?*[11]

In emergency situations, it is important that pregnant women receive appropriate attention throughout their pregnancies and during childbirth. This includes pre- and postnatal care, care of the newborn, breastfeeding support (see also essential attribute 45), and the referral of women with obstetrical complications, including those caused by unsafe abortion. Access to family-planning services and reproductive-health education is equally essential.

The following care components of service delivery have to be considered for mothers and their newborn in emergency situations: antenatal care; delivery care; emergency obstetrical care; postnatal care; and health education.

Regular *antenatal care* plays an important role in ensuring the health of both mother and child throughout pregnancy. It is during antenatal care that health care workers can check for possible complications and/or risk factors on the basis of important health indicators.

To provide *delivery care*, referral systems need to be established or strengthened to ensure 24-hour access to emergency facilities. Interventions associated with delivery care include: the provision of skilled assistance; clean and safe delivery; early detection (recognition) and management of complications; referral and transportation to emergency obstetrical facilities on a 24-hour basis.

Emergency obstetrical care requires various resources: adequate supplies of drugs and equipment; safe blood for transfusion; trained staff (to identify emergency obstetrical conditions); counseling for high-risk mothers; and an appropriate system of referral and transportation for referred obstetrical emergencies.

Postnatal care ensures that the health status of the mother and child is monitored long enough to detect complications, which can occur after delivery. This is particularly important in emergency situations where a woman may be living alone or acting as the head of a household.

Health education can reduce maternal mortality by enabling early recognition of high-risk pregnancies and timely intervention. Most women are unaware of the causes of maternal death or of the danger signs of an obstetrical complication. Ways of implementing maternal-health programs are needed, as well as information, education and communication (IEC) activities to facilitate early of obstetric complications and the implementation of appropriate action, when required.

In an emergency that causes the extensive disruption of routine services, or in the case of temporary settlements, guidelines are needed on establishing, managing, reporting on and terminating temporary or alternate antenatal- and postnatal-care services. Hospital emergency-response plans should contain guidelines for staff on the treatment of obstetrical emergencies. The involvement of public- and medical-transport organizations is needed to improve interhospital transfer and minimize unnecessary delays. Obstetrical staff should be made aware of any temporary arrangements for the postnatal care of patients after an emergency.

RECOMMENDED READING

Abdallah S, Burnham G, eds. *The Johns Hopkins and IFRC public health guide for emergencies. First edition.* Geneva, International Federation of the Red Cross and Red Crescent Societies, 2004 (http://www.terzomondo.org/library /essentials/IFRC_Public_Health_Guide.pdf, accessed 18 April 2004).

---

[10]Further information about MISP is available (http://misp.rhrc.org/, accessed 28 July 2011).

[11]Including measures related to safe motherhood and the prevention of sexually transmitted diseases. These measures are especially important for IDPs.

Minimum initial service package (MISP) for reproductive health in crisis situations: a distance learning module. New York, Women's Refugee Commission, 2006 (http://www.searo.who.int/LinkFiles/Publications_MISP.pdf, accessed 3 May 2011).

Reproductive health during conflict and displacement. A guide for program managers. Geneva, World Health Organization, 2000 [WHO/RHR/00.13] (http://whqlibdoc.who.int/hq/2001/WHO_RHR_00.13.pdf, accessed 3 May 2011).

United Nations Population Fund, United Nations Refugee Agency, World Health Organization. *Reproductive Health in refugee situations an Interagency field manual.* Geneva, UNHCR, 1999 (http://www.unhcr.org/3bc6ed6fa.html, accessed 3 May 2011).

Essential attribute 42 Mental health and psychosocial support

KEYNOTES

Until recently, there has been a general tendency to consider the basic needs of people affected by an emergency in terms of physical injury and material loss rather than mental anguish. Of the scars caused by a disaster, the psychological and social scars are the worst and some are even transgenerational. Mental health is now generally accepted as a priority in any emergency, whether at the individual or the community level. It is not sufficient to have a good knowledge of the plans and related strategies necessary to ensure a successful rescue operation; the rescuers, firefighters and medical staff involved in the pre-hospital and hospital links of the rescue chain must also have a good understanding of the social and psychological needs of those affected both in the immediate aftermath of the event and in the longer term. Furthermore, it is important that the efforts of the mental-health and psychosocial services to provide support are closely linked to those of the social services.

Assessors should verify adherence to the general WHO principles *(27)* with respect to the mental and social aspects of exposure to extreme stressors.

- National-level plans should be developed in *preparation for emergency situations.* They should include a coordination system specifying the focal persons responsible in each of the agencies involved and details of the training planned for relevant personnel in the areas of social and psychological intervention.
- Interventions should be preceded by a broad *assessment* of the local context and careful planning.
- Interventions should involve consultation and *collaboration* with other governmental organizations and NGOs working in the area. The continuous involvement of the government, preferably, or of local NGOs, is essential to ensuring sustainability.
- Mental-health interventions led by the health sector should *be integrated with PHC activities* and maximum use should be made of the care options provided by families and community resources (see also essential attribute 46).

- Setting up separate, vertical mental-health services for special populations is discouraged. As far as possible, these services should be *accessible to the whole community* and not restricted to subpopulations on the basis of their exposure to certain stressors.
- *Training and supervisory activities* should be carried out by mental-health specialists or under their guidance.
- It is preferable to focus on the *medium- and long-term perspectives* of post-emergency psychosocial support (i.e., the development of community-based, primary-care, mental-health services and social interventions) rather than on the provision of immediate, short-term relief of psychological distress during the acute phase.
- Activities should be monitored and evaluated on the basis of predefined *monitoring indicators.*

INDICATOR-RELATED QUESTIONS

a. *Are there mechanisms in place to ensure the continuous treatment of patients in an emergency situation?*
    During the acute phase of an emergency, psychiatric and mentally ill patients may not have access to medication and medical care. Assessors should verify that mechanisms exist for providing continuous treatment (including medication) and for resuming psychiatric care as soon as possible (see also essential attribute 44).

b. *Does capacity exist for of the psychosocial needs of high-risk groups (including bereaved families) and for providing them with the appropriate support?*
    One crucial aspect of mental-health care in emergency situations is the ability to understand stress-related symptoms in the light of the (local) cultural norms. To match the needs of populations affected by emergencies (particularly complex emergencies and those resulting in mass casualties) mental-health programs should, to the extent possible, build on the PHC resources available in the community instead of relying entirely on external expertise. National stakeholders delivering social and psychological services should be strengthened as much as possible (see also essential attributes 46 and 47).

    The community should be regarded as the "golden key" to helping traumatized victims (through social cohesion, social support, traditional networking, etc.). However, in an emergency situation, various external providers of psychosocial support offer their services (e.g., international organizations and NGOs). Since foreign help is often hypothetical, rarely in place, in time and potentially not adapted to the local culture, available local resources should be used before considering external support, whether national or international.

    Assessors should verify that mechanisms exist for regulating and controlling externally provided psychosocial support.

RECOMMENDED READING

Boer J de, Dubouloz M, eds. *Handbook of disaster medicine. Emergency medicine in mass casualty situations.* Utrecht, BRILL, 2000.

IASC guidelines on mental health and psychosocial support in emergency settings. Geneva, Inter-Agency Standing Committee, 2007 (http://www.who.int/mental_health /emergencies/guidelines_iasc_mental_health_ psychosocial_june_2007.pdf, accessed 3 May 2011).

Mental health in emergencies. Mental and social aspects of health of populations exposed to extreme stressors. Geneva, World Health Organization, 2003 (http://www.who.int /mental_health/media/en/640.pdf, accessed 3 May 2011).

Essential attribute 43 Environmental health

KEYNOTES

Strategic planning to increase people's capacity to withstand disaster hazards must address environmental-health concerns. The goal should be not only to respond to disasters but also to reduce their impact on environmental-health infrastructures and systems (e.g., water supplies, sanitation facilities, shelters, and vector-control systems) and strengthen people's ability to withstand the conditions resulting from the disruption of these facilities and to recover rapidly.

Assessors should verify whether emergency-preparedness programs consider environmental-health needs in emergency and disaster situations in terms of action to: reduce community vulnerability; provide guidance on action to be taken at the different stages of the disaster-management cycle (prevention, preparedness, response and recovery) to protect environmental health; provide guidance on simple, practical technical interventions to meet the most important environmental-health needs of communities; address environmental-health needs within PHC (see also essential attribute 46), including training programs, information systems, and community involvement; and promote coordination and collaboration among all sectors.

INDICATOR-RELATED QUESTIONS

a. *Are there mechanisms in place to ensure the availability of adequate amounts of safe water for service providers and the affected population?*
Functional water-supply systems play a major role in emergencies. A systematic vulnerability analysis should be carried out—from the source through the collection works, the transmission and treatment facilities and, finally, the distribution system—to determine whether the water-supply systems can withstand damage in an emergency, taking into account the effect of a disaster on sources, such as surface water (e.g., in the case of wildfires) and groundwater (e.g., in the case of industrial spills). In addition, possible damage to reservoirs and water mains, the effects of power failures, personnel shortages due to lack of transport or injury, and communications' difficulties, all need to be considered. Each water-supply institution in a country (or district) should carry out a review of its resources (both human and material), assess the vulnerability of the components of its system to various hazards and prepare plans for possible repairs needed.

To ensure the provision of adequate amounts of safe water in an emergency, mechanisms should exist for carrying out assessments of unmet needs and of damage to water resources. The assessment of unmet needs should identify: the population affected by insufficient or contaminated water supplies; the quantity of water needed for various purposes (e.g., for humans, livestock, household use, agricultural use, industrial use); how often it will be needed; and any additional treatment, storage and distribution facilities required. Priority should be given to restoring the normal water supply and distribution systems. If these are significantly damaged or there are large groups of people in temporary shelters, arrangements should be made for providing a temporary water supply.

Assessors should verify that mechanisms exist to: enable assessment of unmet needs, damage and water resources; ensure the availability of adequate amounts of safe water for service providers and the affected population; and facilitate the constant monitoring of water quality[12] during an emergency *(28)*. In addition, they should check whether trained staff and technical equipment for testing water quality are in place and can easily be deployed when needed.

b. *Are there mechanisms in place to enable health authorities to identify and control environmental factors that are hazardous to health?*
Assessors should check whether mechanisms exist for performing environmental-health vulnerability assessments, which would enable health authorities to identify hazardous environmental factors and anticipate problems that groups could face in the event of a disaster and during the recovery period.

Firstly, environmental health must be covered in an initial baseline survey of all hazards and patterns of vulnerability affecting the society. The survey should be organized by geographical region and the vulnerabilities of different ethnic and socioeconomic groups (relating, for example, to priority needs, such as water supply, drainage, sanitation, refuse and waste disposal, housing and food hygiene) should be documented. The priority needs of displaced populations should be included (see also essential attribute 47).

Secondly, the location and safety of industrial facilities in relation to settlements should be reviewed, as well as the risk of radiation, fire, explosion, accidental poisonous emissions, and other such incidents.

Assessors should also verify that mechanisms are in place for controlling environmental factors as hazardous to health, such as solid waste, liquid waste and medical waste.

---

[12]**Water quality is usually measured by the absence or presence of** groups of microorganisms. Their presence indicates possible feces contamination. Because human feces typically contain tens of millions of bacteria per gram, even the smallest trace of them in water is often detectable by bacterial monitoring. Fecal coliforms are a category of bacteria that match the characteristics of those found in the stools of warm-blooded mammals. Other indicator bacteria, such as E. coli, fecal streptococci, or total coliforms, are maintained by the same premise—absence implies safe water *(28)*.

c. *Do procedures and facilities exist for the safe disposal of medical waste in emergencies?*

Special care must be taken with medical waste from health care facilities, the main categories of which are: infectious waste, pathological waste, sharps waste, pharmaceutical waste, genotoxic waste, chemical waste; waste with a high content of heavy metal, pressurized containers and radioactive waste *(29)*. Each type of waste requires specific handling, storage, collection, and destruction measures.[13] The deep, compacted burial and, in particular, incineration of medical waste are essential to eliminating the associated health risks.

Assessors should verify that methods used for the safe disposal of medical waste are in accordance with the national guidelines and standards. There should be mechanisms for segregating medical waste according to type and for destroying and disposing of it (e.g., color bags, PVC containers). The same environmental-health considerations are applicable to mobile emergency hospitals.

d. *Do procedures exist for the safe disposal of non-medical waste in emergencies?*

Emergencies can cause transportation problems and disrupt waste-management systems that are inadequate even in normal conditions. Extra quantities or new forms of non-medical waste may be generated in emergencies, which often produce rubble from damaged buildings and other structures that far exceeds the capacity of solid-waste management systems. This waste is not hazardous but it does hamper emergency response by blocking roads (which hinders assessment of the full extent of the damage) and drainage channels (which leads to flooding and overflow of waste-water).

Assessors should verify that procedures and capacity exist for the safe disposal of non-medical waste. In the preparedness phase, each waste-disposal institution in a country (or district) should carry out a review of its resources (both human and material) and of the vulnerability of the components of its system to various hazards, and prepare plans for temporary repairs.

RECOMMENDED READING

Abdallah S, Burnham G, eds. *The Johns Hopkins and IFRC Public Health Guide for Emergencies.* Geneva, International Federation of the Red Cross and Red Crescent Societies, 2004 (http://pdf.usaid.gov/pdf_docs/PNACU086.pdf, accessed 22 July 2011).

Sphere handbook: humanitarian charter and minimum standards in disaster response. Geneva, Sphere Project, 2004

(http://www.unhcr.org/refworld/publisher,SPHERE, 3d64ad7b1,0.html, accessed 3 May 2011).

Essential attribute 44   Chronic and noncommunicable diseases

KEYNOTE

Planning is essential to meeting the special needs of people with chronic and noncommunicable diseases during a disaster. Conditions, such as stress, lack of food or water, extremes of heat or cold and exposure to infection, can contribute to the rapid worsening of a chronic illness that was under control before the event. For instance, chronically ill persons are at risk of dying from an influenza infection during an epidemic or pandemic. Interruptions in medication regimens and medical technology can also exacerbate underlying conditions (e.g., diabetes) and increase the risk of morbidity or mortality.

INDICATOR-RELATED QUESTIONS

a. *Are there mechanisms in place to ensure access to essential medicines and essential medical services?*

b. *Are there mechanisms in place to ensure access to rehabilitation services?*

Assessors should verify the availability of:

- mechanisms to ensure access, through the PHC system, to medications required for the routine, ongoing management of serious chronic diseases;
- mechanisms to ensure continuity of the interfacility transfer and referral system for persons with chronic and noncommunicable diseases who require special hospital treatment (such as dialysis and chemotherapy) on a regular basis;
- hospital capacity, including rehabilitation services (contingency plan, surge capacity, trained personnel, equipment) and continued care for persons with chronic and noncommunicable diseases after an emergency;
- mapping systems for identifying areas with high concentrations of persons with chronic and noncommunicable diseases in the preparedness phase;
- a chronic or noncommunicable diseases and registration system;
- mechanisms for improving pre-disaster coordination and communication between, and response by, public health agencies, services providers, emergency responders and other entities dealing with persons with chronic and noncommunicable diseases;
- appropriate information on emergency preparedness for persons with chronic and noncommunicable diseases;
- an emergency-support system for in-home services, including emergency-care and communications systems for in-home caregivers;
- a formal, standardized, multidisciplinary curriculum for educating health care professionals in working with and responding to the needs of the chronically ill in shelter care;

---

[13]In the case of simple health centers, particularly in rural areas, well-managed onsite burial may be appropriate. In larger centers that produce significant quantities of sharps and infected waste, incineration may also be required. When health facilities operate diagnostic laboratory services, diagnostic radiology and treatment facilities, pharmacies, etc., waste management is a specialized activity requiring trained and well-equipped staff *(29)*.

- mechanisms for implementing special medical-needs shelters that provide a level of medical care beyond that of first aid to medically stable persons who only require shelter:
- private-sector resources (e.g., medical practitioners, private pharmacy suppliers).

RECOMMENDED READING

Aldrich N, Benson WF. Disaster preparedness and the chronic disease needs of vulnerable older adults. *Prevention Chronic Disease*, 2008, 5(1) (http://www.cdc.gov/pcd/issues/2008/jan/07_0135.htm, accessed 3 May 2011).

Jellinek I. *Perspectives from the private sector on emergency preparedness for seniors and persons with disabilities in New York City: lessons learned from our city's aging services providers from the tragedy of September 11, 2001.* New York, Council of Senior Centers and Services of New York City Inc., 2002.

Sphere handbook: humanitarian charter and minimum standards in disaster response. Geneva, Sphere Project, 2004 (http://www.unhcr.org/refworld/publisher,SPHERE,,,3d64ad7b1,0.html, accessed 3 May 2011).

Essential attribute 45   Nutrition and food safety

KEYNOTES

Major disasters, whether natural or human-made, commonly result in the impairment of food supplies and, consequently, in suffering, poor health and high rates of morbidity and mortality. Malnutrition characterizes emergency situations, especially those that are long-lasting and complex, as a result of which general malnutrition rates are often very high. Such emergency situations are also characterized by a marked increase in the incidence of communicable diseases, especially among vulnerable groups, such as infants and young children, resulting in the further deterioration of their nutritional status.

Assessors should verify that the authorities are in a position to review all stages of food supply from production through processing and manufacturing, transport; distribution and sale to preparation in food-service and catering establishments and households. A nutrition policy should exist, which:

- defines roles, responsibilities and limits of authority (see also the section entitled "leadership and governance");
- identifies minimum food-safety standards;
- identifies objectives related to priority public health issues;
- is coordinated with the policies of other sectors to ensure that priorities are met and gaps and overlaps avoided;
- provides measures to ensure that private or foreign agencies work within national guidelines under national supervision and that donated relief assistance meets national standards;
- takes local-development contexts (economic, social, political and environmental) into consideration.

INDICATOR-RELATED QUESTIONS

a. *Are there mechanisms in place to ensure coverage of food and nutrition needs?*

Assessors should verify that mechanisms exist for evaluating the nutritional status of the population during emergencies. This involves carrying out assessments: (i) to identify the nutritional needs of individuals, families, vulnerable groups and populations as a whole; (ii) to monitor the adequacy of the nutritional intake in these groups; and (iii) to ensure that adequate quantities of safe food and appropriate food commodities are procured for use as general rations and in selective feeding programs. The assessments should include an IRA (to provide the basis for planning a food-relief program), individual screening (to identify individuals who need special assistance) and surveillance of the nutritional status of the population *(30)*.

Assessors should also verify the existence of mechanisms for evaluating the level of access to food both at the local administrative level and, in more detail, at the household level. The social and economic situation should also be assessed, taking into account family and school disruption, violence, employment opportunities, displacement of populations, vulnerable minorities and the availability of essential services and commodities, such as fuel.

The existence of food distribution and feeding programs should also be determined. The aim of these programs should be to ensure that the needs of the population are met through the provision of adequate general rations.[14] In certain situations, however, there may be a need to provide additional food for a period of time to groups who are already malnourished and/or at risk of becoming malnourished.[15]

b. *Are there mechanisms in place to ensure capacity for food quality and safety control?*

Assessors should verify that mechanisms exist to assess the effects of an emergency on the quality and safety of food. It should be a requirement that, before resuming their activities after an emergency, food industries (including slaughterhouses) and catering establishments are inspected to establish their ability to ensure food safety.

In an emergency situation, the extent and type of damage to food needs to be assessed and a decision taken regarding the separation and reconditioning of salvageable food. Control procedures should be in place to ensure that irredeemably damaged food is not marketed and that food distributed through markets, retailers or street vendors has not been subjected to time and temperature abuse, or otherwise contaminated.

---

[14]**General food distribution provides enough food to maintain the health** and nutritional status of the affected population. The food supplied in general and supplementary feeding programs must match the food needs and habits of the recipients, be convenient to transport, store and distribute, and be equitably distributed.

[15]Selective food distribution is the provision of additional food to , vulnerable groups and those needing nutritional rehabilitation. It has two subcategories: supplementary food distribution and therapeutic feeding.

Provisions must be in place to ensure that food unaffected by the emergency situation will not be exposed to other sources of contamination or kept where there is a possibility of bacterial growth, such as may be found in warehouses that have been flooded (high humidity encourages the growth of molds and bacteria in foodstuff).

Mechanisms should exist for monitoring the condition of donated or imported food, starting at point of entry. Food that, on inspection and/or through laboratory analysis, is found to be unfit for human consumption should be rejected.

While public education in food safety is important at all times, in emergencies it becomes vital. In such circumstances, the possible contamination of raw foodstuffs, pollution of the environment and disruption of basic health services increase both the risk of epidemics of foodborne diseases and the severity of their consequences to health. Assessors should verify that mechanisms and procedures are in place for intensifying health-education activities and extending channels of communication with the public, if needed.[16]

RECOMMENDED READING

Abdallah S, Burnham G, eds. *The Johns Hopkins and IFRC public health guide for emergencies. First edition.* Geneva, International Federation of the Red Cross and Red Crescent Societies, 2004 (http://www.terzomondo.org/library/essentials/IFRC_Public_Health_Guide.pdf, accessed 18 April 2004).

De Boer J, Dubouloz M, eds. *Handbook of disaster medicine. Emergency medicine in mass casualty situations.* Utrecht, BRILL, 2000.

Guiding principles for feeding infants and young children during emergencies. Geneva, World Health Organization, 2004 (http://whqlibdoc.who.int/hq/2004/9241546069.pdf, accessed 4 May 2011).

Rapid health assessment protocols for emergencies. Geneva, World Health Organization, 1999.

> **Essential attribute 46**   Primary health care

KEYNOTES

Many emergencies are characterized by a large displaced population living under crowded, unhygienic and often unsafe conditions (see also essential attribute 47). A significant proportion of the population may lack access to basic needs, including health care. Under these conditions, setting up curative services alone is unlikely to improve the health of the majority of this population. It is only through a combination of curative care and preventive and public health interventions that a significant

reduction in the disease burden of the affected population can be maintained.

After the acute phase of an emergency, emergency health care typically shifts towards PHC.[17] This shift occurs more rapidly in sudden-impact disasters than in refugee situations. There are notable differences between PHC strategies and those for emergency health care. For instance, emergency health care does not focus much on social and economic development. This is because affected (displaced) populations are expected to return to their pre-disaster origins relatively soon after a disaster. The effectiveness of emergency health care in alleviating the suffering of displaced people and promoting their recovery depends on how closely the strategy for emergency health care reflects the PHC strategy. Humanitarian assistance should be delivered to displaced populations within the PHC framework so that any skills they acquire through community participation, e.g., in the areas of health education, nutrition and preventive health measures, can help them take responsibility for their own health and rebuild their future.

INDICATOR-RELATED QUESTIONS

Are there mechanisms in place to ensure:

a.   *patient access to clinical investigation and treatment and*

b.   *continuity of the referral systems?*
   Assessors should determine the existence of mechanisms to:

- ensure that emergency health care is implemented within the existing PHC framework so that skills acquired through community participation, health education, nutrition and preventive health measures will enable those affected to take responsibility for their own health and rebuild their future;
- ensure that displaced persons have access to basic clinical examinations and treatment (relating, inter alia, to mental health, maternal-and-child health and reproductive health) at PHC facilities during emergencies (see also essential attributes 41 and 42);
- ensure the continuity of the referral system during emergencies from PHC to the next level of health care (see also essential attributes 34 and 36);
- promote collaboration within the referral system with a view to maximizing the use of resources and labor, and to providing the appropriate level of care;
- strengthen the existing public health infrastructure (basic health facilities, community-health network, local referral system, water supply, disease control, etc.);

---

[16]**Golden rules for safe food preparation: cook raw foods thoroughly; eat** cooked food immediately; prepare food for only one meal; avoid contact between raw foods and cooked foods; choose foods processed for safety; wash hands repeatedly; keep all food-preparation areas meticulously clean; use safe water; be cautious with foods purchased outside; breastfeed infants and young children *(31)*.

[17]**PHC is defined as essential health care based on practical, scientifically** sound and socially acceptable methods and technology, which is accessible to individuals and families in the community through their full participation and at a cost that the community and country can afford to maintain, in the spirit of self-reliance and self-determination *(32)*. The ultimate goal of PHC is better health for all. WHO has identified the following five key elements of that goal: reduction of exclusion and social disparities in health (universal coverage reforms); organization of health services around people's needs and expectations (service delivery reforms); integration of health into all sectors (public policy reforms); pursuance of collaborative models of policy dialogue (leadership reforms); and increased stakeholder participation.

- make use of PHC capacities and capabilities to enhance medical surge capacity (see also essential attribute 33).

RECOMMENDED READING

Abdallah S, Burnham G, eds. *The Johns Hopkins and IFRC public health guide for emergencies. First edition.* Geneva, International Federation of the Red Cross and Red Crescent Societies, 2004 (http://www.terzomondo.org/library /essentials/IFRC_Public_Health_Guide.pdf, accessed 18 April 2004).

Essential attribute 47 Health services for displaced populations

KEYNOTES

Within the context of emergencies, displaced people are those who have had to leave their homes as a result of a natural, technological or deliberate event *(33)*. They often end up in large camps where environmental health measures are insufficient. Displaced people include IDP (displaced people who remain in their own countries) and refugees (displaced people who have crossed international borders).

A refugee is defined someone who, owing to a well-founded fear of being persecuted for reasons of race, religion, nationality, membership of a particular social group, or political opinion, is outside the country of his nationality and is unable to or, owing to such fear, unwilling to avail himself of the protection of that country *(34)*.

There is no single universally accepted definition of IDP. The United Nations defines IDP as "…persons or groups of persons who have been forced or obliged to flee or to leave their homes or places of habitual residence, in particular as a result of or in order to avoid the effects of armed conflict, situations of generalized violence, violations of human rights or natural or human-made disasters and who have not crossed an internationally recognized state border." *(35)*.

Unlike refugees, IDP are not the subject of a specific international convention. Though not specifically referred to therein, they are nevertheless protected by various bodies of law, most notably those related to national law, human rights and, if they are in a country affected by armed conflict, international humanitarian law.

The conditions that characterize displacement can have a profound impact on the health and well-being of individuals and communities. Displacement, combined with a lack of adequate shelter, sanitation, food and safe water, can seriously undermine people's ability to prevent and respond to health-related risks in their environment.

Health-related risks impact people in different ways depending on a range of factors, including age and gender. Young children, older persons, pregnant women and persons living with disability or serious illness are generally more vulnerable to disease and may face additional difficulty in accessing health care. It is important that differential risks and needs be assessed and taken into account when planning and implementing health-related interventions.

INDICATOR-RELATED QUESTIONS

a. *Are there mechanisms in place to assure displaced populations have access to essential health programs, including PHC?* (See also essential attribute 47.)
Assessors should verify that mechanisms are in place to guarantee displaced people access to essential health programs, such as those for immunization, reproductive health, maternal- and-child health care, mental-health care, emergency care, curative care, and rehabilitative care.

Once the crisis is over, the displaced population is likely to return to an environment with limited resources for health care. Therefore, assessors should look into whether humanitarian assistance is being delivered within the PHC framework, allowing displaced populations to gain skills through, for example, community participation and health education that could enable them to take responsibility for their own health and rebuild their future.

b. *Are there mechanisms in place to establish mobile teams that operate outside the existing health facilities (with displaced populations)?*
Assessors should verify that mobile teams can be deployed from existing health facilities to provide medical care for displaced populations, if needed. However, the focus should be not only on providing them with medical care but also on building their capacity to deal with humanitarian experiences by affording them training and development opportunities in this area. Having sufficient numbers of skilled staff locally would enable displaced populations to better cope with future disasters and reduce long-term dependence on external expertise.

c. *Are there mechanisms in place to ensure efficient monitoring of the health status of people living in temporary settlements and at ad hoc sites?*
Mortality and malnutrition rates are the most specific indicators of the health status of displaced populations living in temporary settlements and they reflect the adequacy and quality of the overall relief effort. The regular, systematic and reliable collection, collation, and analysis of data are prerequisites for effective planning and monitoring. The segregation of data by gender and age is essential.

Assessors should establish which indicators are used for monitoring, and investigate mechanisms of collection, collation, and analysis. Provision for ensuring the availability of trained staff and equipment should be in place.

d. *Are there mechanisms in place to address cultural barriers?*
Assessors should verify that mechanisms exist for ensuring that health care programs for displaced populations are culturally appropriate, accessible and affordable. To this end, it is essential to involve the displaced populations in such programs.

e. *Are there mechanisms in place to ensure adequate sanitary and personal-hygiene facilities for displaced populations?* (See also essential attribute 44.)

In humanitarian emergencies, establishing a sanitation system for displaced populations should be among the first priorities. Epidemiological studies in developing countries have shown that the use of latrines or other excreta-containment facilities provides greater protection against diarrheal diseases than any other environmental-health measure.

Assessors should verify that mechanisms exist to ensure adequate sanitation facilities for displaced populations, taking cultural factors, access to and education in the proper use of sanitation facilities, as well as the maintenance and protection of surface-water drainage, into account.

Personal hygiene (e.g., hand-washing, bathing, avoiding contaminated articles and clothing) promotes health and limits the spread of infectious diseases transmitted by direct contact. For cultural reasons, local professionals are best suited to develop and deliver education in personal hygiene, which is ultimately the responsibility of the individual.

Assessors should verify that mechanisms are in place (e.g., educational messages) to promote personal hygiene among displaced populations and provide them with the necessary items (e.g., soap) and facilities.

RECOMMENDED READING

Abdallah S, Burnham G, eds. *The Johns Hopkins and IFRC public health guide for emergencies. First edition.* Geneva, International Federation of the Red Cross and Red Crescent Societies, 2004 (http://www.terzomondo.org/library/essentials /IFRC_Public_Health_Guide.pdf, accessed 18 April 2004).

Guiding principles on internal displacement. Geneva, Office for the Coordination of Humanitarian Affairs, 2001 (http:// ochanet.unocha.org/p/Documents/GuidingPrinciplesDispl .pdf, accessed 7 May 2011).

Handbook for the protection of internally displaced persons. Geneva, Inter-Agency Standing Committee, 2007 (http:// www.unhcr.org/refworld/docid/4790cbc02.html, accessed 7 May 2011).

Position on internally displaced persons (IDPs) (May 2006). Geneva, International Committee of the Red Cross, 2006 (http://www.unhcr.org/refworld/category,POLICY,ICRC, 46e943710,0.html, accessed 7 May 2011).

Refugee health. Geneva, The Office of the United Nations High Commissioner for Refugees, 1995 (http://www.unhcr .org/print/3ae68bf424.html, accessed 7 May 2011).

Key component 6.5 Logistics and operational support functions in emergencies

Essential attribute 48 Emergency telecommunications

KEYNOTES

Many emergencies occur in remote areas where telecommunications systems are usually weak. Good communication lies at the heart of an effective response to, and recovery from, an emergency situation (see also essential attribute 36). A well-organized telecommunications system greatly increases the efficiency of relief operations, which makes it essential to set up new telecommunications systems rapidly in an emergency.

INDICATOR-RELATED QUESTIONS

a. *Do guidelines and procedures exist for establishing standardized telecommunications systems across all sectors?*

b. *Do protocols exist for the use of temporary means of telecommunication?*
Resilient telecommunications are able to absorb or mitigate the effects of disruptions, such as an electrical power failure, on normal life. The causes of such disruptions include natural events or circumstances resulting from human intervention. Assessments of their consequences should result in guidance on planning a framework for testing the resilience of responder communications, which can be adapted to local circumstances.

Assessors should verify that a national telecommunications resilience strategy *(36)* (see key component 1.3) is in place, which aims for:

- collaboration among providers and responders to enhance everyday commercially available resilient telecommunications;
- improvement in the management, adoption and resilience of privileged telecommunications schemes that are accessible only to emergency responders;
- the delivery of a high-integrity telecommunications system that provides connectivity between and services for key responder sites at the national, regional and local levels;
- the provision of a secure means of sharing information between all local, regional and national responders, both in preparing for and responding to emergencies;

At the local level, a plan on enhancing telecommunications between responders and their partners should be drawn up, including:

- an assessment to identify key local responders and resilient communication partners, their communication requirements and their telecommunications arrangements;
- an analysis of the current telecommunications arrangements to identify shortfalls in their resilience in the light of communication requirements and local risks for telecommunications;
- steps to enhance telecommunications resilience and establish a timetable for any remedial action necessary;
- liaison with neighboring entities with resilient telecommunications arrangements;
- telecommunications testing and exercises.

c. *Has staff been trained in the use of emergency telecommunications equipment?*

d. *Are adequate human resources available for emergency telecommunications?*
Assessors should check across all sectors whether staff involved in telecommunications receives adequate training in how to set up and use telecommunications equipment. Trained staff and adequate equipment need to be in place.

An updated roster of those trained in setting up the necessary equipment would facilitate rapid deployment in cases of emergency.

RECOMMENDED READING

Abdallah S, Burnham G, eds. *The Johns Hopkins and IFRC public health guide for emergencies. First edition.* Geneva, International Federation of the Red Cross and Red Crescent Societies, 2004 (http://www.terzomondo.org/library /essentials/IFRC_Public_Health_Guide.pdf, accessed 18 April 2004).

Emergency response and recovery. Non statutory guidance accompanying the Civil Contingencies Act 2004. London, Her Majesty's Government, 2010 (http://interim.cabinetOffice .gov.uk/media/353478/err-guidance-050410.pdf, accessed 7 May 2011).

Essential attribute 49 Temporary health facilities

KEYNOTES

Natural and complex emergencies can cause a dramatic increase in the demand for emergency medical care. Local health services can be overwhelmed and damage to clinics and hospitals can render them useless. Temporary health facilities, such as field hospitals, may be used to substitute or complement medical systems in the aftermath of emergencies. A field hospital is defined as "a mobile, self-contained, self-sufficient health care facility capable of rapid deployment and expansion or contraction to meet immediate emergency requirements for a specified period of time" *(37)*.

According to the Pan American Health Organization (PAHO) and WHO, the essential requirements for field hospitals are that:

- they can be operational on site within 24 hours after the impact of a disaster;
- they can be fully operational within 3–5 days;
- they are entirely self-sufficient;
- they offer comparable or higher standards of medical care than were available in the affected country prior to the precipitating event;
- they have minimal need for support from the local communities;
- they have staff with a basic knowledge of the health situation and language of the country and who respect its culture;
- they include selected specialties;
- they are sustainable (have the appropriate technology);
- there is a lack of other more cost-effective alternatives;
- they can be installed and maintained at no cost to the affected country.

The operational criteria defined by PAHO and WHO include a broad range of medical disciplines and require that staff in field hospitals is familiar with the health situation and culture of the affected country *(37)*.

INDICATOR-RELATED QUESTIONS

a. *Do guidelines and procedures exist for the establishment of temporary health facilities?*
Assessors should verify that mechanisms exist for establishing temporary health facilities. Guidelines on field-hospital inventories should be in place. Mechanisms for mobilizing additional resources from the local, regional and national levels should include the integration of all available assets from field hospitals (see also essential attribute 33).

b. *Are the roles of field hospitals and mobile hospitals clearly defined?*
The roles of field and mobile hospitals in emergencies can vary. They may be used to substitute or complement medical systems in the aftermath of sudden-impact events. Assessors should verify the existence of guidelines and procedures that clearly define the roles of field and mobile hospitals in different situations.

c. *Are adequate resources available for establishing temporary basic health facilities?*
Assessors should verify that adequately trained staff, equipment and financial resources are available for establishing mobile and field hospitals.

RECOMMENDED READING

Mass casualty management hospital emergency response plan. Regional training course on mass casualty management and hospital preparedness. Manila, WHO Regional Office for the Western Pacific, 2008 (http://acilafet.org/upload /dosyalar/Hospital_emergency_response_plan_Toolkit_ .pdf, accessed 2 May 2011).

WHO-PAHO Guidelines for the use of foreign field hospitals in the aftermath of sudden-impact disasters. Washington, DC, Pan American Health Organization, 2003 (http://new.paho .org/disasters/index.php?option=com_docman&task=doc_ download&gid=30&Itemid, accessed 8 May 2011).

Essential attribute 50 Logistics

KEYNOTES

Logistics is a set of systems, which provide the necessary means of delivering the right amount of resources of the right quality at the right price to the right place at the right time. Logistics and supply cannot be improvised when an emergency occurs and should, therefore, be one of the corner-stones of emergency planning and preparedness. Logistics should be an active component of the national emergency-response plan, individual subnational plans and plans of key institutions. Logistics must be closely linked to all operational response activities.

INDICATOR-RELATED QUESTIONS

a. *Do guidelines and procedures exist for the management and use of logistics systems in emergency situations?*
There should be procedures in place for assessing needs vis-à-vis logistics and supply in an emergency (needs of

the population; availability of local capacity and resources; complementary capabilities and resources required to meet the needs).

Assessors should verify the availability of guidelines on requesting international assistance. Such requests should only be made if a needs assessment has clearly identified the insufficiency of local resources to deal with the situation. Ideally, such assessments should help in screening offers of assistance, reducing the number of inappropriate donations and ensuring the delivery of appropriate supplies when and where they are most needed (see also essential attribute 5).

b. *Is there a logistics system in place that includes tracking, monitoring and reporting components?*
Managing logistics also involves maintaining records and updating registries of supplies, medicines, consumables and other materials on a regular basis.

Assessors should verify that logistics systems include tracking, monitoring and reporting components.

c. *Has staff been trained in the use of logistics systems in emergencies?*

d. *Are adequate resources available to ensure logistics support in emergencies?*
Assessors should ensure that all components of the logistics and supply chain (procurement, transport, storage, distribution and human resources) have been taken into consideration and are closely linked.

e. *Are agreements in place with partners and/or private companies for the provision of logistics services to ensure continuity of essential functions?*
Logistics plans must define procedures, responsibilities and timetables for implementation. Actors in relief operations are diverse, as are their mandates and working methods.

Assessors should verify the existence of coordination mechanisms (guidelines and procedures) for linking actors in the field. The following action should be considered:

* identification of the specialties and fields of action of all national, international, governmental and non-profit organizations present in the country;
* organization of frequent meetings and carrying out coordination activities to decide on (and even rehearse) action to be taken before, during and after an emergency;
* development of joint plans and collaborative agreements with various organizations on action to be taken before, during and after an emergency;

Establishment and maintenance of an up-to-date inventory (at the national, regional or institutional level, as the case may be) of resources and contacts that would prove useful in the event of an emergency;

* information-exchange among actors about resources that may be useful in the event of an emergency;
* establishment and maintenance of a directory of suppliers and manufacturers (including contact details and

information about manufacturing capacity and production and delivery times).

RECOMMENDED READING

Humanitarian supply management and logistics in the health sector. Washington, DC, Pan American Health Organization, 2001 (http://www.paho.org/english/ped/Humanitarian-Supply-part1.pdf, accessed 8 May 2011).

SUMA. The WHO/PAHO supply management system. Washington, DC, Pan American Health Organization, 2001 (http://www.paho.org/english/ped/suma.pdf, accessed 8 May 2011).

World Health Organization et al. *The interagency emergency health kit 2006. Medicines and medical devices for 10 000 people for approximately 3 months. An interagency document.* Geneva, World Health Organization, 2006 (WHO/PSM/PAR/2006.4) (http://apps.who.int/medicinedocs/en/d/Js13486e/6.10.5.html, accessed 8 May 2011).

Essential attribute 51   Service-delivery support function

INDICATOR-RELATED QUESTIONS

a. *Is the security of health care facilities guaranteed during an emergency?*
It is vital that health care facilities are protected and secure. This is a complex issue, which not only involves the security of the facilities but also that of the staff, patients, visitors and various areas around the facilities.

Assessors should check whether:

* the security and protection of health care facilities, and the use of protective measures, such as PPE, vaccination and prophylactic medication are included in preparedness and response plans;
* the characteristics of possible emergencies and how they may threaten health care facilities have been ;
* heads of security have been appointed within the health care facilities and are part of their incident-command groups;
* procedures, job action sheets, forms and logs have been prepared for the management of security;
* the roads to and from the health care facilities are open and protected and whether procedures for identifying hospital personnel are in place;
* pre-established arrangements, guidelines and procedures exist for collaborating with both internal security personnel and outside security services, such as the police and fire brigades;
* the necessary equipment (vests, arrows, ropes) is available for marking access roads, cordoning off areas and delineating restricted zones;
* joint exercises and drills are carried out in conjunction with the security services (police, fire brigades, etc.).

b. *Is continuity of lifelines in health care facilities planned for in case of an emergency?*

Health care facilities are often directly affected by emergencies with serious consequences, including the death of staff members and patients, the destruction of buildings and the loss of lifelines. Therefore, the restoration of lifelines and critical equipment is of vital importance. Activities, for example, to maintain essential equipment, ensure electrical power and water supplies, assess damage (in cooperation with the security services), and restore lifelines, are the key to the continuity of business operations and the delivery of essential services (see also essential attribute 39).

Assessors should check whether:

- continuity of lifelines is included in preparedness and response plans;
- working contacts have been established with stakeholders and suppliers who could contribute to the efficient operation of critical equipment or action to restore lifelines;
- external technical assistance (e.g., community-relevant services) has been identified and can be deployed rapidly, if necessary;
- constraints have been considered, such as the protection of technicians while they are working in the health care facility (e.g., by supplying PPE in case of a pandemic);
- mechanisms exist for setting up a monitoring system to anticipate problems, such as shortage or overuse;
- technical expertise is available for assessing damage to buildings and the safety and sustainability of lifelines (power and water);
- back-up systems for water supply, power supply, fuel for transport, etc., are in place and regularly tested;
- the main stakeholders inside the health care facilities and partners outside the health care facilities participate in exercises and drills.

c. *Have transportation and fuel requirements for emergencies been taken into consideration in planning?*

Assessors should verify that mechanisms and procedures exist for ensuring that, in emergencies, transportation and fuel requirements can be met. Emergency fuel stocks are essential for the additional interfacility transport and referral involved. Furthermore, fuel is needed for back-up systems (generators) in health care facilities. Agreements with local transport and fuel providers might be considered.

RECOMMENDED READING

Hospital safety index. Guide for evaluators. Washington, DC, Pan American Health Organization, 2008 (http://www.preventionweb.net/files/8974_SafeHosEvaluatorGuideEng1.pdf, accessed 8 May 2011).

Safe hospitals in emergencies and disasters. Structural, non-structural and functional indicators. Manila, WHO Regional Office for the Western Pacific, 2009 (http://www.wpro.who.int/NR/rdonlyres/390133EC-089F-4C77-902D-DFEE8532F558/0/ SafeHospitalsinEmergenciesandDisasters160709.pdf, accessed 8 May 2011).

REFERENCES

1. *Everybody's business: strengthening health systems to improve health outcomes.* Geneva, World Health Organization, 2007 (http://www.who.int/healthsystems/strategy/everybodys_business.pdf, accessed on 1 July 2011).
2. *Hospital safety index. Guide for evaluators.* Washington, DC, Pan American Health Organization, 2008 (http://new.paho.org/disasters/index.php?option=com_content&task=view&id=663&Itemid=924, accessed 1 July 2011).
3. *Health sector self-assessment tool for disaster risk reduction.* Washington, DC, Pan American Health Organization, 2010 (http://new.paho.org/disasters/index.php?option=com_content&task=view&id=1375&Itemid=1&lang=en, accessed 1 July 2010).
4. *Protocol for assessing national surveillance and response capacities for the International Health Regulations (2005) in accordance with Annex 1 of the IHR. A guide for assessment teams. December 2010.* Geneva, World Health Organization, 2010 (http://www.who.int/ihr/publications/who_hse_ihr_201007_en.pdf, accessed 1 July 2011).
5. Resolution WHA58.1. Health action in relation to crises and disasters, with particular emphasis on the earthquakes and tsunamis of 26 December 2004. In: *Fifty-eighth World Health Assembly, Geneva, 16–25 May 2005. Resolutions and decisions. Annex.* Geneva, World Health Organization, 2005 (http://apps.who.int/gb/ebwha/pdf_files/WHA58-REC1/english/Resolutions.pdf, accessed 31 July 2011).
6. Resolution WHA59.22. Emergency preparedness and response. In: *Fifty-ninth World Health Assembly, Geneva, 22–27 May 2006. Resolutions and decisions. Annex.* Geneva, World Health Organization, 2006 (https://apps.who.int/gb/ebwha/pdf_files/WHA59/A59_R22-en.pdf, accessed 31 July 2011).
7. *Hyogo Framework for Action 2005–2015: Building the resistance of nations and communities to disasters. World Conference on Disaster Reduction, 18-22 January 2005, Kobe, Hyogo, Japan.* Geneva, United Nations International Strategy for Disaster Reduction, 2005 (http://www.unisdr.org/wcdr/intergover/official-doc/L-docs/Hyogo-framework-for-action-english.pdf, accessed 1 July 2011).
8. *Communication from the Commission to the Council, the European Parliament, the European Economic and Social Committee and the Committee of the Regions on strengthening coordination on generic preparedness planning for public health emergencies at EU level, Brussels, 28.11.2005.* Brussels, Commission of the European Communities, 2005 (COM(2005) 605; http://eur-lex.europa.eu/LexUriServ/site/en/com/2005/com2005_0605en01.pdf, accessed 8 August 2011).
9. *Interim document: technical guidance on generic preparedness planning for public health emergencies.* Brussels, European Union, 2005 (http://ec.europa.eu/health/ph_threats/Bioterrorisme/keydo_bio_01_en.pdf, accessed on 8 August 2011).

10. Resolution WHA58.5. Strengthening pandemic-influenza preparedness and response. In: *Fifty-eighth World Health Assembly, Geneva, 16–25 May 2005. Resolutions and decisions. Annex.* Geneva, World Health Organization, 2005 (http://apps.who.int/gb/ebwha/pdf_files/WHA58 /WHA58_5-en.pdf, accessed 31 July 2011).

11. *International Health Regulations (2005). Second edition.* Geneva, World Health Organization, 2008 (http://whqlib-doc.who.int/publications/2008/9789241580410_eng.pdf, accessed 1 July 2011).

12. *The world health report 2000. Health systems: improving performance.* Geneva, World Health Organization, 2007 (http://www.who.int/whr/2000/en/, accessed 18 May 2011).

13. *The Tallinn Charter: health systems for health and wealth.* Copenhagen, WHO Regional Office for Europe, 2008 (http://www.euro.who.int/__data/assets/pdf_file/0008/88613/E91438.pdf, accessed 1 July 2011)

14. *Key components of a well functioning health system.* Geneva, World Health Organization, 2010 (http://www.who.int/entity/healthsystems/HSSkeycomponents.pdf, accessed 1 July 2011).

15. *Protocol additional to the Geneva Conventions of 12 August 1949, and relating to the protection of victims of international armed conflicts (Protocol I), 8 June 1977.* Geneva, International Committee of the Red Cross, 2005 (http://www.icrc.org/ihl.nsf/FULL/470?OpenDocument, accessed 1 July 2011).

16. Health Metrics Network, World Health Organization. *Framework and standards for country health information systems. Second edition.* Geneva, World Health Organization, 2008 (www.who.int/healthmetrics/documents/hmn_framework200803.pdf assessed 1 July 2011).

17. Hanoi School of Public Health, WHO Regional Office for the Western Pacific. Rapid health assessment guidelines. *Regional Training course on rapid health assessment, Hanoi, Viet Nam, 27-30 November 2007.* Manila, WHO Regional Office for the Western Pacific, 2007 (http://www.wpro.who.int/internet/files/eha/dir/Regional%20Training%20Course%20on%20Rapid%20Health%20Assessment/RHA%20global%20health%20cluster.pdf, accessed 8 August 2011).

18. *Initial rapid assessment (IRA) guidance notes for country level. Version for field testing.* Geneva, Inter-Agency Standing Committee, 2007 (www.humanitarianreform.org/humanitarianreform/Portals/1/cluster%20approach%20page/clusters%20pages/health%20cluster/RT/IRA_Guidance_Country%20Level_field_test.doc, last accessed 1 July 2011).

19. *Outbreak communication. Best practices for communicating with the public during an outbreak. Report of WHO Expert Consultation on Outbreak Communications, Singapore, 21–23 September 2004.* Geneva, World Health Organization, 2005 (http://www.who.int/csr/resources/publications/WHO_CDS_2005_32web.pdf assessed 1 July 2011).

20. *Effective media communication during public health emergencies. A WHO handbook.* Geneva, World Health Organization, 2005 (WHO/CDS/2005.31) (http://www.who.int/csr/resources/publications/WHO%20MEDIA%20HANDBOOK.pdf, accessed 1 July 2011).

21. Abdallah S, Burnham G, eds. *The Johns Hopkins and Red Cross/Red Crescent public health guide for emergencies. First edition.* Geneva, International Federation of the Red Cross and Red Crescent Societies, 2004 (http://pdf.usaid.gov/pdf_docs/PNACU086.pdf, accessed 1 July 2011).

22. The CNA Corporation Institute for Public Research. *Medical surge capacity and capability: a management system for integrating medical and health resources during large-scale emergencies.* Washington, DC, Department of Health and Human Services, 2007 (http://www.phe.gov/preparedness/planning/mscc/handbook/documents/mscc080626.pdf, accessed 1 July 2011).

23. *Mass casualty management systems. Strategies and guidelines for building health sector capacity.* Geneva, World Health Organization, 2007 (www.who.int/entity/hac/techguidance/MCM_guidelines_inside_final.pdf assessed 1 July 2011).

24. *Establishing a mass casualty management system.* Washington, DC, Pan American Health Organization, 2001 (http://www.paho.org/english/ped/masscas.pdf assessed 1 July 2011).

25. *On-site activities for mass casualty incidents. Regional training course on mass casualty management and hospital preparedness. Toolkit.* Manila, WHO Regional Office for the Western Pacific, 2008 (http://www.gujhealth.gov.in/pdf/on-site-mass-casualty-mg-hospital-preparedness.pdf, accessed 8 August 2011).

26. *Module 3. Emergency medical service systems. Regional training course on mass casualty management and hospital preparedness. Oral Presentation and Workshop, Ho Chi Minh City, Vietnam, October 2010.* Manila, WHO Regional Office for the Western Pacific, 2010.

27. *Mental health in emergencies. Mental and social aspects of health of populations exposed to extreme stressors.* Geneva, World Health Organization, 2003 (www.who.int/mental_health/media/en/640.pdf assessed 1 July 2011).

28. *Guidelines for drinking-water quality. Third edition, incorporating first and second addenda. Volume 1. Recommendations.* Geneva, World Health Organization, 2008 (http://www.who.int/water_sanitation_health/dwq/fulltext.pdf assessed 1 July 2011)

29. Wisner B, Adams J, eds. *Environmental health in emergencies and disasters. A practical guide.* Geneva, World Health Organization, 2002 (http://www.who.int/water_sanitation_health/hygiene/emergencies/emergencies2002/en/, assessed 1 July 2011).

30. *Rapid health assessment protocols for emergencies.* Geneva, World Health Organization, 1999 (http://www.healthlibrary.com/book51.htm, accessed 28 October 2011).

31. *Global Strategy for food safety. Safer food for better health.* Geneva, World Health Organization, 2002 (http://www.who.int/entity/foodsafety/publications/general/en/strategy_en.pdf, accessed 1 July 2011).

32. *Declaration of Alma-Ata.* Copenhagen, WHO Regional Office for Europe, 1978 (http://www.who.int/publications/almaata_declaration_en.pdf assessed 1 July 2011).

33. Environmental health in emergencies-displaced people [web site]. Geneva, World Health Organization, 2011 (http://www.who.int/environmental_health_emergencies/displaced_people/en/, accessed 1 July 2011).

34. *Protocol additional to the Geneva Conventions of 12 August 1949, and relating to the protection of victims of international armed conflicts (Protocol 1), 8 June 1977.* Geneva, International Committee of the Red Cross, 1977 (http://www.icrc.org/ihl.nsf/INTRO/470, accessed 5 August 2011).

35. *Handbook for applying the guiding principles on internal displacement.* Geneva, United Nations Office for the Coordination of Humanitarian Affairs, 2001 (http://www.unhcr.org/refworld/docid/3d52a6432.html, accessed 3 July 2011]).

36. *Emergency response and recovery: non-statutory guidance to complement emergency preparedness.* London, HM Government, 2005 (http://products.ihs.com/cis/Doc.aspx?AuthCode=&DocNum=280662, accessed 1 July 2011).

37. *WHO-PAHO guidelines for the use of foreign field hospitals in the aftermath of sudden-impact disasters.* Washington, DC, Pan American Health Organization, 2003 (http://helid.digicollection.org/en/d/Js8253e/, accessed 8 August 2011).

Note: For additional information on strengthening health system emergency preparedness, as well as the Annex content references mentioned in this appendix, visit http://www.euro.who.int/__data/assets/pdf_file/0008/157886/e96187.pdf

GLOSSARY

accountable care organization (ACO)   a voluntarily created team of health care providers who will care for a patient together, sharing responsibility.

acute care hospital   a facility providing medical care in an inpatient setting to diagnose and treat an injury or illness for a limited duration of time.

acute myocardial infarction (AMI)   an area of dead tissue within the heart, the result of an embolus or thrombus blocking sufficient blood flow; commonly known as a heart attack.

administrator   individual with the responsibility to oversee the workings of an organization and the provision of its services and products.

adverse outcome   an unexpected harmful reaction (harm) to a procedure, service, or treatment, including medications; also known as adverse effect.

advertising   direct methods for calling attention to something or someone.

Affordable Care Act (ACA)   a federal law that provides stronger protections for patients in their acquisition of health care insurance.

ambulatory surgical center (ASC)   facility that provides surgical procedures on an outpatient basis.

Americans with Disabilities Act (ADA)   a federal law that offers protection from prejudice in employment for individuals documented with a disability.

Anti-Kickback Law   a federal law that prohibits facilities from paying referral fees to physicians.

app   short for application, a mini software program used mostly on mobile devices.

assisted living facility   an inpatient facility providing long-term care for individuals requiring help with the activities of daily living (ADL) and requiring limited medical services.

audit   an assessment of specified data points to determine compliance with previously identified standards.

bloodborne pathogens   bacteria and viruses that are transmitted via bodily fluids.

board-certified physician   a credential signifying the completion of additional education in a specific area of health care, as authenticated by the passing of an exam administered by an authorized association.

brand awareness   a marketing term used to describe activities that draw attention to both the name of the company or facility and the product or service itself.

buy-in   obtaining consensus from participants before putting a plan into action.

capitation plan   a payment plan in which a primary care physician receives a monthly stipend for ongoing care of a managed care beneficiary.

case mix   a strategic plan to ensure a health care facility is caring for patients with a variety of diagnoses.

Centers for Medicare and Medicaid Services (CMS)   a federal government agency authorized to manage the Medicare and Medicaid programs.

certified nurse midwife (CNM)   a credential signifying the successful completion of additional specialized training in assisting the delivery of a neonate.

certified registered nurse anesthetist (CRNA)   a credential signifying the successful completion of additional specialized training in the administration of anesthesia.

clinic   a health care facility providing a limited range of services on an outpatient basis.

clinician   an individual trained to directly care for patients in a health care environment.

collateral materials   the term used to identify all printed materials used by your facility to deliver a message.

commercial loan   a loan provided by a bank.

complementary alternative medicine (CAM)   a term used to represent the use of theories and practices not considered to be included in conventional medicine: acupuncture, chiropractics, and physical therapies are included in this grouping.

compliance   observance of laws and policies; behaviors and actions directly following rules and regulations.

comprehensive audit   an assessment of the entire body of data to determine compliance with previously identified standards.

computer physician order entry (CPOE)   interactive electronic documentation of physician's orders and prescriptions electronically sent to pharmacies, imaging centers, and laboratories.

concurrent audit   an assessment conducted at the same time with the creation of data or the performance of the activity.

concurrent phase   the time during a crisis.

consequence   result or outcome of behavior.

continuing education   educational events required for the maintenance of a professional license or certification.

cost-benefit analysis   a mathematical process by which to evaluate whether or not the purchase of something has a value equal to or greater than the amount paid.

covered entities   individuals and organizations obligated to abide by the Privacy Rule of HIPAA.

covert problem   a noncompliant event that is not obvious or easily seen.

credentials   documentation of knowledge and skills as confirmed by an authorized association or agency.

crisis   a circumstance or event that is expected to cause difficulty or danger.

cross-training   orientation and education about job responsibilities in a different role or department.

current   the present time.

deontological   a perspective of ethical decision making that focuses on the obligation of one's oath or duty to care.

Department of Health and Human Services (DHHS)   the principal agency for protecting the health of all Americans.

dietetic technician, registered (DTR)   a credential signifying the successful completion of additional specialized training in nutrition.

doctrine of corporate negligence   a law that states that hospitals can be held liable for the competence, or lack thereof, of their staff.

domiciliary   a place of residence for independent individuals requiring supervision, for example, a halfway house.

due diligence   complete and thorough background checks; proof that everything possible was done, every reasonable precaution was made to prevent a wrong from occurring.

economics   the study of the production, distribution, and consumption of goods and services, often referring to the financial well-being, or lack thereof, of a group.

elective procedures   those procedures typically prompted by the patient's desire to correct a concern; a procedure that is not immediately medically necessary (nonemergency).

electronic health record (EHR)   software used to create and maintain patient charts; a computerized record of health care information and associated processes.

electronic medical record (EMR)   software used by hospitals to create and maintain patient charts; a computerized record of medical information and associated processes.

Emergency Medical Treatment and Active Labor Act (EMTALA)   a federal law binding on only those hospitals who are participating providers with CMS, directing them to care for anyone in an emergency situation without deference to the patient's ability to pay.

employee retention   the ability of an organization to ensure that high-quality staff continue working for their company.

endemic   a disease that spreads throughout a small area, such as a community.

epidemic   a disease that spreads over a large area.

episodic care   a method of paying a provider with one lump sum based on the standard of care for a specific diagnosis.

Equal Employment Opportunity (EEO) Act   a federal law regulating hiring and firing individuals based on race, gender, or age.

ethics   a previously determined set of correct, or right, conducts or behaviors.

evidence-based medicine (EBM)   the process of medical decision making determined by research.

executive summary   the first section of a strategic plan that contains summaries of all other sections within that same plan.

expenditures   money spent or paid out.

exposure control plan (ECP)   a set of policies and procedures designed to protect staff from harmful effects.

external audit   an assessment to determine compliance performed by an authorized agency or organization.

external crisis   an event that is focused outside of the organization.

extrapolation   to determine by projecting existing experience or known data.

extrinsic motivation   inspirational elements derived from outside forces, such as a reward or acknowledgement.

facility maintenance   the upkeep of building and equipment.

False Claims Act   a federal law, with individual states enacting their own versions, making it illegal to submit a claim form to a third-party payer containing information that is untrue.

Family and Medical Leave Act (FMLA)   a federal law directing companies to provide unpaid leave to employees with a personal or family health care crisis.

Federal Register   the daily publication for rules, proposed rules, and notices of the federal government.

fee-for-service (FFS)   a payment plan in which a health care provider receives reimbursement from a third-party payer based on the specific procedure, services, and treatments provided.

fixed costs   expenses that remain the same, month after month.

food preparation area   any surface touched by food.

food safety   all measures taken to ensure edible elements are protected from everything that could cause harm to the individual who consumes them.

foodborne hazard   any biological, physical, or chemical substance that may get into food and cause harm to individuals who consume that food.

foodborne illness   any illness or disease caused by ingesting contaminated food or drink.

for-profit organization   an organization that is structured to share excess revenue with its shareholders.

fraud   using dishonest or inaccurate information with the intention of wrongly gaining money or other benefit.

grant   monies provided under very specific terms.

harm   physical or psychological injury.

health information exchange (HIE)   technical network enabling different providers to access patient information.

Health Insurance Portability and Accountability Act (HIPAA)   a federal law protecting patient confidentiality.

heart failure (HF)   a cardiac condition where the heart cannot pump enough to provide proper blood for circulation.

heating, ventilation, air conditioning (HVAC)   equipment responsible for control of internal environment.

Hill-Burton Act   a federal act that provided loans and federal grants to fund construction for updating of health care facilities in exchange for the free provision of health care to those individuals unable to pay for those services who live in the facility's communities.

home health agency   an organization that provides health care services to a patient in their own home.

hospice   an organization that provides health care services, most often palliative care to those who are terminally ill.

hospital acquired condition (HAC)   an illness or injury that a patient contracts during a stay in an acute care hospital.

inpatient facility   a facility providing room and meals in addition to health care services on a continuous basis.

intellectual capital   the assets provided to an organization by the staff: ideas, innovations, energies, and efforts.

internal audit   an assessment to determine compliance performed by, or initiated by, the organization or facility itself, to look for improprieties, errors, and other wrongdoing.

internal crisis   an event that occurs within the facility and, primarily, affects only those within the organization.

interoperability   the ability for software to communicate and exchange data with other software programs.

intrinsic motivation   incentive derived from one's own desire or enthusiasm for doing a specific job or completing a task.

long-term goal   action scheduled for completion in five to ten years from the plan's implementation.

marketing   activities designed to build awareness, more specifically brand awareness.

marketing plan   a written document containing both short-term and long-term diagrams of how the facility's message will be dispersed, using marketing, advertising, and public relations vehicles.

meaningful use   a set of standards set by the HITECH Act and used by CMS to determine qualification for financial incentives connected to the adoption of electronic healthcare records (EHR).

medical malpractice   a legal concept that identifies negligence by a medical professional.

medical necessity   determination that an individual has need for a procedure, service, or treatment based on the standards of care.

microorganism   a tiny life form, including some parasites, viruses, bacteria, molds, and yeasts.

minimal access surgery (MAS)   the ability to visualize and treat internal aspects of the patient without the need for a large incision.

mission statement   an all-encompassing long-term goal or objective.

mitigating circumstance   an event that partially excuses a wrong or lessens the result.

mitigation   an action taken that will lessen the severity of harm.

mortality   death.

motivation   reason to act; forces that are beneath behavior.

never event   an event that is not supposed to ever happen; also known as a sentinel event.

noninvasive procedure   a health care procedure that does not physically enter the body.

not-for-profit (nonprofit) facility   an organization with a tax status that is designated to reinvest excess revenue into the organization for the betterment of its patients (customers).

nurse practitioner (NP)   a credential signifying the successful completion of additional specialized training, authorizing a registered nurse (RN) to provide basic health care services to patients, including determining diagnosis and treatment plan for common acute injuries and illnesses.

objective   a statement of what is to be accomplished or achieved.

occult problem   a noncompliant event that is deeply hidden and cannot be identified without an in-depth investigation.

Occupational Safety and Health Act (OSHA)   a federal law that requires employers to develop and implement whatever is necessary to ensure a safe and healthy workplace for all staff.

Office of the Inspector General (OIG)   an investigative branch of the U.S. federal government.

other potentially infectious materials (OPIM)   those materials other than bloodborne pathogens that may cause illness.

outpatient facility   a facility that provides health care services alone, without room and board.

outsourcing   contracting with another company to provide food services for the facility.

overt problem   a noncompliant event that is obvious or easily seen.

pandemic   an epidemic that occurs over a very large geographic area.

pathogen   bacterium or virus that can cause illness or disease.

patient population   the group of individuals accepting health care services from a specific organization.

patient safety practice   a behavior or action performed in a manner designed to keep the patient safe.

patient-centered care   a full-circle approach to health care, with the patient in the middle, in full control of the process.

patient-related encounter   an exchange between health care professionals discussing a specific patient when the patient is not present.

performance improvement plan (PIP)   documentation of a staff member's current skills as well as a list of those skills that need to be improved and what action(s) should be taken to ensure that improvement.

physician's office   a private facility in which a licensed health care professional can provide outpatient services.

post-event analysis   an evaluation of how the organization handled each aspect of a crisis.

practice management system (PMS)   the software used to create, submit, and manage claims to third-party payers.

preventive care   health care services intended to keep a patient healthy and avoid illness, disease, or injury.

preventive phase   the opportunity to implement policies and procedures designed to avert a crisis.

primary target market   your most likely customer; the largest group of people with the biggest and most frequent need or want for your product or service.

private health insurance   a third-party payer that is not affiliated with the federal government.

private investment   an individual endowing money to an individual or organization.

proactive strategy   a plan to prevent, or diminish the opportunity for, an adverse outcome.

propensity   a tendency to demonstrate particular behavior.

proprietary facility   an organization owned and operated by a for-profit corporation.

psychographics   four descriptors: geographical location; job title or position; education level; and mind-set used to identify specific groups of consumers.

public health care facility   an organization, established by a government agency, to provide health care services to its citizens.

public relations   the process of building good will and trust with the public.

quality improvement strategies   a group of plans designed to raise the level of benefit derived from the organization.

quality indicators (QI)   specific standard measures of benefit provided.

Qui tam lawsuit   a feature of HIPAA that entitles an individual citizen to file a lawsuit on behalf of the government; used in cases of whistleblowers uncovering fraud.

radio frequency identification (RFID)   wireless technology used to track specific items, such as medications, patient charts, patient identification.

reactive strategy   a plan that specifies what actions staff members should take after an adverse outcome has occurred.

recovery phase   the segment of time, after the crisis has passed, during which the organization, and all its members, must recoup and get back to a pre-crisis state.

redetermination   CMS's (Centers for Medicare and Medicaid Services) term for a review of a claim.

registered dietitian (RD)   a credential signifying the successful completion of additional specialized training in nutrition.

rehabilitation center   a health care facility providing services and therapies designed to restore an individual to an optimal level of physical, mental, and/or vocational health and independence.

remote presence (RP)   use of telecommunication devices, such as robots, enabling a physician to meet with and evaluate a patient without being physically at the location.

retrospective audit   an assessment conducted on activities or events that have occurred in the past.

revenue   income; monies received.

risk   the statistical calculation that an adverse outcome might occur.

risk management   the process by which an organization can reduce the opportunity for an adverse outcome, or harm, to result.

safe harbor   a location protected from storm or other crisis.

sampling audit   an assessment conducted on a statistically valid portion of the entire body of data.

secured bonds   an investment vehicle backed by another asset.

self-operation   procurement, preparation, and delivery of food items managed and performed by employees of the facility.

sentinel event   *See* "never event."

shares of stock   percentage of ownership of a company.

short-term goal   action and accomplishment intended to be realized within one to three years.

skilled nursing facility (SNF)   an inpatient facility providing 24-hour, continuous health care services provided by health care professionals, including registered nurses.

socio-demographic   a collection of specific data related to an individual's age, gender, education, income level, occupation, and other details.

staff satisfaction   when employees feel appreciated and valued for their job performance.

Stark   a federal law that prohibits physicians from making referrals to any facility or other health-related item in which that physician has a financial interest.

strategic goal   a statement of how the organization expects to achieve an objective.

strategic plan   the process of determining direction and guidance for the accomplishment of goals.

subpoena ad testificandum   a court order for an individual to testify under oath.

subpoena duces tecum   a court order for specified documents to be delivered to the authorities.

Surgical Care Improvement Project (SCIP)   a standard of measure used by Hospital Compare to determine the level of effort used to enhance surgical outcomes.

SWOT analysis   an evaluation of the strengths, weaknesses, opportunities, and threats relative to the facility's business activities.

telehealth   any remote telecommunication between health care providers and patients or other providers for the purposes of managing the patient's health care.

teleological   a perspective for ethical decision making based on the outcome of that decision.

teletherapy   the provision of health care services and/or consultation without direct patient contact.

third-party payer   an individual or organization who pays for a health care service yet is neither the provider nor the receiver of these services.

trend analysis   the review and assessment of data taken over a period of time with the intention of identifying patterns.

true need   an evaluation of the level of specific requirement; differentiation between want and need.

upcoding   an illegal practice of reporting a code for a higher level of service than that which was actually performed.

utilization   use; operation and employment of resources including staff time, staff expertise, as well as equipment and supplies.

variable expenditures   expenses or debt that change month to month.

Veterans' Administration (VA)   an agency of the federal government with the authority to care for members of the uniformed services.

wage and hour   regulations that govern how much you pay your staff members (wages) and how that amount is calculated (hours).

workers' compensation   an insurance plan specifically designated to pay for medical care for an individual who was injured or became ill as a result of his or her occupation.

workforce health promotion (WHP)   education and activity efforts to assist staff members in better health methodologies.